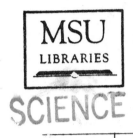

MODERN APPROACHES TO VACCINES

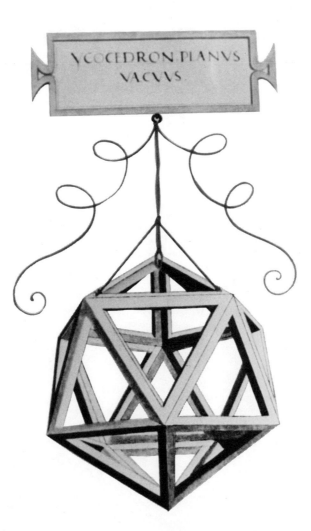

Viruses are composed of a nucleic acid and a number of antigenic subunits, which are arranged in the form of either a helix or an icosahedron. The association of viruses and icosahedra has been known for about thirty years. However, the properties of the icosahedron have been known for rather longer, as demonstrated by this drawing by Leonardo da Vinci. *(Drawing kindly provided by Science Museum, London)*

MODERN APPROACHES TO VACCINES

Molecular and Chemical Basis of Virus Virulence and Immunogenicity

Edited by

Robert M. Chanock
National Institutes of Health

Richard A. Lerner
Research Institute of Scripps Clinic

Cold Spring Harbor Laboratory
1984

MODERN APPROACHES TO VACCINES
Molecular and Chemical Basis of
Virus Virulence and Immunogenicity

©1984 by Cold Spring Harbor Laboratory
Printed in the United States of America
Cover design by Emily Harste

Front cover: High-resolution X-ray diffraction of poliovirus. Photo from J. Hogle, Research Institute of Scripps Clinic, La Jolla, California.

Back cover: Dr. Edward Jenner is here depicted in the act of vaccinating a child. The carving measuring 1.27m. × 1.13m. × 0.97m. is in White Carrara marble and was commissioned by Maria Brignola Sale, Duchess of Galliera in 1873 and executed by the famous Italian sculptor Giulio Monteverde (1837–1917). The sculpture was exhibited in Vienna in 1873 and Paris in 1978. After the death of the Duchess in 1888 it was acquired by the Comune Di Genova for their Museum of Fine Arts. Use of photograph is by courtesy of their Director. Photograph kindly provided by Canon J. Eric Gethyn-Jones.

Library of Congress Cataloging in Publication Data

Main entry under title:

Modern approaches to vaccines.

 Includes index.
 1. Vaccines. I. Chanock, Robert M. II. Lerner, Richard A. [DNLM: 1. Viral vaccines—Congresses. 2. Genes, Viral—Congresses. 3. Virulence— Congresses. W 805 M689 1983]
QR189.M58 1984   615'.372   83-73176
ISBN 0-87969-165-4

All Cold Spring Harbor Laboratory publications are available through booksellers or may be ordered directly from Cold Spring Harbor Laboratory, Box 100, Cold Spring Harbor, New York 11724.

SAN   203-6185

Conference Participants

L. Garry Adams, *Department of Veterinarian Pathology, Texas A & M University, College Station, Texas*

Hannah Alexander, *Scripps Clinic and Research Foundation, La Jolla, California*

E. Amann, *Research Laboratories, Marburg, Federal Republic of Germany*

Guido Antoni, *Sclavo Research Center, Siena, Italy*

Ralph Arlinghaus, *Scripps Clinic and Research Foundation, La Jolla, California*

Jacques Armand, *Institut Merieux, Charbonnieres, France*

Ruth Arnon, *Department of Chemical Immunology, Weizmann Institute of Science, Rehovot, Israel*

D.J.S. Arora, *Department of Virology, Institut Armand-Frappier, Université du Québec, Laval, Canada*

Paul Atkinson, *Department of Developmental Biology, Albert Einstein College, Bronx, New York*

F. Audibert, *Department of Expérimental Immunothérapie, Institut Pasteur, Paris, France*

J. Augstein, *Pharmaceutical Division, Science and Technology Laboratories, Loughborough Leics, England*

Howard Bachrach, *USDA, Plum Island Animal Disease Center, Greenport, New York*

Peter Bailey, *British Technology Group, London, England*

Kalyan Banerjee, *National Institute of Virology, Pune, India*

Richard Bellamy, *Department of Cell Biology, University of Auckland, Auckland, New Zealand*

David D. Bennett, *Veterans Administration Medical Center, Salt Lake City, Utah*

Phillip Berman, *Genentech, Inc., South San Francisco, California*

M. Binns, *Houghton Poultry Research Station, Cambridge, England*

James Bittle, *Scripps Clinic and Research Foundation, La Jolla, California*

Ulf Bjare, *National Bacteriological Laboratory, Stockholm, Sweden*

Fred Bloom, *Bethesda Research Laboratories, Inc., Gaithersburg, Maryland*
Esper Boel, *Novo Research Institute, Bagsvaerd, Denmark*
Clifford Bond, *Department of Microbiology, Montana State University, Bozeman, Montana*
Gerald Both, *Department of Molecular and Cellular Biology, CSIRO, New South Wales, Australia*
Roger Breeze, *Washington State College of Veterinary Medicine, Pullman, Washington*
F. Brown, *Animal Virus Research Institute, Pirbright, England*
B.H. Brownstein, *Department of Molecular Biology, Abbott Laboratories, North Chicago, Illinois*
Doris Bucher, *Department of Microbiology, Mt. Sinai School of Medicine, New York, New York*
W. Neal Burnette, *Amgen, Inc., Thousand Oaks, California*
Jonathan Carlson, *Syngene Products and Research, Inc., Ft. Collins, Colorado*
Nadine Carozzi, *Department of Molecular Biology, Abbott Laboratories, North Chicago, Illinois*
David Cavanagh, *Houghton Poultry Research Station, Cambridge, England*
Hardy Chan, *Syntex Research Corp., Palo Alto, California*
Ding Chang, *Peninsula Laboratories, Inc., Belmont, California*
Robert Chanock, *NIAID, National Institutes of Health, Bethesda, Maryland*
Eugene Chen, *Pitman-Moore, Inc., Washington Crossing, New Jersey*
Andrew Cheung, *Biogen, Inc., Carouge, Switzerland*
Marie Chow, *Center for Cancer Research, Massachusetts Institute of Technology, Cambridge, Massachusetts*
Michael Clarke, *Department of Biochemistry, University of Victoria, Victoria, Canada*
Gary Colgrove, *USDA, National Veterinary Institute, Ames, Iowa*
John Controulis, *Warner-Lambert, Morris Plains, New Jersey*
B. Dale, *California Biotechnology, Inc., Palo Alto, California*
Bill Degrado, *DuPont Center Experimental Station, Wilmington, Delaware*
Philippe Desmettre, *IFFA Merieux, Lyon, France*
Alan H. Deutch, *Research Division, W.R. Grace & Co., Columbia, Maryland*
Dino Dina, *Chiron Corp., Emeryville, California*
Friedrich Dorner, *Immuno Research Center, Orth Donau, Austria*
Gordon Dreesman, *Department of Virology, Baylor College of Medicine, Houston, Texas*
Emilio Emini, *Merck, Sharp & Dohme Research Laboratories, West Point, Pennsylvania*
B.E. Enger-Valk, *Medical Biological Laboratory, Rijswijk, The Netherlands*
Mary Estes, *Department of Virology, Baylor College of Medicine, Houston, Texas*
Bernard Fields, *Department of Microbiology, Harvard Medical School, Boston, Massachusetts*
Anne Flamand, *University of Paris, Orsay, France*
Jorge Flores, *NIAID, National Institutes of Health, Bethesda, Maryland*
Michael Fox, *Amgen, Inc., Thousand Oaks, California*
George French, *Salk Institute, Swiftwater, Pennsylvania*
Y. Furiuchi, *Roche Institute of Molecular Biology, Nutley, New Jersey*
Gary Gallick, *Department of Tumor Virology, University of Texas System Cancer Center, Houston, Texas*
Robert Garvin, *Genetic Engineering Group, Connaught Research Institute, Ontario, Canada*
John Gerin, *Department of Molecular Virology and Immunology, Georgetown University Medical Center, Rockville, Maryland*
H.M. Geysen, *Commonwealth Serum Laboratories, Parkville, Australia*
Richard Giles, *Advanced Genetics Research Institute, Oakland, California*
Lance Gordon, *Connaught Research Institute Laboratory, Swiftwater, Pennsylvania*
John Gorham, *College of Veterinary Medicine, Pullman, Washington*
Harry Greenberg, *Palo Alto Veterans Administration Hospital, Palo Alto, California*

Maurice Guss, *NCI, National Institutes of Health, Bethesda, Maryland*

Charles Hackett, *Department of Anatomy and Biology, Wistar Institute, Philadelphia, Pennsylvania*

Mary Haffey, *Merck, Sharp & Dohme Research Laboratories, West Point, Pennsylvania*

Ted Hall, *Department of Immunology, Walter Reed Army Institute of Research, Washington, D.C.*

Alan Hampson, *Commonwealth Serum Laboratories, Parkville, Australia*

T.J.R. Harris, *Celltech Ltd., Slough, England*

Per Hedman, *Pharmacia Fine Chemicals, Uppsala, Sweden*

Conrad Heilman, *Lederle Laboratories, Pearl River, New York*

Iver Heron, *Statens Serum Institut, Copenhagen, Denmark*

Richard Hjorth, *Wyeth Laboratories, Radner, Pennsylvania*

Robert Hodges, *Department of Biochemistry, University of Alberta, Edmonton, Canada*

Maurice Hofnung, *Unité de Programmation Moléculaire et Toxicologie Génétique, Institut Pasteur, Paris, France*

James Hogle, *Department of Molecular Biology, Scripps Clinic and Research Foundation, La Jolla, California*

Thomas Hopp, *Immunex Corp., Seattle, Washington*

Florian Horaud, *Départment du Virologie Medicale, Institut Pasteur, Paris, France*

C.P. Howard, *London School of Hygiene, London, England*

Shiu-Lok Hu, *Molecular Genetics, Inc., Minnetonka, Minnesota*

Sylvia Hu, *Amgen, Inc., Thousand Oaks, California*

Cinnia Huang, *Center for Laboratory Research, New York State Department of Health, Albany, New York*

Joseph Hughes, *Department of Virus Cell Biology, Merck, Sharp & Dohme Research Laboratories, West Point, Pennsylvania*

Paul Hung, *Wyeth Laboratories, Philadelphia, Pennsylvania*

Mitsunba Imai, *Roche Institute of Molecular Biology, Nutley, New Jersey*

Donald R. Jaffe, *Warner-Lambert Division, Parke-Davis, Morris Plains, New Jersey*

Wolfgang Joklik, *Department of Microbiology, Duke University Medical Center, Durham, North Carolina*

Raymond Jones, *Merck, Sharp & Dohme Research Laboratories, West Point, Pennsylvania*

William Jordan, Jr., *NIAID, National Institutes of Health, Bethesda, Maryland*

Ellen Jorgensen, *Department of Cell Biology, New York University, New York, New York*

Amrit Judd, *Bio-organic Laboratory, Stanford Research Institute International, Menlo Park, California*

Dominic Justewicz, *Institute Armand-Frappier, Université du Québec, Institute Armand-Frappier, Laval, Canada*

D.E. Kahn, *Department of Bio-Research, Pitman-Moore, Inc., Washington Crossing, New Jersey*

Joseph Kates, *Division of Cellular Biology, Scripps Clinic and Research Foundation, La Jolla, California*

Jerry Keith, *National Institutes of Health, Bethesda, Maryland*

Paul Keller, *Merck, Sharp & Dohme Research Laboratories, West Point, Pennsylvania*

Alan Kendal, *Department of Viral Diseases, Center for Disease Control, Atlanta, Georgia*

Ronald Kennedy, *Department of Virology and Epidemiology, Baylor College of Medicine, Houston, Texas*

Olen Kew, *Molecular Virology Branch, Center for Infectious Diseases, Atlanta, Georgia*

Edwin Kilbourne, *Department of Microbiology, Mt. Sinai School of Medicine, New York, New York*

Paul Kimball, *Battelle Columbus Laboratory, Columbus, Ohio*

Per Klemm, *Department of Microbiology, Technical University of Denmark, Copenhagen, Denmark*

C. Komly, *Institut Pasteur, Paris, France*
Ernst Kuechler, *Department of Biochemistry, University of Vienna, Austria*
John LaMontagne, *National Institutes of Health, Bethesda, Maryland*
Martial LaCroix, *Institute Armand-Frappier, Université du Québec, Laval, Canada*
Ching Lai, *NIAID, National Institutes of Health, Bethesda, Maryland*
Terry Landers, *Bethesda Research Laboratories, Inc., Gaithersburg, Maryland*
Larry Lasky, *Genentech, Inc., South San Francisco, California*
J. LeComte, *Department of Virology Research, University of Québec, Laval, Canada*
Sung C. Lee, *Abbott Laboratories, North Chicago, Illinois*
Richard Lerner, *Department of Molecular Biology, Scripps Clinic and Research Foundation, La Jolla, California*
Wai-Choi Leung, *Department of Medicine, University of Alberta, Edmonton, Canada*
Mark Levner, *Wyeth Laboratories, Philadelphia, Pennsylvania*
David Linemeyer, *Department of Biochemical Genetics, Merck, Sharp & Dohme Research Laboratories, Rahway, New Jersey*
Peter LoMedico, *Department of Molecular Genetics, Hoffmann-LaRoche, Nutley, New Jersey*
Douglas Lorenz, *National Institutes of Health, Bethesda, Maryland*
M. MacDonald, *Synergen Associates, Inc., Boulder, Colorado*
Richard MacDonald, *Syntro Corporation, San Diego, California*
R. Macfarlan, *Wistar Institute, Philadelphia, Pennsylvania*
Michael Mackett, *NIAID, National Institutes of Health, Bethesda, Maryland*
Terrence Majewski, *Tri State Center, Smith Laboratories, Northbrook, Illinois*
Jack Makari, *Makari Research Laboratories, Englewood, New Jersey*
Lewis Markoff, *National Institutes of Health, Bethesda, Maryland*
Bernard Meignier, *Institut Merieux, Charbonnieres, France*
Karen Midthun, *National Institutes of Health, Bethesda, Maryland*
J.S. Miller, *Department of Biological Chemistry, Harvard Medical School, Boston, Massachusetts*
Sudha Mitra, *Department of Biochemical Genetics, Merck, Sharp & Dohme Research Laboratories, Rahway, New Jersey*
Tatsuo Miyamura, *Chiron Corporation, Emeryville, California*
Douglas Moore, *USDA, Plum Island Animal Disease Center, Greenport, New York*
Bror Morein, *Institute of Microbiology, National Veterinary Institute, Uppsala, Sweden*
A.J. Morgan, *Department of Pathology, University of Bristol Medical School, Bristol, England*
Donald Morgan, *USDA, Plum Island Animal Disease Center, Greenport, New York*
Bernard Moss, *NIAID, National Institutes of Health, Bethesda, Maryland*
David McCahon, *Department of Genetics, Animal Virus Research Institute, Pirbright, England*
Neville McCarthy, *Commonwealth Serum Laboratories, Parkville, Australia*
Brian Murphy, *NIAID, National Institutes of Health, Bethesda, Maryland*
Fred A. Murphy, *Department of Viral Diseases, Center for Disease Control, Atlanta, Georgia*
Debi Nayak, *Department of Microbiology, University of California, Los Angeles, California*
Paolo Neri, *Sclavo Research Center, Siena, Italy*
Danute Nitecki, *Cetus Corporation, Berkeley, California*
Erling Norrby, *Karolinska Institute School of Medicine, Stockholm, Sweden*
Bodil Norrild, *Department of Medical Microbiology, University of Copenhagen, Copenhagen, Denmark*
Jack Nunberg, *Cetus Corporation, Berkeley, California*
John Obijeski, *Genentech, Inc., South San Francisco, California*
Paul Offit, *Department of Anatomy and Biology, Wistar Institute, Philadelphia, Pennsylvania*
Michael Oldstone, *Scripps Clinic and Research Foundation, La Jolla, California*
Dennis Panicali, *New York State Department of Health, Albany, New York*
Enzo Paoletti, *New York State Department of Health, Albany, New York*

J.M.R. Parker, *Department of Biochemistry, University of Alberta, Edmonton, Canada*
Debbie Parkes, *Chiron Corporation, Emeryville, California*
Andrea Pavirani, *Transgene, S.A., Strasbourg, France*
Olgerts Pavlovskis, *Department of Infectious Disease, Naval Medical Research Institute, Bethesda, Maryland*
Marion Perkus, *New York State Department of Health, Albany, New York*
Stephen Petteway, *E.I. duPont, Wilmington, Delaware*
Eberhgard Pfaff, *Department of Microbiology, University of Heidelberg, Heidelberg, Federal Republic of Germany*
Nina Piccini, *New York State Department of Health, Albany, New York*
Stanley Plotkin, *Children's Hospital of Philadelphia, Philadelphia, Pennsylvania*
Steven Popple, *Department of Microbiology, Mt. Sinai School of Medicine, New York, New York*
Philip Provost, *Merck, Sharp & Dohme Research Laboratories, West Point, Pennsylvania*
Robert Purcell, *NIAID, National Institutes of Health, Bethesda, Maryland*
Tony Purchio, *Molecular Genetics, Inc., Minnetonka, Minnesota*
Jasodhara Ray, *Glasgow Research Laboratory, E.I. duPont, Wilmington, Delaware*
Craig Rice, *Codon Corp., Brisbane, California*
John Rice, *Battelle Columbus Laboratories, Columbus, Ohio*
Bryan Roberts, *Department of Biological Chemistry, Harvard Medical School, Boston, Massachusetts*
Betty Robertson, *USDA, Plum Island Animal Disease Center, Greenport, New York*
James Robertson, *National Institute of Biological Standards, London, England*
Bernard Roizman, *Kovler Viral Oncology Laboratory, University of Chicago, Chicago, Illinois*
Rudolph Rott, *Institut fur Virologie, Justus-Liebig-Universitat, Giessen, Federal Republic of Germany*
D.J. Rowlands, *Animal Virus Research Institute, Pirbright, England*
W. Rutter, *Department of Biochemistry, University of California, San Francisco, California*
Babiu Samal, *Applied Molecular Genetics, Inc., Newbury Park, California*
A.R. Sanderson, *Medical Research Council Immunology Team, Guy's Hospital, London, England*
Virender Sarin, *Department of Molecular Biology, Abbott Laboratories, North Chicago, Illinois*
G.C. Schild, *National Institute of Biological Standards, London, England*
H. Edward Schmitz, *Department of Immunology, Mayo Clinic, Rochester, Minnesota*
Grazia Sessa, *Merck, Sharp & Dohme International Division, Rahway, New Jersey*
Alexis Shelokov, *Department of Hygiene and Public Health, Johns Hopkins University, Baltimore, Maryland*
James Shih, *FDA, Bureau of Biologics, Bethesda, Maryland*
Jacqueline Siegal, *Scripps Clinic and Research Foundation, La Jolla, California*
Geoffrey Smith, *NIAID, National Institutes of Health, Bethesda, Maryland*
Robert Smith, *Department of Molecular Biology, Abbott Laboratories, North Chicago, Illinois*
R.E. Spier, *Animal Virus Research Institute, Pirbright, England*
C. Stratowa, *Max-Planck Institut, Munich, Federal Republic of Germany*
Richard Sublett, *Schering Animal Health, Omaha, Nebraska*
N. Sivasubramanian, *Department of Microbiology, and Immunology, University of California School of Medicine, Los Angeles, California*
Robert Swanson, *Markari Research Laboratories, Englewood, New Jersey*
Jeff Swarz, *Pall Corporation, Glen Cove, New York*
John Sninsky, *Albert Einstein College of Medicine, Bronx, New York*
Rees Thomas, *Tech Innovations, Inc., Lambertville, New Jersey*
G.B. Thornton, *Johnson and Johnson Co., La Jolla, California*

John Ticehurst, *National Institutes of Health, Bethesda, Maryland*

Pierre Tiollais, *Institut Pasteur, Paris, France*

Michel Trudel, *Institut Armand-Frappier, Université du Québec, Laval, Canada*

Bernard Vacher, *Institut Pasteur, Paris, France*

Pablo Valenzuela, *Chiron Corporation, Emeryville, California*

Pieter van der Marel, *Instituut voor de Volksgezondheid, Bilthowen, The Netherlands*

Gary Van Nest, *Chiron Corporation, Emeryville, California*

Leland Velicer, *Department of Microbiology, Michigan State University, East Lansing, Michigan*

Fleming Velin, *Scan Vet, Fredensborg, Denmark*

S. Venkatesan, *NIAID, National Institutes of Health, Bethesda, Maryland*

Eladio Vinuela, *Department of Molecular Biology, University Autonoma, Madrid, Spain*

Roberto Waack, *Department of Biotechnology, Embrabio-Empresa Brasileira, Sao Paulo, Brazil*

D. Eugene Wampler, *Merck, Sharp & Dohme Research Laboratories, West Point, Pennsylvania*

Kenneth Watson, *Department of Molecular Biology, Abbott Laboratories, North Chicago, Illinois*

N.J. Watt, *Department of Veterinary Pathology, University of Glasgow, Glasgow, Scotland*

G. Weddell, *Genentech, Inc., South San Francisco, California*

Robert Weibel, *Children's Hospital of Philadelphia, Philadelphia, Pennsylvania*

Gjalt Welling, *Laboratory of Medical Microbiology, Rijksuniversiteit Groningen, Groningen, The Netherlands*

Douglas Welsh, *USDA, Plum Island Animal Disease Center, Greenport, New York*

C.A. Whetstone, *Biologics Virology Laboratory, National Veterinary Services Laboratory, Ames, Iowa*

Roy Widdus, *National Academy of Sciences, Washington, D.C.*

Nigel Williams, *Nature, London, England*

Ian Wilson, *Scripps Clinic and Research Foundation, La Jolla, California*

Tazewell Wilson, *Bio/Technology, New York, New York*

Eckard Wimmer, *Department of Microbiology, State University of New York, Stony Brook, New York*

Steven Wright, *Veterans Administration Medical Center, Salt Lake City, Utah*

M.D Yavardios, *Berri Balzac, Chalaronne, France*

Tilahum Yilma, *Department of Veterinary Microbiology, Washington State University, Pullman, Washington*

James Young, *Smith Kline & French Laboratories, Philadelphia, Pennsylvania*

Janis Young, *Division of Infectious Diseases, Children's Hospital Medical Center, Boston, Massachusetts*

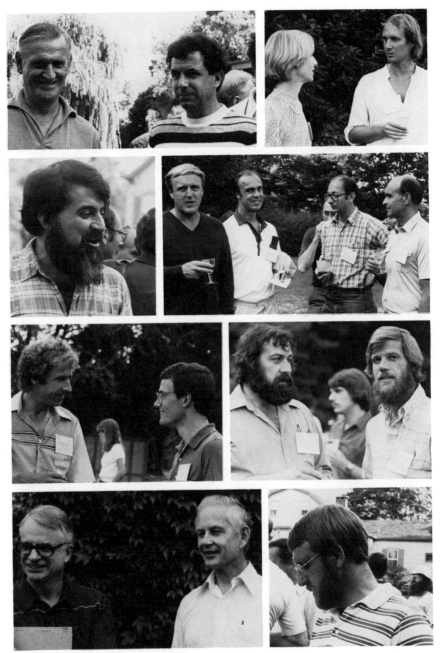

First row: F. Brown, D.J. Rowlands; B. Norrild, P. Klemm
Second row: J. Flores; R. Lerner, E. Norrby, A. Kendal, R. Rott
Third row: J. Robertson, G. Smith; J. Keith, E. Paoletti
Fourth row: R. Chanock, W. Joklik; G. Both

Contents

Section 2   CHEMISTRY OF VIRUS NEUTRALIZATION

Section 3   CLONING AND EXPRESSION OF VIRAL GENES

Section 4   ATTENUATION OF VIRULENCE

Preface

Although vaccination is one of medicine's most time-honored processes, it remains an imperfect solution to the prevention of infectious diseases. Very recently, however, tremendous advances have been made in the design of new vaccines. Accordingly, in September 1983, a meeting was held at Cold Spring Harbor Laboratory to review these results and to discuss new vaccine strategies.

This first meeting on Modern Approaches to Vaccines was a highly successful undertaking that focused on virus vaccines. Sixty-six papers and a poster session provided a broad review of the current knowledge in this field and indicated the direction of future research. In honor of those who have laid the foundation for and influenced our endeavors in the field of virus vaccines, we have dedicated this volume to three eminent scientists, Dr. Wallace Rowe, Dr. Robert Huebner, and Dr. Albert Sabin. The bacterial approach will be the topic of the second meeting in this series, to be held in 1984.

The organizers wish to thank Merck, Sharp and Dohme Research Laboratories, Merieux Institute, Inc., and the Wellcome Foundation, Ltd., for their generous support of this meeting.

We also thank Dr. James Watson for his support and for making the conference and publication facilities of Cold Spring Harbor Laboratory available to us; Gladys Kist and her staff of the Meetings office for their help in organizing the meeting; and Nancy Ford, Director of Publications, Dorothy Brown, Adrienne Guerra, and Laurel Garbarini for their help in preparing this book for publication.

R.M.C.
R.A.L.

A Tribute to Wallace Rowe, Robert Huebner, and Albert Sabin

The first meeting on Modern Approaches to Vaccines was dedicated to three eminent scientists: Drs. Wallace Rowe, Robert Huebner, and Albert Sabin. I have been asked by the editors to write the tribute for this volume, a task I acknowledge with pleasure and respect.

In the modern era of revolutionary developments in molecular biology, there is a certain tendency among scientists to neglect the importance of historical developments. The new techniques allow the accumulation of amazingly detailed knowledge about the structure of molecules, but the molecules only come alive when this knowledge allows a more refined understanding of functional relationships. A considerable body of knowledge of biological phenomena had already accumulated before the current molecular era, and this early information should be recognized.

Of the three scientists to whom this volume is dedicated, Wallace Rowe is no longer with us. His last paper recently appeared in *Science*, ending a long series of outstanding contributions. In his early career, Rowe studied the immunological background of the persistence of LCM virus infections in mice. He was one of the pioneers who used tissue-culture techniques developed in the 1950s to isolate and characterize new viruses. In these studies, he discovered human cytomegalovirus and codiscovered human adenoviruses. Rowe then became interested in oncogenic viruses. He analyzed infection with polyoma virus under natural and laboratory conditions and found that tumors arose only under laboratory conditions. Further studies of DNA tumor virus systems led to the identification of T antigens in cells infected with adenovirus, polyoma virus, and SV40. In this context, Rowe also codiscovered adenovirus-SV40 hybrids.

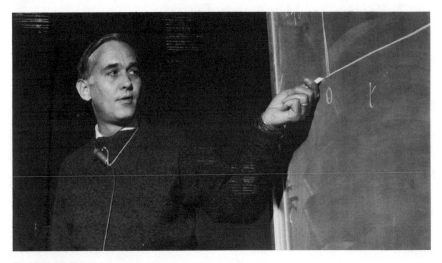

Dr. Wallace Rowe

In the mid-1960s, Rowe became interested in murine retroviruses. His many contributions resulting from studies of these viruses include the description of new techniques for detecting and analyzing these viruses, the elucidation of the genetic bases for the infection of cells by certain retroviruses, the demonstration that halogenated pyrimidins can activate a retrovirus integrated in the host-cell genome to productive infection, the discovery of naturally occurring murine leukemia viruses that are genetic recombinants, and finally the demonstration of the genetics of transmittance of such viruses.

During his last years, Rowe undertook the effort to document the harmlessness of recombinant DNA experiments, an important service to the scientific community. Rowe's generous and low-key personality will always be remembered by colleagues who had the privilege to know him. His experimental proficiency in well-targeted problem solving will forever give him a place in the history of modern virology.

Robert Huebner's approach to research is completely different from that of Rowe. He has always been overflowing with ideas for solving many different virological problems. He started his career by making important discoveries about rickettsial pox and Q fever. Turning to virology in the 1950s, he defined coxsackie viruses and also gave the first description of adenoviruses. Huebner set up the important Junior Village study in Washing-

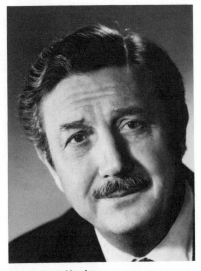

Dr. Robert Huebner

ton D.C., which elucidated the medical importance of many respiratory viruses and mycoplasmas. Later he discovered the T antigen of adenoviruses and consequently became involved in studies of virus oncogenesis. He continued to be active in this field throughout the rest of his career. From relatively limited experimental evidence, he formulated the oncogene theory. Since the recent discovery of oncogenes, this prophetic theory has again become the focus of attention. Because of his many important contributions, Huebner will always be remembered as a devoted scientist of high standing.

Albert Sabin has made important contributions in many fields, although most people associate his name with the development of the live polio vaccine. The

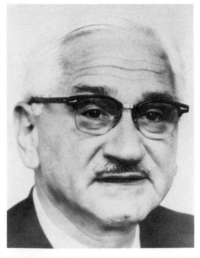

Dr. Albert Sabin

medical impact of this pioneering work is enormous. In his early work, he described the pathogenesis and medical importance of toxoplasmas in man and mycoplasmas in mice. He then embarked on pathogenetic and genetic studies of arboviruses, which were long-time forerunners of later similar studies. He made the first discovery of dengue viruses and sandfly fever viruses, and he demonstrated the hemagglutinating activity of group-A and group-B arboviruses. Sabin is a man of unique character and penetrating intelligence. He has had the privilege of serving (or perhaps dominating is a more appropriate word) the scientific community until now and we hope he will continue to be actively involved in solving virological problems in the future.

Although scientists have different personalities, it is clear that their personalities are influenced by their mentors and also by the leading investigators in their areas of research. Furthermore, the unforseen rapid development of virology, reflected in consecutive paradigmatic shifts, and the richness in the personality gallery of past and present contributors to the field provide a fertile soil for our enthusiasm and joy in the present day endeavors in virology. In this spirit we pay our tribute to Drs. Rowe, Huebner, and Sabin.

Erling Norrby
Karolinska Institutet
Stockholm, Sweden

MODERN APPROACHES TO VACCINES

Three-dimensional Structure of a Viral Antigen: Hemagglutinin Glycoprotein of Influenza Virus

Ian A. Wilson
Department of Molecular Biology
Research Institute of Scripps Clinic
La Jolla, California 92037

John J. Skehel
National Institute for Medical Research
Mill Hill, London NW71AA, England

Don C. Wiley
Department of Biochemistry and
Molecular Biology, Harvard University
Cambridge, Massachusetts 02138

Defense against a variety of viral and bacterial agents depends on the ability of the host immune system to recognize and neutralize antigens on the surfaces of these organisms. Some viruses, such as influenza virus, may in turn evade previous immunization and escape neutralization by altering their own immunogenic properties. Influenza virus, in particular, can cause recurrent epidemics, usually every 3−4 years, by altering the antigenicity of its surface proteins. A precise definition of the antigenic sites or determinants is required in order to understand the molecular basis of the immune response. To understand the structural basis of viral antigen-antibody recognition, the three-dimensional structure of the Hong Kong 1968 influenza virus hemagglutinin was determined. Recurrent epidemics of influenza virus are associated with changes in the antigenicity of this surface glycoprotein. Availability of amino acid sequences of the 1972, 1975, and 1979 strains enabled a detailed evaluation of how, by an accumulation of amino acid mutations, the antigen can change its surface in order to evade neutralization by the immune system. The function of the protein and its antigenic properties are discussed below.

Structure Determination

The bromelain-released hemagglutinin structure was determined to 3-Å resolution using one heavy atom derivative, mercury phenyl glyoxal. Solution of the Patterson gave six heavy atom sites, two per monomer, and the direction of the

1

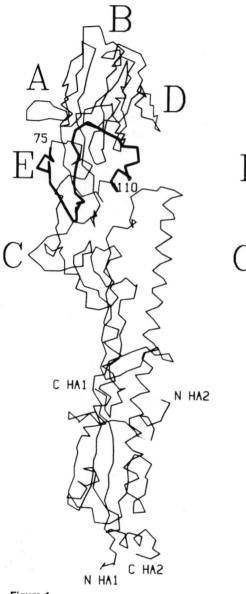
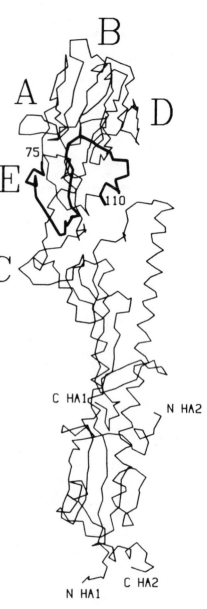

Figure 1

Stereodrawing of the α-carbon chain of an influenza hemagglutinin monomer. The brome-lain-released molecule is 146 Å long and up to 40 Å in radius. N and C indicate the amino and carboxyl termini for HA₁ (328 residues) and HA₂ (175 residues). (*A—E*) Proposed an-tibody-combining sites. The location in the hemagglutinin monomer of a chemically syn-thesized peptide (residues 75—110) against which monoclonal antibodies were raised is shown by the thicker trace. The membrane attachment end of the molecule to the virus surface is at the bottom, and the receptor binding site is at the top (distal end).

2

noncrystallographic threefold axis of the trimer. Phase determination and refinement with noncrystallographic threefold symmetry averaging and solvent flattening (Bricogne 1976) produced an electron density map, which was interpreted in terms of the amino acid sequence (Wilson et al. 1981).

Three-dimensional Structure

The hemagglutinin is synthesized as a single polypeptide chain of 550 residues and 20% carbohydrate by weight. Cleavage activation, by removal of a single arginine residue, gives rise to the fusion activity of the virus. The two polypeptide chains are HA_1 (328 residues) and HA_2 (221 residues). The bromelain-released protein is cleaved from the membrane at Gly-175 of HA_2, leaving behind the hydrophobic membrane-anchoring tail. The structure of the viral spike reveals a globular head of HA_1 residues and a fibrous tail, consisting of both HA_1 and HA_2 (Wilson et al. 1981). The hemagglutinin extends about 146 Å from the membrane in a usual looplike structure (Fig. 1). The globular heads are mainly composed of β-structure in a Swiss-roll-type motif. The fibrous tail has a high percentage of α-helix, and the trimer is stabilized by a 76-Å-long helical triple coiled-coil structure. The fusion peptide, the amino terminus of HA_2, is embedded in the trimer interface. A conformational change in the hemagglutinin has been observed to occur at approximately pH 5, the pH optimal for membrane fusion activity of the virus. At this pH, the fusion peptide appears to be released from the trimer interface, and this conformational change initiates fusion activity (Skehel et al. 1982).

Antigenic Variation

The structure of the Hong Kong strain was analyzed with reference to available amino acid sequence information from natural and laboratory-selected antigenic variants. Four antibody-combining sites on the molecule were identified, and from 1968 to 1975, at least one mutation in each of these sites seemed to be required for the virus to escape neutralization (Fig. 1A–D) (Wiley et al. 1981). These antigenic sites are located on the globular head of the molecule and generally consist of exposed loops on the surface of the molecule (sites A, B, and C). However, one combining site maps in the trimer interface (site D). Change in carbohydrate attachment from residue 81 to residue 63 in the HA_1 1975 Victoria strain appears to have exposed another probable antibody-combining site (E), around an area previously buried by hexose residues. Thus, amino acid mutation and variation in the carbohydrate location seem to modulate antigenicity of the hemagglutinin (Wiley et al. 1981; Wilson et al. 1983).

Carbohydrate

The carbohydrate electron density is not generally as well defined as the protein density. Only approximately 25% of the carbohydrate moieties have been identified clearly (Fig. 2). The density for the high-mannose hexoses, attached to residues 165 and 285, is generally better defined than that for the complex carbohydrate. The carbohydrate buries some potential tryptic and chymotryptic cleavage sites and may help protect against degradation of the protein. Another possible role for the carbohydrate is to stabilize the three-dimensional structure,

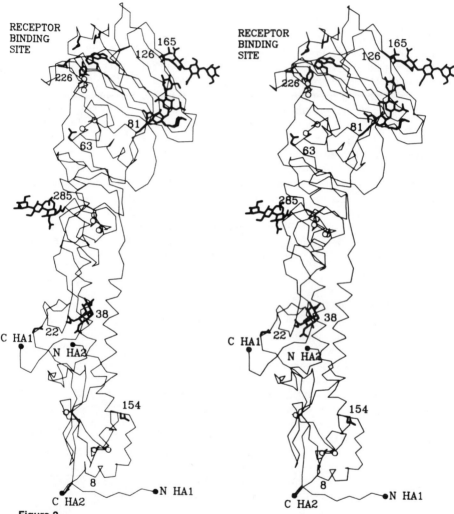

Figure 2
Stereodrawing of the a-carbon chain of the hemagglutinin monomer (Hong Kong, 1968) with location of carbohydrate attachment sites and receptor binding sites. Hexose moieties that are defined best in the electron density are indicated by thicker lines for residues 38, 81, 165, and 285 of HA_1. Asn side chains (22 HA_1, 154 HA_2) for which no carbohydrate has yet been built is shown. Carbohydrate is also attached to residue 8 of HA_2, but weak density is present for the main chain (1–8) and no Asn is shown. Locations of new carbohydrate attachment sites in 1975 at residues 63 and 126 are shown (residue 81 is lost). Side chains of residues implicated in the receptor binding site are shown by thicker lines at the distal end of the molecule as indicated around residue 226.

as, for example, the carbohydrate attached at Asn-165, which interacts with the adjacent monomer (Fig. 2). Modulation of the antigenicity of the virus by altering the number and location of carbohydrate attachment sites and hence masking and unmasking the protein is clearly an important function for the carbohydrate as discussed above.

Receptor Binding Site

The receptor binding site for sialic-acid-containing lipids or proteins was proposed on the basis of a conservation of amino acids in a shallow pocket at the distal end of the molecule from the membiane (Wilson et al. 1981). Chemical identification of this binding site was made by selecting mutants with different binding specificities in the presence of inhibitors (Rogers et al. 1983). Nucleic acid sequence analysis of these variants shows that only a single amino acid change from Leu-226 to Gln-226 alters the specificity of carbohydrate binding for (2-6) NeuAc-Gal to (2-3) NeuAc-Gal. Another mutant that had both binding activities and a Met at residue 226 was identified. This residue is located at the mouth of the previously postulated receptor binding pocket (Fig. 2).

Synthetic Polypeptides

Chemically synthesized peptides have been used to probe the antigenic structure of influenza virus (Green et al. 1982). Twenty peptides with sequences corresponding to the X:47 (1975) strain elicited an immune response. The antisera to most of these peptides showed significant binding to both intact antigen and whole virus. Recently, 20 monoclonal antibodies were raised against a single synthetic peptide (residues 75−110 of HA_1; Fig. 1). The frequency with which antibodies were produced and that were intact-protein-reactive was higher than expected (75%) (Niman et al. 1983). Crystallization of protein-reactive monoclonal antibodies with synthetic peptides is being carried out to evaluate the structural nature of the antibody-antigen complex and to evaluate their potential use as models for synthetic peptide vaccines.

ACKNOWLEDGMENTS

We would like to thank Andrew R. Cherenson for preparation of the illustrations. Acknowledgment is given to grant support for the hemagglutinin structural work from National Institutes of Health grant AI-13654 (D.C.W.) and National Science Foundation grant PC-77-11398 (D.C.W., computing hardware). The monoclonal antibody structure work is being supported by National Institutes of Health grant 1-PO1-A1-19499-01 (I.A.W.).

REFERENCES

Bricogne, G. 1976. Methods and programs for direct-space exploitation of redundancies. *Acta Crystallog.* **A32:** 832.

Green, N., H. Alexander, A. Olson, S. Alexander, T.M. Shinnick, J.G. Sutcliffe, and R.A. Lerner. 1982. Immunogenic structure of the influenza virus hemagglutinin. *Cell* **28:** 477.

Niman, H.L., R.A. Houghten, L.E. Walker, R.A. Reisfeld, I.A. Wilson, J.M. Hogle, and R.A. Lerner. 1983. Generation of protein reactive antibodies by short peptides is an event of high frequency: Implications for the structural basis of immune recognition. *Proc. Natl. Acad. Sci.* **80:** 4949.

Rogers, G.N., J.C. Paulson, R.S. Daniels, J.J. Skehel, I.A. Wilson, and D.C. Wiley. 1983. Single amino acid substitutions in influenza hemagglutinin change receptor binding specificity. *Nature* **304:** 76.

Skehel, J.J., P.M. Bayley, E.B. Brown, S.R. Martin, M.D. Waterfield, J.M. White, I.A. Wilson, and D.C. Wiley. 1982. Changes in the conformation of influenza virus hemagglutinin at the pH optimum of virus-mediated membrane fusion. *Proc. Natl. Acad. Sci.* **79:** 968.

Wiley, D.C., I.A. Wilson, and J.J. Skehel. 1981. Structural identification of the antibody-binding sites of Hong Kong influenza hemagglutinin and their involvement in antigenic variation. *Nature* **289:** 373.

Wilson, I.A., J.J. Skehel, and D.C. Wiley. 1981. Structure of the hemagglutinin membrane glycoprotein of influenza at 3 Å resolution. *Nature* **289:** 366.

Wilson, I.A., R.C. Ladner, J.J. Skehel, and D.C. Wiley. 1983. The structure and role of the carbohydrate moieties of influenza virus hemagglutinin. *Biochem. Soc. Trans.* **11:** 145.

High-resolution Structural Studies of Poliovirus

James M. Hogle
Department of Molecular Biology
Scripps Clinic and Research Foundation
La Jolla, California 92037

For more than 30 years poliovirus has served a role as a model system from which many current concepts of viral molecular biology have been established. The recent introduction of several new technologies, including monoclonal antibodies, rapid nucleic acid sequencing, site-directed mutagenesis, and the use of synthetic peptide antigens as specific probes of antigenic structure have resulted in a renewed interest in poliovirus, including interest in the development of more satisfactory vaccines.

The elegant studies of the influenza hemagglutinin have demonstrated the power of structural studies of viral antigens when coupled with active biochemical and immunological characterization (Wiley et al. 1981; Wilson et al. 1981; Wilson et al., this volume). We have recently obtained crystals of both the Sabin and the Mahoney strains of the type-I serotype of poliovirus (Hogle 1982). The crystals of the Mahoney strain diffract to at least 2.4-Å resolution and are highly suitable for high-resolution X-ray crystallographic analysis. We believe that the structural studies of poliovirus hold great promise, providing for the first time the possibility of studying a well-characterized viral antigen in the context of the intact virus.

At the present time there has only been limited characterization of the structure of poliovirus and other members of the picornavirus family, which also includes the aphthoviruses, such as foot-and-mouth disease virus, and the rhinoviruses. The poliovirus particle diameter is 300 Å, and the particle weight is 8.4 million daltons. In the electron microscope, poliovirus has a rather featureless spherical appearance, which has to date proved refractory to structural analysis. The virus is a naked virus with a capsid that is composed entirely of 60 copies of

7

each of the four coat-protein subunits VP1, VP2, VP3, and VP4 (with molecular weights of 34,000, 30,000, 26,000, and 7,400, respectively) arranged on a $T = 1$ icosahedral surface. Several lines of evidence suggest that VP1 is the major surface protein of the viral capsid and that VP4 occupies an (relatively) interior position. The capsid encloses a single unique molecule of single-stranded RNA with a molecular weight of 2.5 million. The RNA is of positive polarity, is poly-adenylated at its 3' end, and is linked via a uridyl-phosphotyrosine link to the genome-linked protein VPg at its 5' end. The complete nucleotide sequences (~7500 bases) of several strains of poliovirus have now been determined, including both the Sabin and its parent Mahoney strain of the type-I serotype (Kitamura et al. 1981; Racaniello and Baltimore 1981; Nomoto et al. 1982).

Poliovirus apparently has a strong tendency to form ordered arrays. It often forms crystalline inclusions inside infected cells. In the late 1950s, microcrystals of all three serotypes of poliovirus were observed in the insoluble residues of ultracentrifuged pellets. Subsequently, large single crystals of the Mahoney strain were observed to form during prolonged storage (1 year) of concentrated stocks (5–10 mg/ml) of the virus (Steere and Schaffer 1958). This observation was made possible by the availability of large amounts of the virus from contaminated stocks prepared for production of the Salk vaccine. These crystals were char-

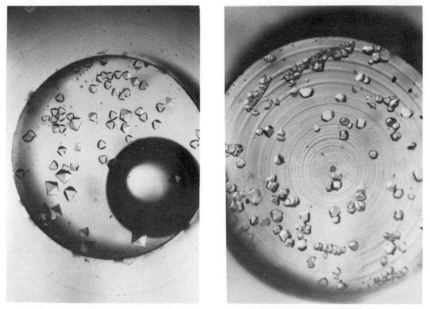

Figure 1
Crystals of the Sabin (*left*) and the Mahoney (*right*) strains of the type-I serotype of polio-virus. The crystals were obtained by dialysis of concentrated stocks (10 mg/ml) of the virus vs. progressively lower concentrations of NaCl in 10 mm phosphate or PIPES buffer at pH 7.0. Crystallization generally occurs between 0.05 M and 0.15 M NaCl, depending on the virus concentration and the quality of the preparation.

acterized crystallographically by Finch and Klug (1959) and were found to diffract to very high resolution. These crystals also provided the first definitive proof that poliovirus was an icosahedral particle. Further characterization of the crystals was not possible due to limitations in data collection and processing technologies. Within the past 5 years, the technology required for the complete characterization of small virus structures has been developed, and the structures of four spherical plant viruses are now known at high resolution (Harrison et al. 1978; Abad-Zapatero et al. 1980; Liljas et al. 1982; J.M. Hogle and S.C. Harrison, in prep.).

When crystallographic studies of poliovirus were resumed, the first concern was to find a means for the reproducible production of large single crystals of the virus. The Sabin and the Mahoney strains of the virus were observed to produce suitably sized crystals under similar conditions, namely, by dialysis versus low-ionic-strength NaCl (<0.1 M) in phosphate or PIPES buffer at pH 7.0. The crystals are shown in Figure 1. Unfortunately, the crystals of the Sabin strain have proved to be exceptionally sensitive to X-irradiation and have not yet been suitable for structural studies. We are currently beginning a reinvestigation of the crystallization conditions of the Sabin strain in the hope of producing more suitable crystals. The crystals of the Mahoney strain are also sensitive to X-irradiation, but by cooling the crystals, it has been possible to prolong their lifetime in the beam sufficiently to obtain high-resolution diffraction photographs. In fact, in an important recent development, improvement in the design of the sample cooling apparatus (and in the size and quality of the crystals) has made it possible to routinely obtain several photographs (up to nine) from a single crystal. This development will considerably accelerate the rate of data acquisition.

A typical oscillation photograph obtained from crystals of the Mahoney strain is shown in Figure 2. The photograph shows discernible intensities out to at least 2.4-Å resolution. There are more than 30,000 intensities within the 2.9-Å limit (the practical limit of our current cameras), and a complete data set will consist of more than 100 such photographs. For technical reasons, the packing of intensity maxima on the poliovirus diffraction photographs is almost twice that of corresponding photographs from crystals of plant viruses whose structures have been determined to date. This has necessitated considerable modification of the methods for scanning these photographs to obtain integrated intensity measurements. These modifications (which are being developed by Dr. D. Filman in our laboratory) are nearly completed, and the processing of the native data is in progress.

The structure of the virus will obviously have important implications in understanding many fundamental properties of the virus, including its assembly, receptor recognition, and mode of entry into cells. In addition, the structure will be relevant to two areas that are particularly important to vaccine technologies, namely, (1) immune recognition and neutralization by antibodies and (2) the factors responsible for neurovirulence and attenuation.

Investigators in several laboratories (including our own) are using a variety of techniques, including synthetic peptides, monoclonal antibodies, and genetic engineering, to define the sites on the poliovirus sequence that are responsible for eliciting neutralizing antibodies (see Schild et al.; Emini et al.; Chow et al.; all

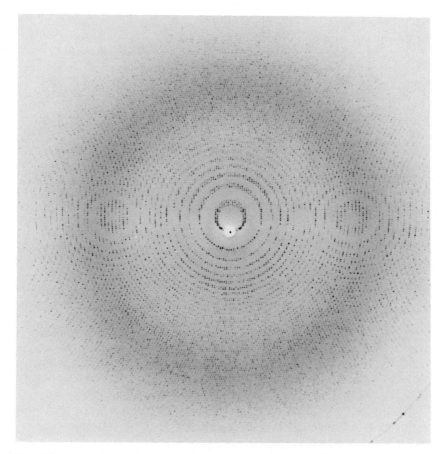

Figure 2
Typical 1/2 degree oscillation photograph from crystals of the Mahoney strain of type-I poliovirus. The space group is $P2_12_12$ with unit cell constants a = 324 Å, b = 359 Å, and c = 381 Å. The exposure time was 12 hr on an Elliot GX-20 rotating anode with a 100-μm focus and Franks mirror focusing optics.

this volume). Placing this inherently one-dimensional information on the three-dimensional structure of the virus may help (1) to define the mechanism of neutralization, (2) to select peptides (or combinations of peptides) for use as synthetic vaccines, and (3) to derive criteria for the rational selection of peptides for screening as synthetic vaccines in other systems.

Similarly, recent experiments suggest that mutations resulting in attenuation of neurovirulence of poliovirus may map preferentially to the capsid region of the genome. In the near future, nucleic acid sequencing and site-directed mutagenesis are expected to provide a map of virulence/attenuation mutations on the protein sequence. Placing the mutations on the three-dimensional structure of the virus will help define the factors responsible for neurovirulence and for attenuation and could aid in the rational design of more satisfactory attenuated strains.

ACKNOWLEDGMENTS

The author would like to thank Drs. Rueckert and Anderegg (University of Wisconsin) for samples of the Mahoney and Sabin strains of type-I poliovirus, Drs. Chow and Baltimore (M.I.T.) for supplying stocks of the Mahoney strain, and Dr. S.C. Harrison (Harvard University) for support and discussion. This work was supported in part by a Charles A. King Trust Fellowship to J.M.H. and in part by National Institutes of Health grant CA-13202 to S.C. Harrison.

REFERENCES

Abad-Zapatero, C., S.S. Abdel-Meguid, J.E. Johnson, A.G.W. Leslie, I. Rayment, M.G. Rossmann, D. Suck, and T. Tsukihara. 1980. Structure of southern bean mosaic virus at 2.8-Å resolution. *Nature* **286:** 33.

Finch, J.T. and A. Klug. 1959. Structure of poliomyelitis virus. *Nature* **183:** 1709.

Harrison, S.C., A.J. Olson, C.E. Schutt, F.K. Winkler, and G. Bricogne. 1978. Tomato bushy stunt virus at 2.9-Å resolution. *Nature* **276:** 368.

Hogle, J.M. 1982. Preliminary studies of crystals of poliovirus type I. *J. Mol. Biol.* **160:** 663.

Kitamura, N., B.L. Semler, P.G. Rothberg, G.R. Larsen, C.J. Adler, A.J. Dorner, E.A. Emini, R. Hanecak, J.J. Lee, S. van der Werf, C.W. Anderson, and E. Wimmer. 1981. Primary structure, gene organization and polypeptide expression of poliovirus RNA. *Nature* **291:** 547.

Liljas, L., T. Unge, T.A. Jones, K. Fridborg, S. Lovgren, U. Skoglund, and B. Strandberg. 1982. Structure of satellite tobacco necrosis virus at 3.0-Å resolution. *J. Mol. Biol.* **159:** 93.

Nomoto, A., T. Omata, H. Toyoda, S. Kuge, H. Horie, Y. Kataoka, Y. Genba, Y. Nakano, and N. Imura. 1982. Complete nucleotide sequence of the attenuated poliovirus Sabin 1 strain genome. *Proc. Natl. Acad. Sci.* **79:** 5793.

Racaniello, V.R. and D. Baltimore. 1981. Molecular cloning of poliovirus cDNA and determination of the complete nucleotide sequence of the viral genome. *Proc. Natl. Acad. Sci.* **78:** 4887.

Steere, R.L. and F.L. Schaffer. 1958. The structure of crystals of purified Mahoney poliovirus. *Biochim. Biophys. Acta* **28:** 241.

Wiley, D.C., I.A. Wilson, and J.J. Skehel. 1981. Structural identification of the antibody-binding sites of Hong Kong influenza haemagglutinin and their involvement in antigenic variation. *Nature* **289:** 373.

Wilson, I.A., J.J. Skehel, and D.C. Wiley. 1981. Structure of the haemagglutinin membrane glycoprotein of influenza virus at 3-Å resolution. *Nature* **289:** 366.

Antigenic Relationships between the Proteins of the Three Serotypes of Reovirus

Wolfgang K. Joklik
Department of Microbiology and Immunology
Duke University Medical Center
Durham, North Carolina 27710

The construction of an antiviral vaccine requires first and foremost a detailed understanding of the nature of the antigenic determinants on the proteins encoded by the virus and its antigenic variants. The purpose of the work discussed in this paper is to examine the antigenic determinants on the various proteins encoded by the three serotypes of reovirus at the gene level. Similar information will be required to construct vaccines against other members of the Reoviridae family such as the rotaviruses and orbiviruses, which include human and animal pathogens of medical and economic importance.

On Which Viral Structural Proteins Are Antigenic Determinants Located That Give Rise to Neutralizing Antibodies?

Reoviral particles comprise an inner capsid shell or core that contains the viral genome and is surrounded by an outer capsid shell. The outer capsid shell comprises three structural proteins; there are about 500 molecules of protein $\mu1C$ (m.w. 72,000), about 1000 molecules of protein $\sigma3$ (m.w. 34,000), and 24 molecules of protein $\sigma1$ (m.w. 40,000). The latter is the reoviral cell-attachment protein, the reoviral hemagglutinin, and the protein primarily responsible for specifying the interaction between reoviral particles and the immune mechanism, on the one hand, and tissue tropism, on the other. Monoclonal antibodies directed against all of these proteins have been isolated (Lee et al. 1981a). Antibodies against protein $\sigma1$ strongly neutralize reoviral particles in an almost completely type-specific manner; of the four monoclonal antibodies examined in detail, three neutralized in a totally type-specific manner while one was also capable of neu-

13

tralizing viral particles of another serotype. Antibodies against protein $o3$ possess weak neutralizing activity that is partially type-specific. Antibodies against protein $\mu1C$ do not neutralize infectivity. Interestingly, however, antibodies against a protein that has long been regarded as a core component do give rise to powerful neutralizing antibodies; this is protein $\lambda2$, the constituent of the core projections or spikes, which evidently project through the outer capsid shell to the surface of reoviral particles. Monoclonal antibodies against $\lambda2$ neutralize infectivity very efficiently and in a group-specific manner (i.e., monoclonal antibodies against serotype-3 $\lambda2$ protein neutralize particles of serotypes 1 and 2 with equal efficiency). The nature of an antiserum against any given serotype of reovirus depends on the relative proportions of antibodies against these three proteins. Usually, antibodies against $o1$ predominate, because antisera against the three serotypes of reovirus are mostly type-specific; but they do also contain group-specific components, which are no doubt due to antibodies against $\lambda2$ and $o3$. It should be pointed out that these antibodies also possess hemagglutination inhibition (HI) activity and that HI activity is much more type-specific than neutralizing activity (in other words, monoclonal antibodies against $\lambda2$ proteins, which exhibit group-specific neutralizing activity, possess mostly type-specific HI activity).

Are Antibodies against Antigenic Determinants on Other Reoviral Proteins Group- or Type-specific?

To determine the relatedness of the antigenic determinants on other reoviral proteins, antisera against serotypes 1, 2, and 3 were reacted with extracts of cells that had been infected with each of the three serotypes and labeled with radioactive amino acids. Antigen-antibody complexes were collected on Staph A, and the proteins present in such complexes were analyzed by quantitative autoradiography following electrophoresis in polyacrylamide gels (Gaillard and Joklik 1980).

The results are shown in Table 1. The ability of a given antiserum to react with any particular protein was quantitated by determining the concentration of antiserum that precipitated 50% of the maximum amount of protein that could be precipitated. As pointed out above, the most type specific of all reoviral proteins is indeed $o1$. There are several other isolated examples of type specificity, but the antigenic determinants of most proteins cannot be differentiated by antisera against any of the three serotypes. In other words, in most cases, a protein of a given serotype reacts as well with the two heterologous antisera as with homologous antiserum. Thus, the antigenic determinants on most reoviral proteins have been greatly conserved during evolution.

Extent of the Relatedness of the Three Serotypes of Reovirus at the Gene Level

The conservation of antigenic determinants on most reoviral proteins is remarkable because the three serotypes are not very closely related. As measured by the ability of their total genomes to hybridize with each other, serotypes 1 and 3 are related to the extent of about 70%, and both are only about 10% related to

Table 1
Quantitation of the Serologic Relatedness of Reovirus-coded Proteins

Protein	M_r	Approximate number of molecules per viral particle	Location	Coded by serotype	Antiserum against strain Abney serotype 1	Antiserum against strain D/5 Jones serotype 2	Antiserum against strain Dearing serotype 3
λ1	155,000	100	core	1	250	180	160
				2	190	200	240
				3	110	140	120
λ2	140,000	100	core spike/	1	230	60	120
			virion surface	2	260	160	200
				3	80	240	1000
μ1	80,000	24	core?	1	660	140	520
				2	420	200	660
				3	200	410	700
μ1C	72,000	500	virion surface	1	1420	80	700
				2	1000	1100	1220
				3	700	1780	1100
μNS	85,000	—	nonstructural	1	40	30	30
				2	40	40	30
				3	60	30	40
σ1	42,000	24	virion surface	1	1240	60	<10
				2	100	200	<10
				3	<10	<10	2000
σ2	38,000	200	core	1	280	100	1100
				2	280	1250	2300
				3	320	400	820
σ3	34,000	1000	virion surface	1	1000	260	1060
				2	1060	2400	1700
				3	860	1660	680
σNS	36,000	—	nonstructural	1	40	40	45
				2	30	45	30
				3	50	40	50

Numbers are the reciprocals of the antiserum dilutions at which 50% of the maximum amount of each protein reacted. Numbers in boxes indicate significant type specificity.

strains of serotype 2. We have carried out an extensive analysis to quantitate the genetic relatedness of the ten cognate gene sets. Hybrid genes were constructed in which the plus strand was that of a gene of one serotype and the minus strand that of the same gene but of another serotype. The extent of sensitivity to ribonuclease was then measured, using appropriate limits of resistance (homologous hybrids being taken to be completely resistant and single-stranded RNA molecules as completely sensitive, under the conditions used). The results are shown in Table 2 (Gaillard and Joklik 1982). The reoviral gene that has diverged to the greatest extent is gene *S1*, serotype-1 and -2 *S1* genes being no more than about 2% related; the genes that have diverged least are the *L* genes,

Table 2
Percentage Homology among the Genes of Reovirus Serotypes 1, 2, and 3

Gene	$\dfrac{+(1)^a}{-(2)}$	$\dfrac{+(1)}{-(3)}$	$\dfrac{+(3)}{-(1)}$	$\dfrac{+(3)}{-(2)}$	$\dfrac{+(2)}{-(1)}$	$\dfrac{+(2)}{-(3)}$
L1	15	86	84	18	21	11
L2	23	85	94	13	12	7
L3	12	88	79	13	15	14
M1	9	66	69	5	8	3
M2	5	31	42	9	11	8
M3	10	63	67	5	6	8
S1	4	12	6	1	1	4
S2	14	56	44	9	6	13
S3	12	69	81	14	8	12
S4	11	57	51	11	11	15

Data from Gaillard and Joklik (1982).
[a]Percentage of ribonuclease-resistant material (adjusted and corrected) in hybrid genes consisting of serotype-1 plus strands and serotype-2 minus strands.

serotype-1 and -3 L2 genes still being related to the extent of about 90%. Other genes show intermediate degrees of relatedness. The remarkable point is that in all cases, genes of serotypes 1 and 3 are much more closely related to each other than to genes of serotype 2. This suggests that the gene sets of the three reovirus serotypes have evolved as independent gene pools. It is within the context of these results that the results presented above assume significance. It is seen that the antigenic determinants on the proteins of even serotype 2 are still very closely related to those of serotypes 1 and 3, whereas their genes are by now only very distantly related. In other words, the regions of genes that encode the antigenic determinants of proteins have been highly conserved, but other regions have not.

Sequence Relationships among the Genes
of the Three Reovirus Serotypes

We have sequenced regions 70—100 residues long at both ends of four sets of cognate serotype-1, -2, and -3 genes; these are the L3 genes that encode the major core component λ1, the M3 genes that encode the nonstructural protein μNS, the S1 genes that encode the highly type-specific protein σ1, and the S2 genes that encode another major core component, protein σ2. The sequences at the ends of the L3, M3, and S1 genes that contain the 5' termini of the plus strands are shown in Figure 1 (Gaillard et al. 1982). It is remarkable how similar these sequences are in genes L3 and M3 (and also in gene S2; sequences not shown), not only for the closely related serotypes 1 and 3, but also for the much more distantly related serotype 2 (note that of the 11 differences in gene L3, 8 are in third codon positions, and the other 3 result in the substitution of an Arg codon for a Lys codon). In contrast, the sequences of the three S1 genes are very different, except for a 5'-terminal hexanucleotide and an octanucleotide several residues downstream. Clearly, both the sequences that encode the anti-

Gene L₃ (major core protein λ₁)

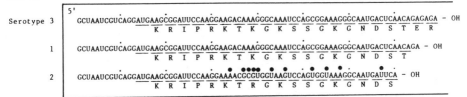

Gene M₃ (nonstructural protein μ_NS)

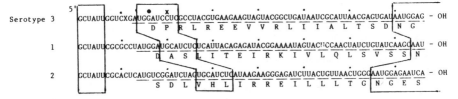

Gene S₁ (minor outer shell protein σ₁; type-specific protein)

Figure 1
Sequences of the 5'-terminal regions of the plus strands of genes *L3*, *M3*, and *S1* of reoviral serotypes 1, 2, and 3. (●) Base changes (the odd base out of three being indicated); (X) insertions (i.e., bases inserted into the sequence of one gene, but not into that of the other two). (Reprinted, with permission, from Gaillard et al. 1982.)

genic determinants and the sequences at the ends of reoviral genes have been highly conserved (the sequence relationships at the 3' termini, not shown here, are very similar to those at the 5' termini).

Sequencing of Cognate Genes of the Three Serotypes

We have cloned intact copies of all genes of all three reovirus serotypes. We have sequenced the *S1* genes of serotypes 1 and 3 and are in the process of sequencing the serotype-2 *S1* gene (unpubl.). The serotype-3 *S1* gene comprises 1416 nucleotides and possesses a single, long open reading frame of 345 codons starting at the first initiation codon that begins at position 13, and a long untranslated region at the 3' end. Interestingly, the first initiation codon of this gene provides a weak initiation signal, since it has C in position −3 (Kozak 1981). Kozak (1982) has found that ribosomal subunits protect two *S1* initiation codons, one that starts at position 13 and another that starts at position 71 and provides a strong initiation signal since it possesses A in position − 3 (Li et al. 1980; Antczak et al. 1982). However, initiation at that second initiation codon is followed by an open reading frame of only 360 nucleotides. The protein that could be encoded by this reading frame has not yet been identified. Clearly, however, protein σ1 is initiated at the first, weak initiation codon.

Whereas the amino acid sequences of the three S1-gene proteins are quite different, their tertiary structures as determined by computer analysis are remarkably similar. Thus, although their sequences have diverged greatly, their functions have been conserved: All three σ1 proteins are still the cell-attachment proteins (in fact, they still combine with the same cellular receptor [Lee et al. 1981b]); all three σ1 proteins are still the reoviral hemagglutinin; and they all still react with the immune mechanism and specify tissue tropism.

DISCUSSION

These studies lay the groundwork for the construction of antireovirus vaccines. They provide essential information concerning the nature of the relatedness of the antigenic variants of reovirus. Similar studies will be required for preparing vaccines against human rotaviruses and the various medically and economically important orbiviruses.

ACKNOWLEDGMENTS

The work described in this paper resulted from the collaboration of numerous colleagues, among them Jim Antczak, Rich Chmelo, Dick Gaillard, Ed Hayes, Jack Keene, Patrick Lee, Joe Li, and David Pickup. The expert technical assistance of Sherry Montgomery, Pat McClellan-Green, and Lilly Lou is also gratefully acknowledged. This work was supported by grants 1R01-AI-08909, 1-P01-CA-30246, and 5T32-AI-07148.

REFERENCES

Antczak, J.B., R. Chmelo, D.J. Pickup, and W.K. Joklik. 1982. Sequences at both termini of the ten genes of reovirus serotype 3 (strain Dearing). *Virology* **121:** 307.

Gaillard, R.K., Jr. and W.K. Joklik. 1980. The antigenic determinants of most of the proteins coded by the three serotypes of reovirus are highly conserved during evolution. *Virology* **107:** 533.

―――. 1982. Quantitation of the relatedness of reovirus serotypes 1, 2, and 3 at the gene level. *Virology* **123:** 152.

Gaillard, R.K., Jr., J.K.-K. Li, J.D. Keene, and W.K. Joklik. 1982. The sequences at the termini of four genes of the three reovirus serotypes. *Virology* **121:** 320.

Kozak, M. 1981. Possible role of flanking nucleotides in recognition of AUG initiator codon by eukaryotic ribosomes. *Nucleic Acids Res.* **9:** 5233.

―――. 1982. Analysis of ribosome binding sites from s1 message of reovirus. *J. Mol. Biol.* **156:** 807.

Lee, P.W.K., E.C. Hayes, and W. K. Joklik. 1981a. Characterization of anti-reovirus immunoglobulins secreted by cloned hybridoma cell lines. *Virology* **108:** 134.

―――. 1981b. Protein σ1 is the reovirus cell attachment protein. *Virology* **108:** 156.

Li, J.K.-K., J.D. Keene, P.P. Scheible, and W.K. Joklik. 1980. Nature of the 3'-terminal sequences of the plus and minus strands of the *S1* gene of reovirus serotypes 1, 2, and 3. *Virology* **105:** 41.

Morphology and Immunogenicity of Purified Measles Virus Peplomer Components

Erling Norrby, Tamas Varsanyi, and Goran Utter
Department of Virology
Karolinska Institute, School of Medicine
SBL, 10521 Stockholm, Sweden

Max Appel
Department of Microbiology
New York State College of
Veterinary Medicine, Cornell University
Ithaca, New York 14853

Measles and distemper viruses are two members of the genus *Morbillivirus* in the family Paramyxoviridae. The envelope of paramyxovirus contains two different kinds of peplomers. One kind of peplomer can react with viral adsorption proteins on cells that can be infected and with receptors on erythrocytes. It is referred to as hemagglutinin (HA), and in the case of paramyxoviruses other than morbilliviruses, it also carries a neuraminidase activity. The other kind of peplomer can induce fusion of cytoplasmic membranes and can lyse erythrocytes. For this fusion (F) component to show biological activity, it has to be cleaved into F_1 and F_2 products by proteolysis. The activity of the component can become expressed only when it is placed in proximity to the peripheral membrane of cells by HA component receptor binding. Each peplomer is composed of a few, probably 3–4, copies of either the HA 79K glycoprotein or the disulfate-bonded 41K nonglycosylated F_1 protein and 18K–22K glycosylated F_2 protein.

Circulating antibodies are capable of mitigating or completely preventing the development of a measles virus infection, as evidenced by the effectiveness of treatment with immunoglobulin. Measles-virus-specific antibodies can be induced by the use of live or inactivated measles vaccines. However, although the live measles vaccine has been found to give effective immunity, the inactivated vaccines (formalin-treated material or envelope components prepared from Tween 80 ether-treated material) did not give long-term protection against disease.

Some vaccinated individuals instead were found to develop an atypical form of measles. These findings were explained by the observation (Norrby et al. 1975) that the procedures of inactivation employed caused a selective destruc-

21

tion of biologically essential immunogenic parts of the F component. Thus, the humoral immunity induced by the HA component did not by itself provide long-term protection. The antibodies induced could neutralize the virus in vitro, but prevention of in vivo dissemination of the infection required the presence of antibodies against the F component. So far, it has not been possible to study the degree of protection provided by a humoral immunity against the F component alone.

The present studies encompassed (1) high-degree purification of measles virus peplomers by affinity chromatography using monoclonal antibodies (Norrby et al. 1982), (2) characterization of the morphology of the purified components, (3) preparation of rabbit hyperimmune sera against the purified components and evaluation of the antibody activity of these sera, and finally (4) analysis of the serological response in dogs immunized with live measles vaccine and challenged with highly pathogenic distemper virus. Since the F peplomers of measles and distemper viruses are closely related antigenically, whereas the HA components of the two viruses are distinct (H. Sheshberadaran et al., unpubl.), the latter study was considered to allow an evaluation of the effect of selective anti-F humoral immunity.

Purification of Measles Virus HA and F Components

The virus peplomers were isolated from a common detergent (2% Triton X-100)-solubilized cell antigen preparation. One cycle of adsorption-elution of material on a Sepharose column coupled with monoclonal antibodies against the HA component sufficed to give a degree of purification that allowed the detection of a single 79K protein by SDS-polyacrylamide gel electrophoresis (Varsanyi et al. 1984). To obtain a corresponding degree of purification of the F_1 and F_2 components, two consecutive chromatography steps were required. Washing with 1 M guanidine-HCl facilitated elimination of contaminating cellular proteins, especially actin.

Ultrastructural Analysis of Purified Measles Virus Peplomers

The peplomers showed a varying tendency to aggregate via their hydrophobic ends depending on the conditions employed. The two kinds of peplomers had different morphologies. The HA peplomers had the appearance of a truncated cone with a gradually narrowing width about 6.5 nm in diameter at the distal end and about 4 nm close to the hydrophobic part. The overall length was about 22 nm. The F peplomers were dumbbell-shaped, with an oval head 6 nm by 9 nm connected by a slender shaft to a smaller spherical structure about 8 nm in diameter. Aggregation occurred via the latter structure, which is therefore interpreted to be hydrophobic. The total length was 23 nm.

Antibody Activity of Rabbit Hyperimmune Sera against Purified HA and F Peplomers

Radioimmunoprecipitation assays (RIPA) demonstrated that the rabbit polyclonal antisera specifically precipitated each of the envelope polypeptides (Fig. 1). Ad-

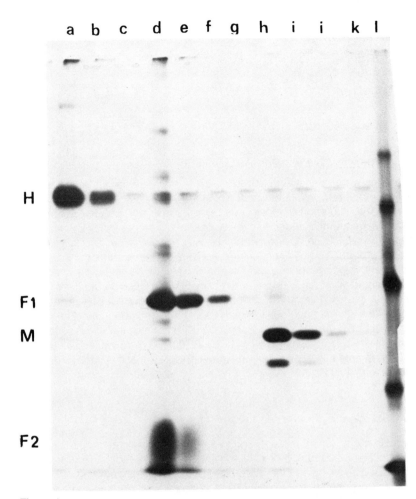

Figure 1
Autoradiograph of SDS-polyacrylamide gel electrophoresis showing results of RIPA using rabbit hyperimmune sera from animals immunized with purified HA (dilutions 1:2, 1:10, and 1:50; *a–c*), F (dilutions 1:10, 1:50, 1:250, and 1:1250; *d–g*), and M components (dilutions 1:10, 1:50, 1:250, and 1:1250; *h–k*). (Lane *l*) Molecular-weight markers. All samples contain a small amount of contaminating 80K host-cell protein.

ditional serological tests (Table 1) showed that the sera reacted to about equal titers in ELISA and complement fixation (CF) tests. The antiserum against HA peplomers inhibited hemagglutination (HI) and as a consequence also blocked hemolysis. The two antisera against F peplomers did not interfere with the hemagglutinating activity but showed high activity in hemolysis-inhibition (HLI) tests. Both antisera against HA and F peplomers neutralized virus infectivity. However, only antisera against F peplomers could prevent cell-to-cell transmission in infected tissue cultures.

Table 1
Antibody Activities of Rabbit Hyperimmune Sera against Measles Virus Peplomers

Antigen used for immunization	Hyperimmune serum no.	Antibody activity in different tests				
		ELISA	CF	neutralization	HLI	HI
HA	1	10^3	80	14	80	80
F	1	10^4	80	14	320	<10
	2	10^4	160	14	320	<10

Immunization with Live Measles Vaccine in Dogs

Pairs of dogs were immunized with live canine distemper or live measles vaccines, and after 4 weeks these animals, together with a pair of control dogs, were challenged with virulent distemper virus. The control dogs became severely ill, whereas the immunity provided by the live canine distemper vaccine completely blocked virus replication. Dogs immunized with the live measles vaccine were only partially protected against the disease. They showed a transiently elevated body temperature, lymphopenia, and period of weight loss.

Dogs immunized with live distemper vaccine showed high serum titers of distemper-virus-neutralizing and CF antibodies and also a low titer of measles virus HLI antibodies. In contrast, dogs immunized with live measles vaccine did not produce distemper-virus-neutralizing antibodies, but a low titer of CF antibodies and a moderate titer of measles virus HLI antibodies. In postchallenge sera, the latter dogs had high titers of distemper-virus-neutralizing and CF antibodies and very high titers of HLI antibodies.

CONCLUSIONS

Measles virus envelope components can be obtained in highly purified form by use of affinity chromatography employing monoclonal antibodies. The HA and F peplomers were elongated structures (22–23 nm long) with different morphologies. Rabbit hyperimmune sera against immunoadsorbent purified components only reacted with the homologous antigen in RIPA. Antisera against HA and F components neutralized virus infectivity and blocked hemolysis. These effects were mediated by different reactions, since, on the one hand, only anti-HA serum blocked hemagglutination and, on the other hand, only anti-F serum prevented cell-to-cell spread in infected tissue cultures.

It has been found that immunization of humans with only the HA surface component of measles virus did not lead to establishment of long-term immunity. A simultaneous immunization against the F component was required for effective protection. The immunity provided by immunization with only the latter surface component has not been evaluated. It would be interesting to perform such an analysis to determine whether it might suffice for a possible future synthetic vaccine to include only parts of this peplomer. Since the F components of measles and distemper viruses are closely immunologically related, whereas their HA components are distinct, immunization of dogs with live measles vaccine can provide some information on the protection efficacy of immunization with the F component alone. It was found that dogs immunized with such a vaccine only developed transient symptoms after exposure to virulent canine distemper virus.

ACKNOWLEDGMENT

This work was supported by a grant from the Swedish Medical Council (Project no. B84-16X-00116-20A).

REFERENCES

Norrby, E., G. Enders-Ruckle, and V. terMeulen. 1975. Differences in the appearance of antibodies to structural components of measles virus after immunization with inactivated and live virus. *J. Infect. Dis.* **132:** 262.

Norrby, E., S.-N. Chen, T. Togashi, H. Sheshberadaran, and K.P. Johnson. 1982. Five measles virus antigens demonstrated by use of mouse hybridoma antibodies in productively infected tissue culture cells. *Arch. Virol.* **71:** 1.

Varsanyi, T.M., G. Utter, and E. Norrby. 1984. Purification, morphology, and antigenic characterization of measles virus envelope components. *J. Gen. Virol.* (in press).

Molecular Basis for the Antigenicity and Virulence of Poliovirus Type 3

**Geoffrey C. Schild, Philip D. Minor,
David M.A. Evans, and Morag Ferguson**
National Institute for Biological Standards
and Control, Holly Hill, London NW3 6RB

Glyn Stanway and Jeffrey W. Almond
University of Leicester, Leicester, England

Modern biotechnologies offer prospects for radical innovation in the development of safer, cheaper, and more effective vaccines against viral diseases. The design of novel vaccines based on antigenic peptides will require detailed information on the molecular basis of antigenicity. Knowledge of the precise molecular basis of virulence will provide prospects for the construction of attenuated vaccines of improved safety and efficacy.

We have studied the molecular aspects of antigenicity and virulence of poliovirus type 3 (PV-3). An eight-amino-acid sequence, positions 93–100 from the amino terminus of the viral capsid protein VP1, was identified as a major antigenic site involved in virus neutralization and type specificity. Virus-neutralizing antibodies were stimulated by synthetic peptides containing sequences from this site. Point mutations that accompanied attenuation and reversion to neurovirulence of PV-3 (Sabin vaccine strain) were identified and were few in number. We have concluded that virulence is critically affected by changes in one to three codons of the virus.

Monoclonal Antibodies as Tools for Analysis of Antigenic Structure Involved in Neutralization

Two populations of polioviral particles predominate in tissue-culture harvests: infectious virus that sediments at 155S and empty 80S capsids (Mayer et al. 1957; Minor et al. 1980). These particles possess distinct antigenic characteristics and have been termed D and C antigens, respectively. To characterize the antigenic determinants on infectious and empty particles, we have developed hybridoma cell lines of rat or mouse origin that secrete monoclonal antibodies to

27

PV-3 (Minor et al. 1982; Ferguson et al. 1984). The antibodies were tested for virus-neutralizing activity, for their ability to bind to D- and C-antigen particles, and for their reactivity with isolated denatured polioviral capsid proteins in immunoblot tests.

Of the 51 antibodies characterized, 31 were of the IgG class and 20 were IgM. Assays for neutralizing activity against PV-3, according to the method of Domok and Magrath (1979), revealed neutralizing activity in 21 of the 51 antibodies tested. Among antibodies that neutralized efficiently were examples of the IgG and IgM classes. The antibodies were tested to determine their binding reactivities with D and C antigens of PV-3 by a modification of the autoradiographic single radial diffusion (SRD) method of Schild et al. (1980) (Table 1). Eight of the 51 monoclonal antibodies reacted with both D and C antigens, indicating that they had affinity for determinants common to both infectious and empty poliovirus particles. Of the remaining 43 antibodies, 19 bound exclusively D antigen and only 12 of these had neutralizing activity. Twenty-four antibodies bound exclusively C antigen and, unexpectedly, one of these (antibody NIB 198) had apparent virus-neutralizing properties. Detailed studies on NIB 198 (P.D. Minor, unpubl.) suggested that it did not prevent initial infection of cells but acted at a late stage in replication, inhibiting release of infectious virus from the cell.

Antibodies that bound to the determinants common to D- and C-antigen particles possessed neutralizing activity against a wide range of PV-3 strains and, in some cases, against all of the 30 strains tested. In contrast, D-specific antibodies often reacted with a narrow range of strains in neutralization and antigen-blocking tests. Thus, some antigenic determinants involved in neutralization appeared to be widespread within PV-3, whereas others were apparently unique for individual strains.

The reactivity of the 51 monoclonal antibodies with individual denatured PV-3 capsid polypeptides separated on polyacrylamide gels was investigated using the immunoblot method of Thorpe et al. (1982). None of the neutralizing antibodies that were specific for D antigen, or those that reacted with antigenic determinants common to D and C antigens, were found to bind to separated capsid polypeptides of PV-3 (Table 1). This suggests that the antigenic sites on the

Table 1
Neutralization Titers and Immunoblot Activity of Monoclonal Antibodies against PV-3

D + C antigen specificity of antibody[a]	No. of antibodies tested[b]	No. of antibodies with virus neutralizing activity at stated titers[c]					Immunoblot reactivity
		< 10	$10^1 - < 10^2$	$10^2 - < 10^3$	$10^3 - < 10^4$	$\geq 10^4$	
D + C-reactive	8	0	0	3	0	5	0
D-specific	19	7	8	3	0	1	0
							5 VP1
C-specific	24	23	0	0	1	0	1 VP3
Total	51	30	8	6	1	6	6

[a]Based on autoradiographic SRD antigen blocking assays.
[b]Each antibody was obtained from an independent hybridoma clone in fusions involving the lymphocytes of mice or rats immunized with PV-3 strains (Minor et al. 1982).
[c]Dilution of antibody just neutralizing 100 $TCID_{50}$ of virus in microtiter assays.

infectious particle, including those involved in virus neutralization, are dependent on secondary or tertiary conformation of viral polypeptides at the virus surface. In contrast, six of the C-specific antibodies reacted with denatured proteins, five with VP1 and one with VP3. Antigenic determinants on empty particles therefore appear more likely to be specified simply by a contiguous amino acid sequence.

Selection of Mutants and Sequencing for Identification of the Antigenic Site(s) Involved in Neutralization

Work with antigenic mutants resistant to neutralizing monoclonal antibodies indicated a single antigenic site for the neutralization of PV-3. Evidence based on oligonucleotide mapping (Minor et al. 1983) suggested that this single site, which was defined operationally, corresponded largely to one physicochemical site whose approximate location in the capsid protein VP1 could be defined. To locate and identify this proposed site, mutants of a single parental PV-3 strain (P3/Leon/USA/37) resistant to neutralization were selected by growth in the presence of several of the individual virus-neutralizing monoclonal antibodies referred to above. Sixteen mutant groups were identified by their distinct patterns of resistance against 11 monoclonal antibodies (Evans et al. 1983). The RNAs of representative strains from each mutant group were sequenced to define the positions of amino acid substitutions in VP1 that conferred resistance. This was done by the dideoxy sequencing method (Caton et al. 1982; see Table 2). A sequence of at least 60 bases, and in most cases up to 150 bases, was identified for each mutant encompassing the site defined by oligonucleotide mapping. The sequences of all the mutants only varied in the single point mutations shown in Table 2. Where mutations were detected, there was only one per mutant and all would result in amino acid substitutions (Evans et al. 1983).

Base changes were detected in viruses of 15 of the 16 mutant groups and were concentrated into a single region of only 8 codons (Table 2) located 93–100 codons from the beginning of the genomic region coding for VP1. We thus conclude that a region of VP1 93–100 amino acids from its amino terminus represents a major antigenic site involved in virus neutralization. Confirmation that a closely analogous region of VP1 of poliovirus type 1 (PV-1; residues 93–104) is a neutralization epitope has been reported by Wychowski et al. (1983). Other reports have suggested the existence of multiple antigenic sites for PV-1 (Emini et al. 1982, 1983b).

Only one mutant group (group 9) had an amino acid substitution at position 1 (glutamic acid to glycine). The amino acid at position 2 was conserved in all of the mutant groups. The remaining mutations were distributed between positions 3 and 8. For example, mutants of groups 1, 2, and 14 showed different point mutations in position 4 and at least two distinct mutations were located in each position from 5 to 8. Furthermore, different mutations that occurred in the same position resulted in different patterns of resistance to neutralization. Single base changes at the seven variable codons could generate 39 possible different mutants. Therefore, nearly half of the total number of theoretically possible mutants had been isolated during the studies. In only one group (group 6) was no mutation detected in the 150 bases sequenced by primer extension, indicating that in

Table 2
Neutralization of PV-3 Mutant Viruses by Antipeptide Sera

Codon position:	93[a]	94	95	96	97	98	99	100
Codon no.:	1	2	3	4	5	6	7	8
Type 1 (Mahoney)	CCA Pro	GCU Ala	UCG Ser	ACC Thr	ACG Thr	AAU Asn	AAG Lys	GAU Asp
Type 3 (Leon)	GAA Glu	CAA Gln	CCA Pro	ACC Thr	ACC Thr	CGG Arg	GCA Ala	CAG Gln
Mutant group 1				AUC Ile				
2				GCC Ala				
3					AAC Asn			
4						CAG Gln		
5								CUG Leu
6								
7							ACA Thr	
8			CUA Leu					
9	GGA Gly							
10								CCG Pro
11							GUA Val	
12								CGG Arg
13								CAC His
14				AAC Asn				
15						UGG Trp		
16					AUC Ile			

The RNA of representative strains of each mutant group derived from Leon PV-3 was sequenced in the region 393–240 bases downstream from the 5′ end of the VP1-coding region of the genome. The dideoxy sequencing method was used, using a restriction fragment primer prepared from cloned polioviral cDNA. The primer was prepared by digesting plasmid DNA with EcoRI and SphI and labeling it by incubation with 1 unit of Klenow fragment from DNA polymerase I and 100 μCi of [a-^{32}P]dATP (3000 Ci/mmole; Amersham). The products were denatured and loaded onto a preparative slab polyacrylamide gel. After electrophoresis, the 47-base restriction fragment was detected by autoradiography, excised, and eluted from the gel. The primer was purified by exclusion chromatography and then annealed onto the virion RNA and incubated with dideoxyribonucleotides and deoxyribonucleotides in appropriate proportions together with 5 units of avian myeloblast reverse transcriptase (Life Sciences, Inc.). Following incubation at 37°C for 25 min, the reaction products were denatured and loaded onto sequencing gels. After electrophoresis, the gels were fixed in 10% acetic acid, washed, dried, and subjected to autoradiography.

[a]Amino acid position from amino terminus of VP1.

this instance, the mutation was elsewhere in the genome. Nevertheless, the mutation exhibited by viruses of group 6 conferred resistance to antibodies that had been shown to recognize the eight-amino-acid sequence, which we propose as a major antigenic site. Thus, the mutations of the group-6 virus appear to be within the same operationally defined antigenic site as those of the other 15 groups.

Evans et al. (1983) have attempted to identify the precise amino acids required for the neutralization of poliovirus by 11 specific monoclonal antibodies. For example, it was concluded that one antibody (25-1-14) required glutamic acid at position 1, threonine at position 4, threonine at position 5, and arginine at position 6 for its neutralizing activity. Amino acids at positions 1, 5, and 6, in particular, affected neutralization of the mutant viruses.

The amino acid sequence of VP1 of PV-1 (Mahoney strain) in the region analogous to that of the proposed antigenic site of PV-3 is also shown in Table 2. There are only two positions within this region that are conserved between PV-3 and PV-1, and one of these is not conserved between the wild type-1 vaccine progenitor strain (Mahoney) and the Sabin type-1 vaccine strain, LSc. In contrast, the amino acid at position 2 (glutamine) was conserved in all mutants derived from the Leon type-3 virus, the Sabin type-3 vaccine, and a strain (119) associated with a virulent type-3 vaccine (A.J. Cann, unpubl.). However, it is not conserved between type 3 and type 1 virus. The same position is conserved between the wild type-1 vaccine progenitor strain (Mahoney) and the Sabin type-1 vaccine strain (LSc). Thus, the proposed antigenic site shows low overall sequence homology between these two serotypes of poliovirus. Recent studies (D. Evans, unpubl.) on the amino acid sequence of the eight-amino-acid antigenic site region of VP1 of different wild strains of PV-3 isolated between 1937 and 1982 show a very high degree of conservation of this region.

As discussed above, none of the 21 monoclonal antibodies we have characterized that neutralize virus infectivity were capable of binding to isolated VP1 that had been denatured during its preparation (Ferguson et al. 1984). However, the genetic and molecular studies of a large collection of over 200 mutants of PV-3 selected for resistance to 16 of the 21 antibodies (Evans et al. 1983; Minor et al. 1983 and unpubl.) indicate that all 16 antibodies react with epitopes specified by the same eight-amino-acid region of VP1. In addition, resistant mutant viruses with identical point mutations within this antigenic site could be isolated by selection in the presence of monoclonal antibodies that reacted only with D antigen or with both D and C antigens. Thus, neutralizing monoclonal antibodies with both types of specificities appear to react with the same antigenic region of VP1. In addition, some of the viruses that have point mutations in this region were resistant to a C-specific antibody with neutralizing activity (antibody NIB 198; Ferguson et al. 1984), suggesting that this antibody also reacts with the same antigenic site on VP1 as the other neutralizing antibodies. However, nonneutralizing C- or D-specific antibodies may be directed against other sites (e.g., antibody NIBp 176, which reacted with VP3).

A synthetic oligopeptide 18 amino acids in length comprising 16 residues (positions 89–104) of VP1 of PV-3 (Leon strain) (of which the sequence 93–100 is the proposed antigenic site), with an additional cysteine residue at its amino and

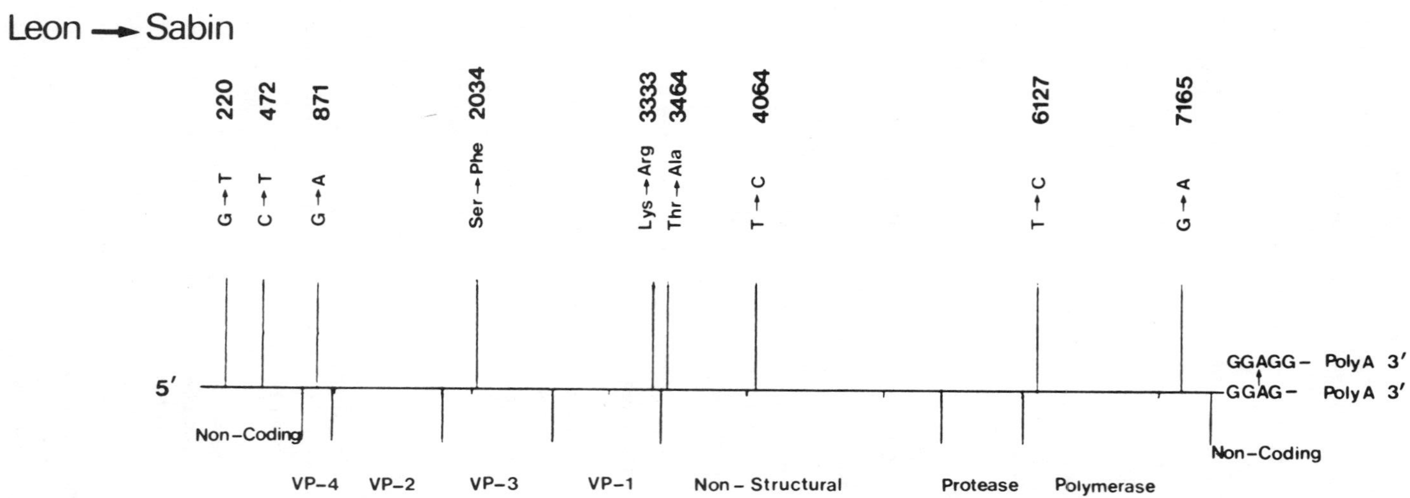

Figure 1

Comparison of the gene sequences of P3/Leon/USA/37, the vaccine progenitor, and the Sabin vaccine virus derived from it. The positions of base differences between the virulent progenitor strain and the vaccine strain are indicated and any amino acid changes that result are identified. For example, the alteration in sequence produced at position 2034, in deriving the Sabin strain from Leon, changed a serine in the coat protein VP3 of Leon into a phenylalanine in the coat protein VP3 of the Sabin strain. Base changes that would not produce amino acid changes are also indicated.

carboxyl termini, was tested for immunological properties in rabbits. The sequence was as follows: amino terminus Cys-Glu-Val-Asp-Asn-Glu-Gln-Pro-Thr-Thr-Arg-Ala-Gln-Lys-Leu-Phe-Ala-Cys carboxyl terminus. The peptide was coupled using glutaraldehyde to bovine thyroglobulin at a molecular ratio of approximately 50:1, and 250–700 μg of coupled product was injected intramuscularly into rabbits with Freund's complete adjuvant. Two weeks after receiving a single dose of coupled peptide, the rabbits developed neutralizing antibody titers for PV-3 ranging from 1:4 to 1:16. After a booster injection of conjugate, neutralization titers ranging from 1:32 to 1:1000 were detected. Neutralizing activity was detectable against a wide range of PV-3 strains but was type-specific; no neutralization was detected with PV-1 and PV-2. The antipeptide sera produced clear precipitin reactions in immuno-double-diffusion tests against purified D or C antigens of a wide range of PV-3 strains, but not with PV-1 or PV-2 antigens. These findings provide confirmatory evidence of the involvement of the eight-amino-acid sequence of VP1 in the type-specific immunological reactivity of poliovirus and suggest it to be relevant to the design of novel polio vaccines. Emini et al. (1983a) have reported that an oligopeptide containing amino acid sequences from a region of VP1 of PV-1, which corresponds to the eight-amino-acid region we have identified for PV-3, was capable of inducing neutralizing antibodies in rabbits. This suggests the existence of a structural and antigenic analogy of the same region of VP1 in both poliovirus serotypes.

Molecular Basis for Virulence

The complete nucleotide sequence has been determined for a cloned DNA copy of the genome of P3/Leon/37, the neurovirulent progenitor of the type-3 Sabin vaccine strain, P3/Leon/12a₁b (G. Stanway et al., in prep.). Comparison of the sequence with that previously obtained for the vaccine strain (Stanway et al. 1983a) indicates that attenuation of the Leon virus to produce the Sabin vaccine strain is brought about by a maximum of ten point mutations.

Strain P3/Leon/37 was plaque-purified, and its highly neurovirulent phenotype was confirmed in monkeys prior to gene cloning (Stanway et al. 1983b). P3/Leon/12a₁b, plaque isolate no. 411, was similarly tested and shown to be attenuated. It is therefore highly likely that nucleotide sequences derived from cloned cDNAs of these strains reflect their neurovirulence properties. A cloned DNA copy of the genome of P3/Leon/37, plaque isolate no. 960, was subjected to random shearing by sonication and subcloned into bacteriophage M13. Nucleotide sequences were determined by the dideoxynucleotide chain-termination method (Sanger et al. 1977). This 7431-nucleotide sequence, excluding the poly(A) tract, is one base shorter than that derived from P3/Leon/12a₁b and differs from it at only ten positions (Fig. 1). Of the ten differences between the Leon and Sabin vaccine strain sequences, seven do not result in an amino acid change and, consequently, are likely to be of no significance to the attenuation of the phenotype. We conclude that the mutations most likely to determine the attenuated phenotype are those at positions 2034, 3333, and 3464, which give rise to amino acid substitutions in VP3, VP1, and a nonstructural protein P2-3b, respectively. The distribution and nature of nucleotide and amino acid sequence differences suggest that a single base substitution may be responsible for the attenuation of the phenotype of the vaccine strain.

Our results contrast with the results obtained in a study comparing the PV-1 strains, Sabin vaccine P1/ LSc,2ab and its neurovirulent precursor P1/Mahoney (Nomoto et al. 1982). Fifty-seven point-mutation differences were observed between these strains, 21 of which gave rise to amino acid changes scattered generally throughout the genome. Although the predicted amino acid sequences of PV-1 and PV-3 show close homology (~90%; Stanway 1983a), none of the mutations observed in the type-3 vaccine strain have an identical counterpart in the type-1 vaccine strain, indicating that the mutational events responsible for attenuation are different in these two serotypes.

The nucleotide sequences of neurovirulent revertants of the Sabin type-3 vaccine, isolated from persons with persistent paralysis temporally associated with vaccination, are currently being determined in an attempt to shed further light on the change(s) associated with reversion to virulence. One such revertant has been studied in detail (J.W. Almond, unpubl.) and showed eight point-mutation differences in its gene sequence from the Sabin vaccine strain, three of which coded for changes in capsid proteins, two in VP2 and one in VP1. However, these changes were not simple back mutations to the wild virulent genotype of Leon virus.

It is likely that a parallel genetic approach based on construction of recombinants from cDNA in vitro (Racaniello and Baltimore 1981) will also be required to fully define the genetic basis for virulence and reversion. A precise definition of attenuating mutations in Sabin vaccine viruses of types 1, 2, and 3 and an explanation of their mechanism of action may raise the possibility of designing derivatives that are incapable of reverting to neurovirulence.

REFERENCES

Caton, A.J., G.G. Brownlee, J. Yewdell, and W. Gerhard. 1982. The antigenic structure of the influenza virus A/PR/8/34 haemagglutinin (H1 subtype). *Cell* **31**: 417.

Domok, I. and D.I. Magrath. 1979. Guide to poliovirus isolation and serological techniques for poliomyelitis surveillance. *WHO Offset Publ.* **46**.

Emini, E.A., B.A. Jameson, and E. Wimmer. 1983a. Priming for and induction of anti poliovirus neutralizing antibodies by synthetic peptides. *Nature* **304**: 699.

Emini, E.A., B.A. Jameson, A.J. Lewis, G.R. Larsen, and E. Wimmer. 1982. Poliovirus neutralization epitopes: Analysis and localization with monoclonal antibodies. *J. Virol.* **43**: 997.

Emini, E.A., S.-Y. Kao, A.J. Lewis, R. Crainic, and E. Wimmer. 1983b. Functional bases of poliovirus neutralization determined with monospecific neutralizing antibodies. *J. Virol.* **46**: 466.

Evans, D.M.A., P.D. Minor, G.C. Schild, and J.W. Almond. 1983. Critical role of an eight-amino acid sequence of VP1 in neutralization of poliovirus type 3. *Nature* **304**: 459.

Ferguson, M., P.D. Minor, D.I. Magrath, Y.-H. Qui, M. Spitz, and G.C. Schild. 1984. Neutralization epitopes on poliovirus type 3 particles: An analysis using monoclonal antibodies. *J. Gen. Virol.* **65**: (in press).

Mayer, M.M., H.J. Rapp, B. Roizman, S.W. Klein, K.M. Cowan, D. Lukery, C.E. Schwerdt, F.L. Schaffer, and J.J. Charnmey. 1957. The purification of poliomyelitis virus as studied by complement fixation. *J. Immunol.* **78**: 435.

Minor, P.D., G.C. Schild, J.M. Wood, and C.N. Dandawate. 1980. The preparation of specific immune sera against type 3 poliovirus D antigen and C antigen, and the demonstration of two C antigenic components in vaccine strain populations. *J. Gen. Virol.* **51:** 147.

Minor, P.D., G.C. Schild, M. Ferguson, A. Mackay, D.I. Magrath, A. John, P.J. Yates, and M. Spitz. 1982. Genetic and antigenic variation in type 3 polioviruses: Characterization of strains by monoclonal antibodies and T1 oligonucleotide mapping. *J. Gen. Virol.* **61:** 167.

Minor, P.D., G. Schild, J. Bootman, D.M.A. Evans, M. Ferguson, P. Reeve, M. Spitz, G. Stanway, A.J. Cann, R. Hauptmann, L.D. Clarke, R.C. Mountford, and J.W. Almond. 1983. Location and primary structure of a major antigenic site for poliovirus neutralization. *Nature* **301:** 674.

Nomoto, A., T. Omata, H. Toyoda, S. Kuge, H. Horie, Y. Kataoka, Y. Genba, Y. Nakano, and N. Imura. 1982. Complete nucleotide sequence of the attenuated poliovirus Sabin 1 strain genome. *Proc. Natl. Acad. Sci.* **79:** 5793.

Raceniello, V.R. and D. Baltimore. 1981. Cloned poliovirus complementary DNA is infectious in mammalian cells. *Science* **214:** 916.

Sanger, F., S. Nicklen, and A.R. Coulson. 1977. DNA sequencing with chain-terminating inhibitors. *Proc. Natl. Acad. Sci.* **74:** 5463.

Schild, G.C., J.M. Wood, P.D. Minor, C.N. Dandawate, and D.I. Magrath. 1980. Immunoassay of poliovirus antigens by single-radial-diffusion: Development and characteristics of a sensitive autoradiographic zone size enhancement (ZE) technique. *J. Gen. Virol.* **51:** 157.

Stanway, G., A.J. Cann, R. Hauptmann, P. Hughes, L.D. Clarke, R.C. Mountford, P.D. Minor, G.C. Schild, and J.W. Almond. 1983a. The nucleotide sequence of poliovirus type 3 Leon 12 A₁ 43B: Comparison with poliovirus type 3. *Nucleic Acids Res.* **11:** 5629.

Stanway, G., A.J. Cann, R. Hauptmann, R.C. Mountford, L.D. Clarke, P. Reeve, P.D. Minor, G.C. Schild, and J.W. Almond. 1983b. Nucleic acid sequence of the region of the genome encoding capsid protein VP1 of neurovirulent and attenuating type 3 polioviruses. *Eur. J. Biochem.* **135:** 529.

Thorpe, R., P.D. Minor, A. Mackay, G.C. Schild, and M. Spitz. 1982. Immunochemical studies of polioviruses: Identification of immunoreactive virus capsid polypeptides. *J. Gen. Virol.* **63:** 487.

Wychowski, C., S. van der Werf, O. Siffert, R. Crainic, P. Bruneau, and M. Girard. 1983. A poliovirus type 1 neutralization epitope is located within amino acid residues 93 to 104 of viral capsid polypeptide VP1. *EMBO J.* **2:** 2019.

Organization and Expression of Human Respiratory Syncytial Virus

Sundararajan Venkatesan,
Narayanasamy Elango, Masanobu Satake,
Ena Camargo, and Robert M. Chanock
Laboratory of Infectious Diseases
National Institute of Allergy and Infectious
Diseases, National Institutes of Health
Bethesda, Maryland 20205

Human respiratory syncytial (RS) virus was isolated initially from a young child with pneumonia. Subsequent epidemiological studies have established this virus to be the most important etiologic agent of severe lower respiratory disease among infants and young children. The impact of RS virus is greatest during early infancy when most infants still possess appreciable amounts of maternally derived serum-neutralizing antibodies. Efforts at development of immunoprophylaxis have met with failure. For example, formalin-inactivated virus vaccine did not protect against infection; instead, it induced a potentiated response to infection that resulted in more serious disease. Also, attempts to develop conditional lethal, temperature-sensitive mutants for use as a live attenuated vaccine also failed because of the problem of genetic instability (Chanock et al. 1982).

Our interest in RS virus stems from its important role as a respiratory tract pathogen during early life and from our failure to develop an effective strategy for prevention of disease. Because of this failure and the deficiency of knowledge concerning the basic organization and expression of the viral genome, our efforts have been redirected toward achieving a better understanding of the structure and function of this virus with the expectation that this information will prove useful in developing an effective vaccine.

DISCUSSION

Biochemical Characterization of RS Virus

RS virus is a negative-strand unsegmented RNA virus with properties similar to those of the paramyxoviruses. It has, however, been placed in a separate genus,

37

Pneumovirus, based on morphologic differences and lack of hemagglutinin and neuraminidase activities. The viral RNA is 5000 kD and encodes eight or nine poly(A)-containing RNAs (Collins and Wertz 1983). This is consistent with the earlier genetic analysis of temperature-sensitive mutants that identified seven or eight nonoverlapping complementation groups (Gimenez and Pringle 1978).

Eight or nine virus-encoded polypeptides have been identified in infected cells as well as in purified extracellular virus; these have apparent molecular masses of 160, 84, 68, 46, 36, 28, 22, and 18 kD. The 84- and 68-kD proteins are glyco-proteins, as indicated by specific incorporation of [^{3}H]glucosamine and fucose (Venkatesan et al. 1983). In addition, they appear to be present on the viral envelope, since they were solubilized readily by nonionic detergents. One of these (84 kD) probably represents the major envelope glycoprotein (G), the equivalent of the paramyxoviral HN protein that is responsible for adsorption to cell-surface receptors. The 68-kD glycoprotein probably represents the putative fusion factor (Fo) responsible for entry of virus and cell fusion. Under reducing electrophoretic conditions, the 68-kD protein is replaced by two proteins of 48 kD and 16 kD. This is analogous to the paramyxovirus fusion factor (Fo) that is synthesized as a precursor and subsequently cleaved by a cellular protease into two subunits (F_1 and F_2) that are held together by disulfide bonds (Kingsbury 1977). Proteins associated with detergent-solubilized cores include the major nucleocapsid protein (NC, 46 kD), a phosphoprotein (P, 36 kD), a matrix protein (M, 28 kD), a 160-kD protein (L), and two nonstructural proteins (NS_1, and NS_2, 22 kD and 18 kD). Intracellular viral nucleocapsids purified by isopycnic banding on cesium chloride gradients contain only the NC, P, and L proteins. The nature of the other proteins is presently not clear. They have been referred to as non-structural proteins, since they are usually not packaged in mature virions. They may be analogous to the nonstructural proteins of the influenza virus or to the C and S proteins of Sendai and Newcastle disease viruses, respectively. Poly(A) RNA from virus-infected cells was translated in a messenger-dependent reticu-locyte lysate system, and the translation products included NC, P, M, and the nonstructural proteins. A 59-kD polypeptide was also detected occasionally. It has been shown that a viral mRNA 2200 bases long is translated to yield a pro-tein of 59 kD (Huang and Wertz 1983). Whether this protein is a precursor of the fusion factor is not clear.

Analysis of RS Virus Transcriptional Units

In an attempt to analyze the genome of RS virus, cDNA clones were constructed in Escherichia coli (HB101) using plasmid pBR322 as a vector. Our strategy avoided the traditional self-priming reaction for second-strand cDNA synthesis that requires nuclease S1 to remove the resulting hairpin. Discrete-sized, single-stranded cDNAs were used separately to construct double-stranded cDNAs that were inserted into plasmid pBR322 prior to transformation (Venkatesan et al. 1983). A substantial proportion (77%) of transformants hybridized to ^{32}P-labeled poly(A) RNA from infected cells that was synthesized in the presence of actino-mycin D (5 μg/ml). A sublibrary of 75 positive transformants was selected based on the size of their cDNA inserts. Several rounds of hybrid selection of viral mRNAs using recombinant DNA immobilized on nitrocellulose filters and subsequent cell-free translation of selected mRNAs allowed us to identify several independent cDNA clones that encoded the RS virus NC, P, M, or NS_2 gene (Fig. 1). Two-dimensional tryptic fingerprinting and partial protease V8 cleavage patterns of the translation products were indistinguishable from those of the authentic viral proteins. Several independent cDNA clones adequate in size to accommodate the coding sequences of the NC, P, M, or NS_2 gene were thus identified.

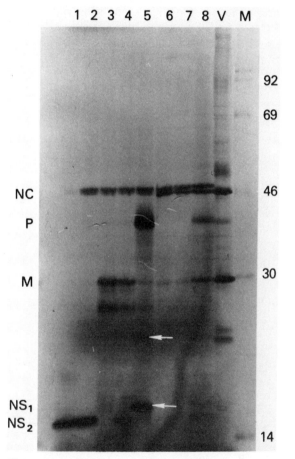

Figure 1
Cell-free translation products of mRNA from RS-virus-infected cells selected by hybridization to putative recombinant RS virus cDNA plasmids. An endogenous band migrating slower than 46 kD (NC protein) was variably present (lanes *2–8*). The recombinant plasmids used were $pRSB_8$ (lane *1*), $pRSC_6$ (lane *2*), $pRSB_7$ (lane *3*), $pRSD_3$ (lane *4*), $pRSC_1$ (lane *5*), $pRSB_{10}$ (lane *6*), and $pRSB_{11}$ (lane *7*). Translation products of polyadenylated RNA from infected cells are displayed in lane *8*. RS virion polypeptides labeled in vivo with [^{35}S]methionine are shown in lane *V*. Molecular-mass markers (M) shown in kilodaltons were obtained commercially from Amersham.

The cDNA library was screened further in duplicate with ^{32}P-labeled cDNA reverse-transcribed from infected-cell or uninfected-cell poly(A) RNAs. Approximately 85% of the recombinants reacted only with cDNA prepared from infected-cell RNA. Several of the recombinants identified in this manner were also confirmed by colony hybridization using as a probe viral genomic RNA extracted from intracellular nucleocapsids and 3'-end-labeled by the RNA ligase reaction or 5'-end-labeled by polynucleotide kinase reaction after partial degradation.

Substractive screening of the positive transformants allowed us to identify additional RS-virus-specific cDNA clones that did not represent the four genes described above. Such plasmids in groups of five were radioactively labeled by nick translation and used to detect poly(A) RNAs from infected cells by Northern blot analysis. When individual recombinants from positive groups of five were analyzed, two additional plasmids (pRS$_4$ and pRSA$_2$) were identified that reacted with poly(A) RNAs containing 2200 and 1100 bases, respectively (Fig. 2). The cDNA insert in one of these plasmids (pRS$_4$) was shorter than the RNA to which

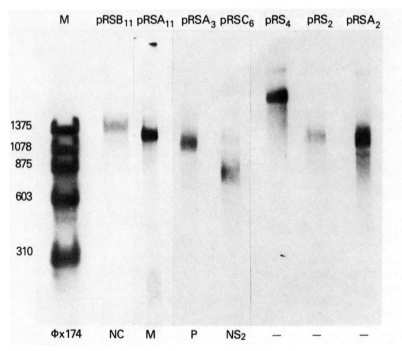

Figure 2
Hybridization of ^{32}P-labeled recombinant plasmids to poly(A) RNA from RS-virus-infected cells. The RNAs were resolved by formaldehyde agarose (1.5%) gel electrophoresis and subsequently transferred to nitrocellulose paper. The individual cDNA plasmids used as hybridization probes are indicated in lanes labeled pRSB$_{11}$, pRSA$_{11}$, pRSA$_3$, pRSC$_6$, pRS$_4$, and pRS$_2$ at the top. The viral genes identified to be within these plasmids are indicated at the bottom of each lane. Lane *M* represents the *Hae*III fragments of ΦX174 that serve as molecular-weight markers with the size of relevant fragments in bases shown at left.

it hybridized. We have since identified additional cDNA plasmids containing larger inserts. One of these containing a 2000-bp insert reacts with a poly(A) RNA of about 2200 bases. This clone may be a full-length cDNA copy of an RNA species that codes for the putative fusion factor. Recently, we have recovered additional cDNA clones containing the coding sequences for the major glycoprotein (G) of RS virus.

DNA Sequence Analysis of RS Virus Genes

We have determined the complete cDNA sequence of inserts encoding the RS virus NC, M, or NS_2 protein. The NC and M clones hybridized to discrete viral mRNAs almost identical in size to the cloned RS virus sequence (Fig. 2). Both have poly(A) tails at their 3' end, and by primer extension analysis these clones were found to lack only 6–7 nucleotides corresponding to those present at the 5' end of their respective mRNA templates. The recombinant plasmid encoding the NS_2 gene, however, hybridized to mRNA about 400 bases shorter than the cloned RS virus insert.

The DNA sequence of the NC-gene insert of plasmid $pRSB_{11}$ (Elango and Venkatesan 1983) contains a single open reading frame that encodes a protein of 467 amino acids. The other two reading frames are blocked extensively (Fig. 3). The sequence AAGAUGG containing the initiator codon AUG is similar to the conserved eukaryotic initiation signal PXXAUGG. This 51-kD protein is relatively rich in basic amino acids but poor in cysteine. It has no sequence homology with the capsid proteins of other viruses, implying that the RS virus has undergone extensive evolutionary divergence. There is no clustering of basic amino acid residues within specific domains.

DNA sequencing of a recombinant plasmid $pRSA_{11}$ containing the RS virus M gene revealed one open reading frame with a potential to encode a 28-kD protein containing 256 amino acids (M. Satake, unpubl.). This protein is rich in hydrophobic residues and is relatively basic. It has no homology with other viral matrix proteins. A second open reading frame, partially overlapping the first reading frame by 62 bases, has the potential to encode a polypeptide of 75 amino acids. This is of interest because some recombinant plasmids containing the matrix protein gene hybrid-select mRNAs that are translated in vitro to yield the matrix protein and a smaller protein of about 15 kD (Fig. 1). The biological significance of the second open reading frame is not clear at this time.

A recombinant plasmid ($pRSC_6$) that hybrid-selected mRNA that encoded a viral nonstructural protein (NS_2) was also sequenced. As seen in Figure 3, the DNA sequence has two different nonoverlapping reading frames capable of encoding proteins containing 124 and 139 amino acids, respectively. The calculated molecular weights of these proteins are similar to the observed molecular weight of the NS_2 protein. Both reading frames have competent translational initiation signals, implying that one or both frames could be used for translation. The presence of the cloned poly(A) tail at one end of the insert establishes the 3' end of the template mRNA used for reverse transcription. Whether one or both proteins are expressed in infected cells is now being investigated by a combination of two-dimensional gel analysis and hybrid-arrested translation of mRNAs,

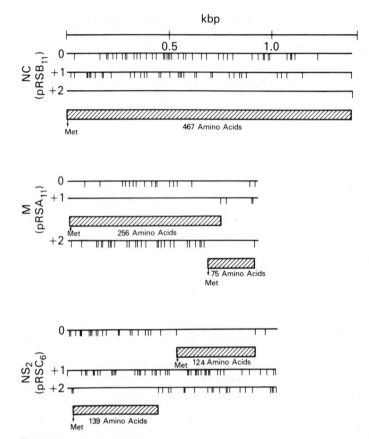

Figure 3
Schematic illustration of open reading frames within cDNA inserts of recombinant plasmids containing RS virus NC, NS_2, or M gene. Each plasmid and the gene contained within it is identified at the left. Vertical lines denote stop codons, and hatched rectangles represent the potential polypeptides encoded within the open reading frames. The number of amino acids for each polypeptide is shown below the rectangles.

using restriction fragments that span only one of the two reading frames. Although the precise gene order of the RS virus has not been established with certainty, Collins and Wertz (1983) have proposed a transcriptional map in which two viral nonstructural protein genes are 3' proximal. Also, it is not known whether an untranslated leader RNA is synthesized as in the case of other nonsegmented negative-strand RNA viruses. If the first reading frame codes for the NS_2 protein, we may have fortuitously cloned a linked transcript containing this gene and upstream sequences for a second NS protein. It is also possible that the second open reading frame codes for the NS_2 protein (Fig. 3).

The codon usage of the RS virus genes showed an inherent bias against the CG dinucleotide within the coding region similar to what has been observed with vesicular stomatitis virus (VSV), influenza virus, and eukaryotic genomes. Each of the RS virus genes lacks the canonical eukaryotic polyadenylation signal AAUAAA upstream of the 3′ poly(A) sequence. In addition, these genes lack homologous sequences upstream of the poly(A) tail, unlike VSV and Sendai virus which have a conserved four-nucleotide sequence AUAC and AUUC, respectively, upstream of the poly(A) tail of each gene transcript (Gupta and Kingsbury 1982).

Plasmid pRSA$_3$ contains a P-gene cDNA insert that hybrid-selects a viral mRNA similar in size to the insert. We are in the process of sequencing this insert. Certain recombinants containing this gene hybrid-select mRNAs that translate P protein and a nonstructural protein (Fig. 1, lane 5, lower arrow). A similar situation has been observed with Sendai virus, where P and C proteins are encoded by the same mRNA either as a tandem nonoverlapping dicistronic RNA or as an mRNA with overlapping reading frames (Dowling et al. 1983). The C protein is derived from a second open reading frame near the 5′ end of the mRNA. DNA sequence analysis of RS virus P-gene cDNA clones should allow us to determine whether this is the case with RS virus.

SUMMARY

A start has been made in elucidating the structure and function of the RS virus genome. Recombinant DNA techniques allowed us to identify at least six distinct classes of cDNA clones containing RS virus sequences. These classes do not share sequence homology with one another. cDNA clones containing almost complete copies of the NC, M, or NS$_2$ viral gene were sequenced, and protein-coding sequences were identified. Future studies should allow us to determine the exact gene order for this virus and obtain complete cDNA clones of the viral surface glycoprotein genes. The latter could then be used to achieve expression in both prokaryotic and eukaryotic cells, allowing us to study antigenicity and immunogenicity of the polypeptides involved in immunity.

REFERENCES

Chanock, R.M., H.W. Kim, C.D. Brandt, and R.H. Parrott. 1982. Respiratory syncytial virus. In *Viral infections of humans: Epidemiology and control* (ed. A.S. Evans), p. 471. Plenum Press, New York.

Collins, P.L. and A.W. Wertz. 1983. cDNA cloning and transcriptional mapping of nine polyadenylated RNAs encoded by the genome of human respiratory syncytial virus. *Proc. Natl. Acad. Sci.* **80:** 3205.

Dowling, P.C., C. Giorgi, L. Roux, L.A. Dethelfsen, M.E. Galantowicz, B. Blumberg, and D. Kolakofsky. 1983. Molecular cloning of the 3′-proximal third of Sendai virus genome. *Proc. Natl. Acad. Sci.* **80:** 5213.

Elango, N. and S. Venkatesan. 1983. Amino acid sequence of human respiratory syncytial virus capsid protein. *Nucleic Acids Res.* **11:** 5941.

Gimenez, H.B. and C.R. Pringle. 1978. Seven complementation groups of respiratory syncytial virus temperature-sensitive mutants. *J. Virol.* **27:** 459.

Gupta, K.C. and D.W. Kingsbury. 1982. Conserved polyadenylation signals in two negative strand RNA virus families. *Virology* **120:** 518.

Huang, Y.T. and G.W. Wertz. 1983. Respiratory syncytial virus coding assignments. *J. Virol.* **43:** 150.

Kingsbury, D.W. 1977. Paramyxoviruses. In *The molecular biology of animal viruses* (ed. D.P. Nayak), p. 349. Marcel Dekker, New York.

Venkatesan, S., N. Elango, and R.M. Chanock. 1983. Construction and characterization of cDNA clones for four respiratory syncytial virus genes. *Proc. Natl. Acad. Sci.* **80:** 1280.

Use of Genetic Recombination for Constructing Novel Strains of a Picornavirus

David McCahon, Andrew M.Q. King,
Keith Saunders,* William R. Slade,
and John W.I. Newman
*Genetics Department, Animal Virus Research
Institute, Pirbright, Woking, Surrey, England*

Picornaviruses have the apparently unique ability among RNA viruses to undergo recombination of their RNA to produce viable recombinant viruses without the involvement of a DNA intermediate (for review, see McCahon 1981). However, it has been difficult to exploit the phenomenon because of its rarity and variability. Recently, we described a sensitive infectious center method (McCahon and Slade 1981), which we have used to isolate recombinants between two biochemically distinguishable strains of foot-and-mouth disease virus (FMDV), thus providing the first clear molecular evidence for recombination in RNA (King et al. 1982).

FMDV undergoes extensive antigenic variation; seven types and numerous subtypes have been described. One of our interests in studying recombination has been the possibility of using it to construct new viruses for use in vaccines. These would, it is hoped, combine the stability and growth properties of an efficient vaccine strain with appropriate antigenic regions from other strains. In the present studies, we have explored recombination between different serotypes and between different subtypes within a serotype in order to obtain some idea of the limitations of the technique to manipulate the genome.

RESULTS

Recombination Can Occur between Different Serotypes

Intertypic crosses were performed between strains belonging to three of the seven FMDV serotypes, O, A, and SAT2. O and A are both European types,

*Present address: Biophysical Laboratory, 1525 Linden Drive, University of Wisconsin-Madison, Madison, Wisconsin 53706.

whereas SAT2 is a representative of the more distantly related South African types (Robson et al. 1977). The strategy adopted was to infect cells with a mixture of two viruses having temperature-sensitive (*ts*) mutations at opposite ends of the genome and to select *ts*+ progeny using the infectious center method. Recombinants were initially identified by electrofocusing virus-induced proteins, and the RNA genomes of these viruses were then characterized by RNase T1 fingerprinting.

In both of the O/SAT2 crosses (Fig. 1b,c), there was no significant increase in the production of *ts*+ virus from mixedly infected cells compared with that from controls. Nevertheless, when the progeny of the SAT×O cross (Fig. 1b) were examined by electrofocusing, 2 out of 15 *ts*+ isolates gave protein patterns that might be expected of recombinants, i.e., Rec E85 had structural proteins (VP0,

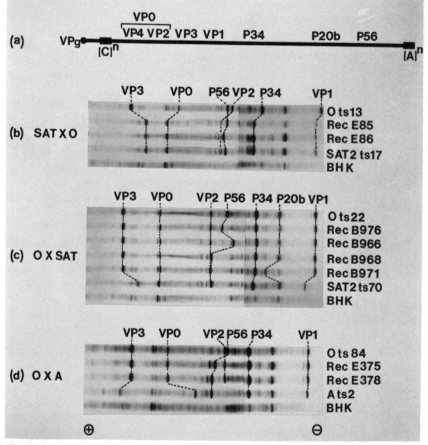

Figure 1

Electrofocusing of ^{35}S-labeled cytoplasmic extracts of virus-infected cells. (*a*) Gene order of polypeptides detected in electrofocusing gels; (*b,c,d*) examples of recombinant patterns obtained in three intertypic crosses.

VP3, and VP1) and polypeptide P34 of type SAT2 and a P56 resembling that of the type-O parent. Rec E86 was identical except that its P56 resembled neither parent, suggesting that it may have been generated by a genetic crossover within the P56 gene. Likewise, in the O × SAT cross (Fig. 1c), 9 out of 15 *ts*+ isolates gave four possible recombinant patterns, represented by Rec B976, B966, B968, and B971. They were essentially the reciprocals of Rec E85 and E86 in that they were principally type O (structural and P34 proteins) but with a P56 that resembled that of the SAT2 parent (e.g., B971) or neither parent. Rec B971 was interesting in that the protein encoded next to P56, P20b, was altered, suggesting that the crossover may have taken place within the P20b gene.

The cross between the two European types, O × A (Fig. 1d), resulted in a significant increase (fivefold) in the production of *ts*+ virus over that of the controls. All eight *ts*+ isolates examined gave protein patterns expected of recombinants, seven (e.g., Rec E378) having the structural proteins of type O and a P56 of type A, and one (Rec E375) having a P56 that resembled neither parent.

When the RNAs of the putative recombinants were examined by RNase T1 fingerprinting, they were found to be recombinant and distinguishable from each other. An example from each of the O/SAT2 crosses is shown in Figure 2A. The fingerprint of Rec B971 resembled that of the type-O parent except that there were three oligonucleotides inherited from the type-SAT2 parent, and six type-O oligonucleotides missing. The latter included oligonucleotides 21 and 41 known from genetic mapping studies (Fig. 3) to be located at the 3' end of the genome. The other recombinant shown in Figure 2A, Rec E85, appeared to have been generated, as expected, by a crossover close to that of Rec B971 but in the opposite direction. The fingerprint of Rec E85 RNA resembled that of type SAT2, but with five SAT2 oligonucleotides substituted by four type-O oligonucleotides. Significantly, the latter belong to the group of oligonucleotides derived from the 3' end of the type-O RNA that were missing from Rec B971.

Figure 2B shows the RNA fingerprints of two of the O × A recombinants. It can be seen that Rec E375 contained two type-A oligonucleotides and Rec E378 contained eight type-A oligonucleotides, all the others being inherited from type O. According to the mapping data of Harris et al. (1980), these type-A oligonucleotides are all derived from the 3' end of the genome. Thus, the oligonucleotide compositions of all four recombinants in Figure 2 are consistent with the protein analyses described earlier. They are also consistent with what we know of the parental temperature-sensitive mutations; for example, the parent that contributed the 5' end of its genome to the recombinant progeny had, in all three crosses, a temperature-sensitive mutation near the 3' end of the genome in the P56 gene.

Recombination Can Occur at Many Different Sites

The most extensive series of crosses that we have performed between any pair of allogenic viruses utilized two type-O strains of different subtypes, O_1 and O_6. Thirteen crosses were performed between these subtypes, using a variety of temperature-sensitive mutants. Nearly all (46/48) of the recombinants identified by electrofocusing appeared to have been generated by crossovers at one of two sites, between VP1 and P34 and between P34 and P56. Of the remaining two

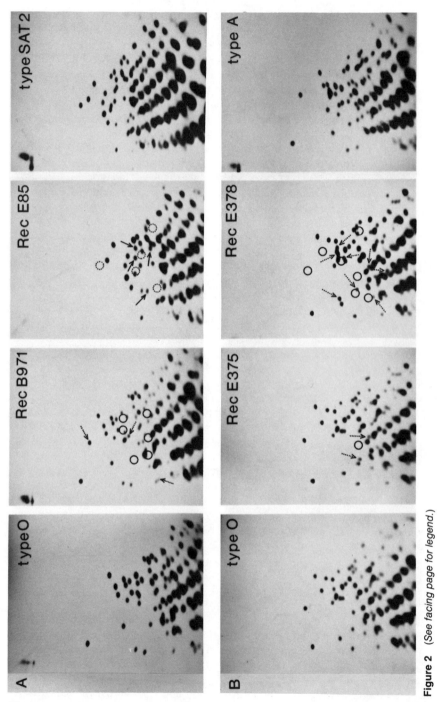

Figure 2 *(See facing page for legend.)*

48

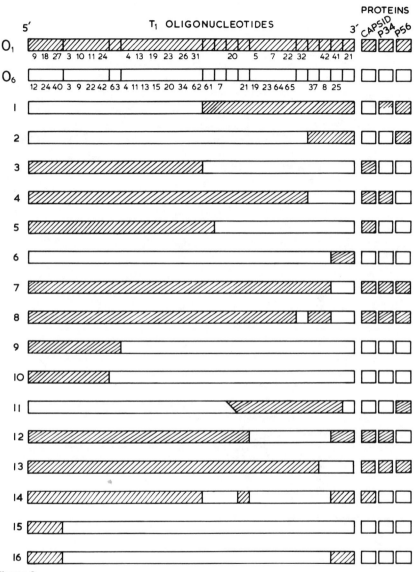

Figure 3
Oligonucleotide and protein compositions of recombinants formed between subtypes O₁ and O₆.

Figure 2
RNA fingerprints of intertypic recombinants and their parents. Arrows (oligonucleotides gained) and circles (oligonucleotides lost) highlight differences between each recombinant and the parent that it most closely resembles. (A) Type-O/type-SAT2 recombinants. Solid arrows indicate O gains; solid circles, O losses; dotted arrows, SAT2 gains; dotted circles, SAT2 losses. (B) Type-O/type-A recombinants. Dotted arrows indicate A gains; solid circles, O losses. Note that different type-O strains were used in A and B.

isolates, one appeared to have a crossover within P34, resulting in a non-parental P34, and the other, a crossover between VP2 and VP3.

A much greater variety of recombinants was revealed by RNA fingerprinting. To date, no less than 16 different oligonucleotide patterns have been identified among the 38 recombinants that have been analyzed. Their compositions are shown in Figure 3 in parallel with their protein compositions. The oligonucleotides are arranged in a linkage map that assumes the minimum number of crossover events per recombinant. The resulting map of O_6 oligonucleotides correlates well with their approximate locations determined by Harris et al. (1980).

Several points emerge from the RNA analyses shown in Figure 3. First, half of the recombinant forms (e.g., Rec 6) had crossovers near one or both termini that could not be detected by electrofocusing virus-induced proteins. Second, recombination occurs at many sites; Figure 3 depicts 13 different sites, although up to three of these could in theory be explained by a point mutation causing the loss of an oligonucleotide from each of Rec 8, 11, and 14. Third, although most of the fingerprints can be reconciled with single crossovers, at least two recombination events, each, are required to form Rec 12, 14, and 16.

DISCUSSION

The successful crosses between the O and SAT2 serotypes suggest that it ought to be possible to recombine almost any pair of FMDV strains with each other. However, the exchange of genetic information between these distantly related serotypes appears to have been limited to relatively small regions at the 3' end of the genome. In contrast, the two subtype strains, O_1 and O_6, were able to recombine at a great many sites throughout the genome, but even here, the very rare occurrence of hybrid capsids, or of recombinant proteins having an altered pI, indicates that crossovers may not have been located entirely at random. We should expect potential sites of recombination to be limited not only by a requirement for homology between the parental RNA molecules, but also, bearing in mind the polycistronic nature of the RNA, by the need to preserve protein function. Despite such limitations, RNA recombination clearly has the potential to provide a wide variety of recombinants that would be suitable for analysis as vaccine strains.

ACKNOWLEDGMENT

We thank A. Cleary for his excellent technical assistance.

REFERENCES

Harris, T.J.R., K.J.H. Robson, and F. Brown. 1980. A study of the level of nucleotide sequence conservation between the RNAs of two serotypes of FMDV. *J. Gen. Virol.* **50:** 403.

King, A.M.Q., D. McCahon, W.R. Slade, and J.W.I. Newman. 1982. Recombination in RNA. *Cell* **29:** 921.

McCahon, D. 1981. The genetics of aphthovirus. *Arch. Virol.* **69:** 1.

McCahon, D. and W.R. Slade. 1981. A sensitive method for the detection and isolation of recombinants of FMDV. *J. Gen. Virol.* **53:** 333.

Robson, K.J.H., T.J.R. Harris, and F. Brown. 1977. An assessment by competition hybridization of the sequence homology between the RNAs of the seven serotypes of FMDV. *J. Gen. Virol.* **37:** 271.

Analysis of Cloned Genes Encoding Rotaviral Type-specific Neutralizing Antigens

Gerald W. Both and Linda J. Siegman
CSIRO, Molecular and Cellular Biology Unit
North Ryde, NSW 2113, Australia

**Paul H. Atkinson, Marianne S. Poruchynsky,
and Ailsa Kabcenell**
Department of Developmental Biology and Cancer
Albert Einstein College of Medicine
Bronx, New York 10471

**Jeanette E. Street, Peter R. Gunn,
Fumiyasu Sato, Kevin F.H. Powell,
and A. Richard Bellamy**
Department of Cell Biology
University of Auckland, New Zealand

Rotaviruses are one of the most important causes of acute diarrheal disease in young children, and the development of an effective vaccine deserves high priority. Recent successes in the cultivation of human isolates may permit the eventual production of a vaccine incorporating suitable attenuated viruses. However, our efforts have been focused recently on producing cloned DNA copies of genes encoding rotaviral antigens with the aim of expressing these for eventual vaccine production. Comparison of protein sequences inferred for the serotype-specific antigens may also permit identification of antigenically important regions of the virus and enable a vaccine based on synthetic peptides to be developed.

Rotaviral Antigenic Proteins

Rotaviruses have at least two surface proteins, VP3 and VP7, and an inner core protein VP6, which are capable of eliciting antibodies when presented in the form of intact viral particles. We have used Western transfer analysis to assess the array of antibodies produced in response to several virus preparations. In our experience the method of virus preparation appears crucial to the integrity of the viral particles and to the retention of VP7 in the preparation. This glycoprotein is easily lost, presumably through particle breakdown and nonspecific adsorption. However, when care is taken to recover dissociated VP7 by ultracentrifugation, antibodies produced against these virus preparations are directed primarily

53

against VP7 (Fig. 1). Others are directed against VP6 and against VP3 and its cleavage products, p55 and p25. This observation tends to confirm the results obtained with recombinant viruses and neutralization tests with monospecific antisera that VP7 is the protein conferring serotype specificity and the major neutralizing antigen.

Cross-reactivity between Serotype Antigens

Western transfer analysis was used to determine whether there was any cross-reactivity between rotaviral proteins from separate neutralization serotypes. Hyperimmune sera against SA11 or Wa showed both homologous and heterologous reactivities with VP7 proteins from these viruses. Both sera also reacted with VP7 from NCDV (Nebraska calf diarrhea virus). However, little or no reactivity was observed with either sera against VP7 from rotavirus S2 (Fig. 1B,C). In view of the serotype specificity associated with VP7, the cross-reactivity between Wa, SA11, and NCDV is presumably due to nonneutralizing antibodies directed against regions of VP7 conserved in viruses from the three serotypes (see below). The implication is that VP7 from rotavirus S2 does not share these common antigenic determinants, presumably because its protein sequence differs substantially from those of the other viruses. Confirmation of this awaits sequence data. The existence of two "families" of viruses was inferred from nucleotide sequence cross-hybridization studies among these and similar strains (Street et al.

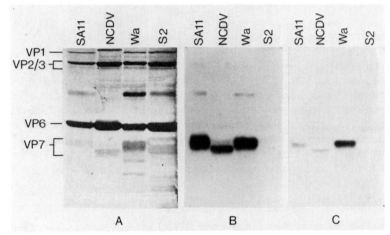

Figure 1
Western blot analysis of antigenic cross-reactivity between VP7 proteins of rotavirus strains. Equal amounts of viral protein were resolved on 10% SDS-polyacrylamide gels and transferred to Schleicher and Schuell BA83 nitrocellulose by transverse electrophoresis. Nitrocellulose strips were incubated overnight with a 10^2 dilution of appropriate antiserum prepared in New Zealand white rabbits using purified double-shelled virus, and bound antibody was detected by autoradiography after exposure of the strips to ^{125}I-labeled protein A. (A) Silver-stained gel (10 μg of virus was loaded into each track); (B) blotted proteins treated with anti-SA11 antiserum; (C) blotted proteins treated with anti-Wa antiserum.

1982; Flores et al. 1983). These Western data may provide stronger support for the idea, since base differences affecting nucleic acid sequence hybridization do not necessarily result in changes in the protein sequence.

Comparison of Rotaviral VP7 Proteins

Recently, a general strategy for cloning rotaviral genes was developed (Both et al. 1982) that enabled us to obtain DNA copies for several rotaviral double-stranded RNA segments, including gene 9. Figure 2 presents a comparison of the inferred sequences for VP7 antigens from our own SA11 (Both et al. 1983) and NCDV rotavirus clones and of UK bovine VP7 sequenced by the Melbourne group (Elleman et al. 1983). The NCDV sequence presently is incomplete and terminates at nucleotide 616.

There is 77.1% nucleic acid sequence homology between genes encoding VP7 for SA11 and UK viruses. Thus, there is striking homology between SA11 and UK bovine VP7 proteins (Fig. 2), with 86% of amino acid residues con-

```
            • • • • •   • • • • • • • • • •   • • •       • • • • • • • • • •   • • • • • • • •              60
SA11    MYGIEYTTVL  TFLISIILLN  YILKSLTRIM  DCIIYRLLFI  IVILSPFLRA  QNYGINLPIT
NCDV             I   I  T            M   I      Y    F L  V   ATIIN            V
UKBOV            I   I  T                I      Y    F L  V V ATMIN            V


                                                                                120
SA11    GSMDTAYANS  TQEETFLTST  LCLYYPTEAA  TEINDNSWKD  TLSQLFLTKG  WPTGSVYFKE
NCDV             D     S P              V  S  N  A TE                         L
UKBOV          _ _     S P            V  S   N  A TE,


                                                                                180
SA11    YTNIASFSVD  PQLYCDYNVV  LMKYDATLQL  DMSELADLIL  NEWLCNPMDI  TLYYYQQTDE
NCDV    AD  A   E            L       S QE
UKBOV    D   A   E           L       S QE,


                                                                                240
SA11    ANKWISMGSS  CTIKVCPLNT  QTLGIGCLTT  DATTFEEVAT  AEKLVITDVV  DGVNHKLDVT
NCDV        T    .  . . .
UKBOV            V                I  NPD  T,        T                      N


                                                                                300
SA11    TATCTIRNCK  KLGPRENVAV  IQVGGSDILD  ITADPITAPQ  TERMMRINWK  KWWQVFYTVV
NCDV
UKBOV                       I        ANV


SA11    DYVDQIIQVM  SKRSRSLNSA  AFYYRV
NCDV
UKBOV    N    T            S
```

Figure 2
Comparison of VP7 amino acid sequences for SA11, NCDV, and UK bovine rotaviruses. Only those residues that differ from the SA11 sequence are shown. The NCDV sequence terminates at amino acid 189. Potential glycosylation sites are underlined. Residues that may contribute to the differences in neutralization serotypes between SA11 and bovine strains are bracketed. The amino acids constituting the dual hydrophobic regions near the amino terminus are indicated by overlined dots.

served. This is in contrast to the influenza hemagglutinins where, for example, H3 and H7 subtypes have only 38% homology in the HA_1 region.

The two regions of hydrophobic amino acids described for the aminoterminal region of SA11 VP7 (Both et al. 1983) are conserved in character in both bovine viruses (Figs. 2 and 3) despite several amino acid differences present between residues 32 and 49. Although there is extensive conservation of amino acid sequence between SA11 and bovine VP7 proteins throughout the remainder of the molecule, blocks of conserved residues are interrupted by clusters of amino acid changes, e.g., residues 87–97, 146–149, and 209–217 (Fig. 2). These all fall in regions of VP7 likely to have surface locations due to their relatively hydrophilic nature (Fig. 3). Determination of VP7 sequences for other rotaviruses, e.g., Wa, should indicate whether or not amino acid differences between antigenically distinct VP7 proteins are confined to these locations. In view of the overall similarity between these proteins, it must be considered likely that some or all of these amino acids contribute to differences in neutralization serotype between bovine and SA11 rotaviruses (Wyatt et al. 1982). This is consistent with the observation that NCDV and UK strains are identical in the two bracketed regions for which data are available (Fig. 2). Whether some of the remaining scattered amino acid differences, e.g., residues 75, 123, and 267, contribute to antigenic epitopes formed by discontinuous regions of the VP7 polypeptide is difficult to assess without structural data.

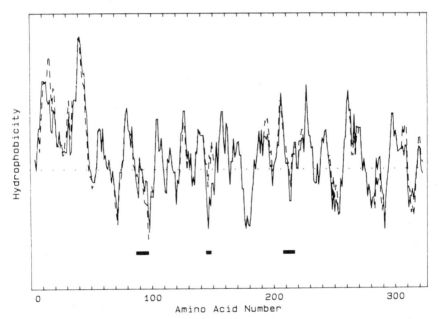

Figure 3
Comparison of hydrophobicity profiles for VP7 proteins from SA11 and UK bovine rotaviruses. Computer-generated plots of a seven-point moving average were generated using the method of Kyte and Doolittle (1982). Regions above the datum line are hydrophobic. Dashed line indicates SA11, and solid line indicates UK bovine. Locations of regions bracketed in Fig. 2 are indicated by black bars.

There are also differences between SA11 and the bovine strains with respect to potential carbohydrate-attachment sites (Fig. 2). The UK bovine strain has potential glycosylation sites at residues 69–71, 238–240, and 318–320. Which of these is used is not known, although for NCDV, the site at Asn-69 is missing due to an Asn→Asp change caused by an A→G mutation of nucleotide 253. This site is almost certainly used in SA11, being the only Asn-X-Ser/Thr sequence in the protein (Fig. 2). Whether the presence of carbohydrate on VP7 can mask an epitope capable of inducing neutralizing antibodies, as occurs for influenza hemagglutinin, remains to be determined.

Possible Novel Approaches to Rotavirus Vaccine Development

One of the major difficulties confronting any future application of recombinant DNA work on rotaviruses to vaccine development is the nature of the virus infection itself. Virus multiplication appears to be restricted to the epithelial cells of the small intestine, and animal studies have demonstrated that it is probably secretory IgA, rather than IgG, antibody that is involved in preventing or reducing illness due to rotavirus infection (Estes et al. 1982; Holmes 1983). Thus, if generation of a protective response requires oral administration of antigen to stimulate production of secretory antibody, then practical difficulties are likely to be encountered in administering cloned protein or antigenic peptides to the appropriate site.

For some animal systems the alternative approach of hyperimmunizing the dam could prove to be of value, particularly since some studies have indicated that "hyperimmune" milk can exert a protective effect (Holmes 1983). Cloned protein or peptides could be of particular value in this situation, since they would be readily prepared and could be administered parenterally.

For the human infant where susceptibility to infection is at its greatest between 6 months and 3 years of age, active immunization is likely to be necessary. It may be that novel routes for delivery of antigen could be investigated, for example, by incorporating the appropriate rotaviral genes into a bacterium capable of colonizing the human gut. Alternatively, the incorporation of genes into other live viral vector systems may provide an opportunity for delivery of antigenic protein and the stimulation of gut immunity.

ACKNOWLEDGMENT

We thank Dr. I. Holmes and colleagues for exchanging sequence data prior to publication.

REFERENCES

Both, G.W., J.S. Mattick, and A.R. Bellamy. 1983. The serotype-specific glycoprotein of Simian 11 rotavirus: Coding assignment and gene sequence. *Proc. Natl. Acad. Sci.* **80:** 3091.

Both, G.W., A.R. Bellamy, J.E. Street, and L.J. Siegman. 1982. A general strategy for cloning double-stranded RNA: Nucleotide sequence of the Simian-11 rotavirus gene 8. *Nucleic Acids Res.* **10:** 7075.

Elleman, T.C., P.A. Hoyne, M.L. Dyall-Smith, I.H. Holmes, and A.A. Azad. 1983. Nucleotide sequence of the gene encoding the serotype-specific glycoprotein of UK bovine rotavirus. *Nucleic Acids Res.* **11:** 4689.

Estes, M.K., E.L. Palmer, and J.F. Obijeski. 1982. Rotaviruses: A review. *Curr. Top. Microbiol. Immunol.* **11:** 4689.

Flores, J., M. Sereno, C.J. Lai, E. Boeggman, I. Perez, R. Purcell, A. Kalica, H. Greenberg, R. Wyatt, J. Hansen, A. Kapikian, and R. Chanock. 1983. Use of single-stranded rotavirus RNA transcripts for the diagnosis of rotavirus infection, the study of genetic diversity among rotaviruses, and the molecular cloning of rotavirus genes. In *Double stranded RNA viruses* (ed. R.W. Compans and D.H.L. Bishop), p. 115. Elsevier Science Publishing Co., New York.

Holmes, I.H. 1983. Rotaviruses. In *The reoviridae* (ed. W.K. Joklik), p. 359. Plenum Press, New York.

Kyte, J. and R.F. Doolittle. 1982. A simple method for displaying the hydropathic character of a protein. *J. Mol. Biol.* **157:** 105.

Street, J.E., M.C. Croxson, W.F. Chadderton, and A.R. Bellamy. 1982. Sequence diversity of human rotavirus strains investigated by Northern blot hybridization. *J. Virol.* **43:** 369.

Wyatt, R.G., H.B. Greenberg, W.D. James, A.L. Pittman, A.R. Kalica, J. Flores, R.M. Chanock, and A.Z. Kapikian. 1982. Definition of human rotavirus serotypes by plaque reduction assay. *Infect. Immun.* **37:** 110.

Approaches to the Development of Hepatitis-A Vaccines: The Old and the New

Robert H. Purcell, Stephen M. Feinstone,
Richard J. Daemer, John R. Ticehurst,
and Bahige M. Baroudy
Laboratory of Infectious Diseases
National Institute of Allergy and Infectious
Diseases, National Institutes of Health
Bethesda, Maryland 20205

Hepatitis-A virus (HAV) is a human pathogen with a worldwide distribution. It is a picornavirus with many of the characteristics of an enterovirus and is spread by fecal-oral contamination. Its host range is limited to man and a few other primate species, principally the chimpanzee and certain South American marmoset species. Its host range in vitro is similarly limited to cells of primate origin, principally primary, secondary, and continuous kidney cells and diploid fibroblasts. The virus was first isolated in tissue culture in 1979.

The isolation of HAV in tissue culture made the development of hepatitis-A vaccines feasible for the first time (Provost et al. 1979, 1982; Daemer et al. 1981, 1982). Until recently, growth of the virus in tissue culture has been relatively poor, characterized by long replicative cycles and low yield of virus and viral antigen. This has made development of an inactivated hepatitis-A vaccine difficult and expensive and has directed research efforts toward the development of live attenuated vaccines, on the one hand, and vaccines derived from molecular cloning experiments, on the other. Significant progress has been made with both approaches, making type-A hepatitis possibly one of the last diseases to be prevented by "classical" vaccines and one of the first to yield vaccines prepared by genetic engineering. The following is a status report on their development.

DISCUSSION

Animal Models

Because of the limited host range of HAV, studies of vaccine safety and efficacy must be carried out in nonhuman primates. Two models have proven useful:

South American marmoset monkeys (*Saguinus mystax* or *Saguinus labiatus*) and chimpanzees (*Pan troglodytes*). Both regularly develop hepatitis following exposure to wild-type HAV. Because of the closer biological relationship between man and chimpanzees than between man and marmosets, we have chosen the former for more detailed studies of infection with wild-type HAVs. Three strains, obtained from epidemiologically and geographically diverse sources, were studied (see Daemer et al. 1981). These included the MS-1 strain derived from endemic hepatitis-A infections among residents of a home for the mentally retarded in New York, the SD-11 strain from an epidemic of hepatitis among Naval recruits in California, and the HM-175 strain from a family outbreak of hepatitis in Melbourne, Australia. All produced hepatitis in chimpanzees. The three strains of HAV did differ in virulence: The SD-11 strain was the least virulent, and the HM-175 strain produced the most severe hepatitis.

Isolation and Propagation of HAV in Tissue Culture

Titered stool pools of the three strains of HAV described above were injected into primary African green monkey kidney (AGMK) cell cultures, a cell type suitable for vaccine development. Only the HM-175 strain of HAV was successfully recovered from primary AGMK cultures. Propagation was difficult and characterized by long replicative cycles measured in weeks and the absence of cytopathogenic effect. Staining of cultures with fluorescein-labeled anti-HAV (human convalescent serum) revealed the presence of discrete fluorescent foci that slowly enlarged with time, suggesting that the virus was mostly cell-associated and not readily released into the tissue-culture medium. This cell association was confirmed by detection of viral antigen in lysed cells but not in the tissue-culture medium by radioimmunoassay. Infectivity titers of HAV were generally low, especially in early passages. To date, the virus has been serially passaged 30 times in primary AGMK cells; at that passage level, it still required up to 3 weeks for 100% infection of cells, as judged by immunofluorescence. Infectivity titers ranged from approximately 10^7 to 10^9 TCID$_{50}$ per milliliter of lysed cells. Although preliminary biological characterization of tissue-culture-adapted HAV described here was carried out with uncloned HAV, the virus was recently triply cloned by terminal dilution.

Biological Characterization of
Tissue-culture-adapted HAV in Primates

Tissue-culture-adapted HAV at passage levels 10 and 20 was evaluated for evidence of attenuation in chimpanzees (Feinstone et al. 1983). Infectivity titrations of the two virus inocula were performed, the recipient chimpanzees were monitored for serologic evidence of infection and biochemical evidence of hepatitis, and the results were compared with those obtained from chimpanzees inoculated with the wild-type parent virus (positive controls) or noninfectious inocula (negative controls). All of the chimpanzees infected with the wild-type HAV developed hepatitis. In contrast, none of the chimpanzees infected with the tissue-culture-adapted HAV developed hepatitis when compared with the negative control animals (Table 1). Furthermore, the anti-HAV response to the attenuated tissue-culture-passaged HAV was comparable to the response in chimpanzees that developed hepatitis following inoculation with the virulent wild-type virus. When chimpanzees previously infected with the attenuated strains were rechallenged with the virulent strain, they were protected from hepatitis unless the rechallenge occurred during early convalescence when the primary immune response was still developing.

The stability of the attenuation of tissue-culture-passaged HAV was examined by attempting to transmit the virus from acute-phase stools of experimentally infected chimpanzees to other chimpanzees. Both the virulent and attenuated strains of HAV were much less transmissible by the oral route than by the intravenous route of inoculation, suggesting that a live attenuated HAV vaccine would not readily spread to contacts of vaccinees. When acute-phase stool samples from chimpanzees infected with attenuated HAV were injected intravenously into other chimpanzees, infection without hepatitis was observed. Thus, even following three passages in chimpanzees, the tissue-culture-passaged HAV retained its attenuation.

In contrast to results obtained in chimpanzees, preliminary studies in marmosets of the tissue-culture passage-20 HAV revealed that it was still virulent for marmosets. Thus, attenuation of HAV was shown to be species-specific.

Molecular Virology of HAV

Because of the relatively poor growth of HAV in tissue culture, HAV RNA for molecular cloning was purified from the livers of experimentally infected marmosets. Eight livers yielded approximately 1 μg of highly purified HAV RNA. In collaborative studies with Drs. Racaniello and Baltimore (Ticehurst et al. 1983), cDNA was prepared from the HAV RNA with reverse transcriptase. The second strand of cDNA was synthesized with *Escherichia coli* DNA polymerase I, and the

Table 1
Attenuation of HAV Strain HM-175 in Tissue Culture

Inoculum (i.v.)	Number chimpanzees infected	Hepatitis: mean max. ALT	Anti-HAV: mean max. N/S[a]
HM-175 wild type	7	314(109–419)	20.4
HM-175, pass 10	7	53(39–71)	17.7
HM-175 pass 20	5	47(44–61)	9.0[b]
No HAV[c]	6	57(41–81)	<2.1

[a]Negative control/sample cpm (Havab; Abbott Labs Inc.). Positive ≥2.1.
[b]Challenged with wild-type HM-175 before reaching maximum titer.
[c]Dilutions beyond endpoint of above pools.

double-stranded DNA was cloned into pBR322. Approximately 3000 clones were selected, of which 18 clones were extensively characterized by restriction endonuclease analysis. The results of these studies have yielded a restriction map of the HAV genome (Fig. 1). At least 99% of the genome is represented by these clones. Sequence analysis of the clones is in progress. Preliminary results support the existence of a single, large open reading frame thought to code for a polyprotein analogous to the polyprotein of other picornaviruses.

Cloning and characterization of HAV genes coding for viral coat proteins may permit the development of "engineered" vaccines to HAV. These might consist of the products of one or more viral-coat-protein genes expressed in prokaryotes or eukaryotes or, alternatively, synthetic peptides composed of amino acid sequences predicted from nucleotide sequences of the coat-protein genes. Both approaches are currently being pursued.

SUMMARY

The hepatitis viruses have been among the most difficult human pathogens to study. To date the etiologic agent of only one form of human viral hepatitis (HAV) has been isolated in tissue culture; this was achieved as recently as 1979. As a result, live, attenuated hepatitis-A vaccines are being developed. And with the recent advances in the molecular cloning of HAV cDNA described here, it becomes feasible to prepare vaccines either by the synthetic peptide approach or by the expression of the viral antigens in prokaryotic or eukaryotic vectors.

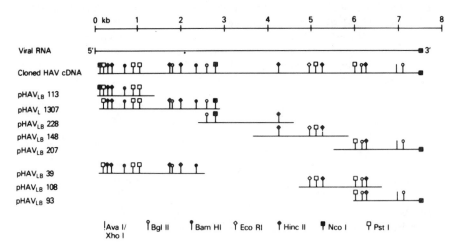

Figure 1
Restriction map of HAV cDNA clones. Viral RNA is estimated to be 7450 nucleotides in length excluding 3' poly(A), which is shown at the right (thicker line). A composite map of cloned HAV cDNA and positions of the inserts from clones pHAV$_{LB}$ 113, pHAV$_L$ 1307, pHAV$_{LB}$ 228, pHAV$_{LB}$ 148, and pHAV$_{LB}$ 207 are shown immediately below the viral RNA. Recombinant plasmids pHAV$_{LB}$ 39, pHAV$_{LB}$ 108, and pHAV$_{LB}$ 93 have been used for DNA sequencing, to confirm regions of overlap or to prepare insert probes (Ticehurst et al. 1983).

REFERENCES

Daemer, R.J., S.M. Feinstone, I.D. Gust, and R.H. Purcell. 1981. Propagation of human hepatitis A virus in African green monkey kidney cell culture: Primary isolation and serial passage. *Infect. Immun.* **32:** 388.

―――. 1982. Titration in cell culture and chimpanzees of hepatitis A isolated and serially passaged in primary African green monkey kidney. In *Viral hepatitis: International symposium 1981* (ed. W. Szmuness et al.), p. 755. The Franklin Institute Press, Philadelphia.

Feinstone, S.M., R.J. Daemer, I.D. Gust, and R.H. Purcell. 1983. Live attenuated vaccine for hepatitis A. In *Proceedings of 2nd International IABS Symposium on Viral Hepatitis, Athens, Greece,* vol. 54, p. 429.

Provost, P.J. and M.R. Hilleman. 1979. Propagation of human hepatitis A virus in cell culture *in vitro. Proc. Soc. Exp. Biol. Med.* **160:** 213.

Provost, P.J., F.S. Barker, P.A. Giesa, W.J. McAleer, E.B. Buynak, and M.R.Hilleman. 1982. Progress toward a live, attenuated human hepatitis A vaccine. *Proc. Soc. Exp. Biol. Med.* **170:** 8.

Ticehurst, J.R., V.R. Racaniello, B.M. Baroudy, D. Baltimore, R.H. Purcell, and S.M. Feinstone. 1983. Molecular cloning and characterization of hepatitis A virus cDNA. *Proc. Natl. Acad. Sci.* **80:** 5885.

Identification of Multiple Neutralization Antigenic Sites on Poliovirus Type 1 and the Priming of the Immune Response with Synthetic Peptides

Emilio A. Emini,* Bradford A. Jameson, and Eckard Wimmer
Department of Microbiology
State University of New York
Stony Brook, New York 11794

The immune response to poliovirus that confers protection against poliomyelitis has been studied for decades. Apart from the enigma of specific antibody formation, little is known about the mechanism by which antibodies neutralize the infectivity of the nonenveloped ("naked") virion. How do antibody molecules prevent the deadly path of penetration and intracellular replication of the virus?

The primary structure of the poliovirion (type 1, strain Mahoney and the corresponding Sabin vaccine strain LSc, 2ab) has recently been determined by a combination of nucleic acid sequence analyses (Kitamura et al. 1981; Racaniello and Baltimore 1981; Nomoto et al. 1982) and partial protein sequence analyses (Semler et al. 1981a,b, 1982; Larsen et al. 1982; Dorner et al. 1982; Emini et al. 1982a). Thus, the amino acid sequences of the four capsid proteins, VP1, VP2, VP3, and VP4, are known. It is the folding of the four capsid polypeptides in the icosahedral shell surrounding the single-stranded RNA genome that determines the antigenic properties of the virion. Poliovirus antigenic sites and their epitopes involved in neutralization (referred to originally as D antigen) are largely lost when the structure of the virion is disturbed, as, for example, when the virion is heated to 55°C or when the virion is disrupted altogether (for review, see Mandel 1979). Each of the large isolated capsid proteins VP1, VP2, and VP3, however, can elicit a neutralizing antibody response, albeit inconsistently or very weakly (Blondel et al. 1982; Chow and Baltimore 1982; Dernick et al. 1983; Emini et al. 1983c; van Wezel et al. 1983). These results are significant in that they show that multiple neutralization antigenic sites exist on the surface of the poliovirion. The objective

---

*Present address: Division of Virus and Cell Biology, Merck, Sharp and Dohme Research Laboratories, West Point, Pennsylvania 19486.

of the study described here is to identify neutralization antigenic sites and the mechanism(s) of the neutralization of poliovirus and to investigate whether on the basis of this information new strategies of vaccination can be developed.

DISCUSSION

Genetic Analysis of Neutralization Epitopes

The first biochemical evidence that neutralization epitopes (N-Eps)[1] are present on capsid protein VP1 of poliovirus type 1 (PV-1) was obtained by chemically cross-linking F(ab) fragments of two different neutralizing monoclonal antibodies (N-mAbs) to the virion (Emini et al. 1982b). The two N-mAbs used recognized two different N-Eps that appear to overlap slightly and belong to the same neutralization antigenic site (N-Ag)[1] (Emini et al. 1982b; 1983a,d). That VP1 harbors N-Eps did not come as a surprise since VP1 (m.w. 34,000) is the largest capsid protein of poliovirus, and it is extensively exposed to the surface of the virion (for references, see Emini et al. 1982b).

The use of several N-mAbs and an anti-VP4/VP3 serum (see below) permitted the selection of many spontaneous genetic variants of poliovirus that were resistant to neutralization. Cross-neutralization data identified at least seven different N-Eps (Emini et al. 1982b, 1983c,d). As discussed below, these epitopes divide among three different N-Ags. It is important to note that N-Eps of a single N-Ag do not necessarily overlap functionally; i.e., mutants in one N-Ep may be completely neutralized by monoclonal antibodies that recognize another N-Ep of the same N-Ag (Emini et al. 1983d).

The selection of spontaneous mutants to resistance of neutralization was carried out in a single-step growth cycle under conditions that made the presence of preexisting variants in the inoculum unlikely (Emini et al. 1982b, 1983c,d). The apparent rate at which variants resistant to neutralization with monoclonal antibodies arose upon passage in HeLa cells was surprisingly high (-3.1 to -4.8 $\log_{10}$ variant per wild-type virus pfu; Emini et al. 1982b, 1983c,d), a phenomenon also observed in other virus systems. It remains to be seen whether this apparent high rate is due to the simultaneous selection of more than one variant that has changed the primary sequence of the N-Ep itself or that has changed the folding of the N-Ep (by distant mutation) such that binding to the selecting N-mAb no longer occurs.

We have fingerprinted (Lee and Wimmer 1976) the RNase T1 oligonucleotides of the genomic RNA of most of the neutralization-resistant variants and have

---

[1]We define an N-Ep as the conformation of a structural element at the surface of a virus to which a monospecific (e.g., monoclonal) antibody can bind, an interaction leading to the neutralization of the virus. The structural element may consist of a linear sequence of amino acids or of complete sequences formed by distant regions in the capsid protein(s). Several N-Eps may be clustered in a specific region of the structural protein of the virus. The N-Eps in a cluster may or may not overlap functionally. That is, a genetic variant of the virus resistant to neutralization by one monoclonal antibody directed to a single N-Ep of a cluster may or may not be resistant to monoclonal antibodies directed to other N-Eps of that same cluster (Emini et al. 1983d). We define a cluster of N-Eps as a neutralization antigenic site (N-Ag).

compared the fingerprints to that of the parental strain. Unfortunately, none of the fingerprints showed any changes in the pattern of large oligonucleotides (E.A. Emini et al., unpubl.), a result that prevented the quick localization of any of the N-Eps. In the case of poliovirus type 3 (PV-3), Minor et al. (1983) were more fortunate in that a major N-Ag of PV-3 is encoded by a nucleotide sequence void of guanosine residues. Nevertheless, we have mapped several N-Ags and their N-Eps of PV-1 making use of synthetic peptides (see below).

Selection and Synthesis of Synthetic Peptides Corresponding to N-Ags

Of the four capsid proteins of poliovirus, the three largest (VP1, VP2, and VP3) are exposed to the surface of the virion and are thus potential carriers of N-Ags. As has been reviewed elsewhere (Lerner 1982; Walter and Doolittle 1983), hydrophilic regions of a polypeptide are the most likely to be antigenic. Computer analyses of the amino acid sequences using programs by Hopp and Woods (1981) and D. Davidson (unpubl.) have guided us to select such hydrophilic sequences on VP1, VP2, and VP3 of PV-1 (Emini et al. 1983a). Equally important for the selection of hydrophilic regions of capsid proteins, however, was the assumption that the major antigenic sequences involved in neutralization should differ from serotype to serotype of poliovirus, since there is little or no cross-neutralization with hyperimmune serum among serotypes.

Fortunately, the entire primary nucleotide and amino acid sequences of all three types of poliovirus have recently been established (Toyoda et al. 1984) and have been generously communicated to us prior to publication. In the course of studying the biological properties of peptides, we have observed the following interesting phenomenon: PV-1 and PV-3 share a certain sequence of hydrophilic amino acids in their respective capsid protein VP1 (amino acids 70–75). In PV-1, this sequence is part of an N-Ag, whereas in PV-3, it is part of an antigenic site to which antibodies bind but fail to neutralize the virus (see below) (Emini et al. 1983a). Thus, the comparison of sequences between serotypes may lead to an erroneous elimination of a true N-Ag in a given serotype.

Peptides corresponding to selected regions were synthesized by the solid-phase method (Erickson and Merrifield 1976). We have added to the virus-specific amino acid sequences two additional aminoterminal glycine residues that serve as spacers when the peptide is linked to the carrier polypeptides, as well as one tyrosine or one cysteine residue to facilitate linkage to bovine serum albumin (BSA) (Walter and Doolittle 1983) or to keyhole limpet hemocyanin (Lerner 1982), respectively (Fig. 1).

Peptide Recognition by N-mAbs

The synthetic peptides 1–4 were found by ELISA to interact specifically with representatives of the groups of N-mAbs (Table 1) (Emini et al. 1983a). Inspection of the data allowed us to define two N-Ags (amino acids 70–80 and 93–103 of VP1) on the surface of PV-1 that harbor clusters of N-Eps. Interestingly, the chain length of the peptide influences its ability to bind to N-mAbs, but the results show that the longer peptides do not necessarily interact with more N-mAbs than the shorter

PEPTIDES OF VP1

No.

1   Y – G – G – $\underline{\text{R – S – R – S – E – S}}$ – G$_{\text{COOH}}$ (70 ... 75)

4   C – G – G – $\underline{\text{R – S – R – S – E – S – S – I – E – S – F}}_{\text{COOH}}$ (70 ... 80)

2   Y – G – G – $\underline{\text{S – T – T – N – L – D – L}}$ – G$_{\text{COOH}}$ (97 ... 103)

3   Y – G – G – $\underline{\text{D – N – P – A – S – T – T – N – L – D – L}}_{\text{COOH}}$ (93 ... 103)

5   Y – G – $\underline{\text{D – N – T – V – R – E – T}}_{\text{COOH}}$ (11 ... 17)

PEPTIDE OF VP2

9   Y – G – G – $\underline{\text{T – P – D – N – N – Q – T – S – P – A – R – R}}_{\text{COOH}}$ (132 ... 143)

PEPTIDE OF VP3

8   Y – G – G – $\underline{\text{R – L – S – D – K – P – H – T – D – D – P – I}}_{\text{COOH}}$ (71 ... 82)

Figure 1
Sequences (in single letter code) of synthetic peptides used in ELISA or, after linking them to carrier proteins via the aminoterminal cytosine or tyrosine residues, used to immunize rabbits. The underlined sequences are those colinear with sequences of capsid proteins VP1, VP2, and VP3 of PV-1 (Mahoney). The amino acid sequences correspond to those published by Nomoto et al. (1982), which we use as a consensus sequence of the sequences obtained by Kitamura et al. (1981), Racaniello and Baltimore (1981), and Nomoto et al. (1982). For experimental details, see Emini et al. (1983a).

Table 1
Recognition of Synthetic Peptides by N-mAbs

Antibody[a]	Peptide				
	1	2	3	4	5
H3 (B)	+	–	–	+	–
I CJ 31-10 (E)	+	–	–	–	–
D3 (A)	+	–	–	–	–
A13 (C)	+	–	–	–	–
I CJ 27 (D)	–	–	+	–	–
1 BM 55-6 (F)	–	+	+	–	–

+ indicates positive response by ELISA using a 1:10 dilution of monoclonal-antibody-containing hybridoma culture supernatant, as described by Emini et al. (1983a). – indicates that ELISA reaction was not significantly above background control.
[a]Neutralizing monoclonal antibody raised against PV-1 (Mahoney strain) (Emini et al. 1982b, 1983b). The epitope grouping to which the antibody belongs (Emini et al. 1983b) is given in parentheses.

peptides (Table 1). This observation indicates the complexity of peptide folding and of peptide binding to the hypervariable region of the antibody, a problem that can currently be solved only empirically. Peptide 5, whose sequence originates near the amino terminus of VP1, did not bind to any N-mAbs available to us. As we shall see, peptide 5 nevertheless is part of an N-Ag distinct from the other two sites. Failure of the poliovirion to elicit N-mAbs against this third N-Ag in mice may be a statistical problem; the other two sites located at amino acids 70–80 and 93–103 of VP1 appear to be more immunopotent.

N-Ags on Capsid Polypeptides VP2 and VP3

As mentioned above, regions of capsid proteins VP2 and VP3 (but not of VP4) of poliovirus are exposed to the outside of the virion albeit to a lesser extent than VP1. Immunization of rabbits with purified VP4 has led in one case to the discovery of neutralizing antibodies directed against VP3 (Emini et al. 1983c) (the gel-purified VP4 [7000 daltons] used for the immunization was probably contaminated with fragmented VP3 [26,000 daltons]). We henceforth call this serum anti-VP4/VP3. Genetic variants resistant to neutralization with anti-VP4/VP3 were selected, and they arose at an apparent rate similar to that of variants resistant to the N-mAb discussed above. Thus, the neutralization activity in anti-VP4/VP3 appears to be monospecific. We have synthesized peptide 8, shown in Figure 1, that corresponds to a hydrophilic hypervariable sequence in VP3. We have found that this peptide reacts specifically with the anti-VP4/VP3 serum in an ELISA (unpubl.). These data confirm our previous claim (Emini et al. 1983c) that VP3 is a carrier of at least one poliovirus N-Ag. Other biological properties of peptide 8, such as the induction of neutralizing antibodies in rabbits, are currently being tested.

Similarly, we have selected by criteria outlined above a hydrophilic sequence within VP2 and have synthesized a peptide corresponding to this sequence (Fig. 1, peptide 9). This peptide elicited neutralizing antibodies in rabbits and was capable of priming a neutralizing immune response (see below), two observations that identify VP2 as a carrier of a poliovirus N-Ag.

van Wezel et al. (1983) have found that all three large capsid proteins of poliovirus can elicit a weak neutralizing immune response provided the capsid proteins were isolated from formalin-inactivated virus. These authors speculate that the formalin treatment stabilized the N-Ags prior to disruption of the virus. If, on the other hand, the capsid polypeptides were isolated by high-performance liquid chromatography of acid-disrupted virus, there would appear to be no requirement for the chemical stabilization of the N-Ags, since all three large capsid polypeptides yielded a weak neutralizing immune response (Dernick et al. 1983). These data agree with our identification of an N-Ag each on VP2 and VP3.

Peptide Induction of Neutralizing Antibody

Of all peptides tested so far in our laboratory, only peptide 3 (Emini et al. 1983a; Wimmer et al. 1983) and peptide 9 (E.A. Emini et al., unpubl.) (Fig. 1) have induced a significant level of neutralizing antibodies in rabbits (Table 2). Although the neutralizing titers are low (values similar to those obtained by others with

Table 2
Anti-type-1 Poliovirus Neutralizing Antibody Titers Obtained with
Conjugated Peptides 3 and 9

		Plaque titer reduction (log_{10} pfu/ml)	
Peptide	Rabbit	prior to virus inoculation	5 weeks after virus inoculation
3	A	0.9	n.d.[a]
	B	1.2	>8.0
	C	2.1	>8.0
	D	0.5	>8.0
9	A	1.0	3.0[b]
	B	0.9	4.0
	C[c]	<0.5	<0.5
	D	0.8	4.1

[a]n.d. indicates not done.
[b]This value was taken 1 week after the virus inoculation.
[c]Rabbit C never produced an antipeptide antibody response.

purified capsid polypeptides), they confirm that the peptide sequences correspond to those of N-Ags of the poliovirion. At present, it is impossible to explain
why the antibodies elicited in response to injection with peptides 1, 2, 4, and 5
do not neutralize poliovirus. Presumably, the peptides fold preferentially into configurations that differ from the configurations into which the exact same sequence is preferentially found in the icosahedron of the virion. Induction of weak
neutralizing antibodies in rats with peptides corresponding to selected regions of
VP1 of PV-1 has also been observed by M. Chow and D. Baltimore (pers. comm.).

Peptide Priming of the Immune Response

The failure of peptides 1, 2, 4, and 5 to elicit a neutralizing antibody response
does not mean that an immunological memory to them would not be activated if
the immune system were to be presented with a small amount of poliovirus. We
tested this hypothesis as follows. Rabbits were inoculated once or three times
with the carrier-linked peptide followed by an inoculation of a small amount
(10^5 pfu) of poliovirus (for details, see Emini et al. 1983a). We found that peptides
1–5 (Emini et al. 1983a) and also peptide 9 (unpubl.) are capable of priming a
neutralizing immune response, the immune sera having a high neutralizing titer
(Emini et al. 1983a; Wimmer et al. 1983). For brevity, we discuss here only the
data for peptide 1 (see Fig. 2).

The nine columns in Figure 2 describe different experiments in which sera
from rabbits that had gone through immunization schedules were tested for neutralization. The rabbits were inoculated three times with peptide 1, except in experiments 2 (a single inoculation), 6 (inoculation was with a control peptide unrelated to poliovirus), and 5 and 7 (no inoculation with peptide). One week after
the last inoculation with peptides, the rabbits were challenged with a single dose
of 10^5 pfu poliovirus (for type see Fig. 2, bottom line). Sera were collected 1, 5,
or 9 weeks after virus inoculation. All sera were tested for their ability to immu-

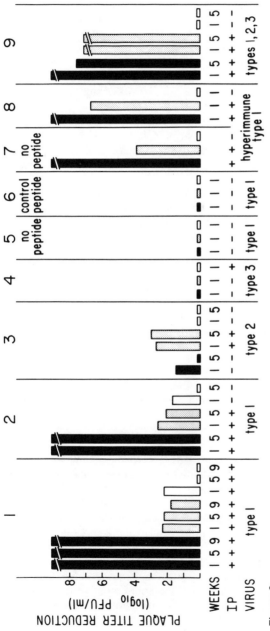

Figure 2

Priming of an anti-poliovirus immune response with peptide 1 (Fig. 1). Rabbits were inoculated (see below) with BSA-conjugated peptide (1 mg/inoculation), followed by a single challenge with 10^5 pfu of poliovirus of either type 1, type 2, or type 3 (VIRUS). One, five, or nine weeks later (WEEKS), immune sera were assayed for their ability to neutralize PV-1(closed bars), PV-2 (shaded bars), or PV-3 (open bars), respectively, or tested whether they can immunoprecipitate the serotypes (IP). (1) Three inoculations with peptide, challenged with PV-1; (2) one inoculation with the peptide, challenged with PV-1; (3,4) three inoculations with the peptide, challenged with PV-2 and PV-3, respectively; (5) no inoculation of peptide, single inoculation with PV-1; (6) single inoculation with a peptide unrelated to poliovirus, challenged with PV-1; (7) no inoculation with peptide, but three inoculations with 50 μg each of PV-1; (8) three inoculations of 50 μg each of PV-1, followed by a single inoculation with peptide; (9) same as 1, but challenged with all three types of polioviruses. For details, see Emini et al. (1983a).

71

noprecipitate the three types of polioviruses (Fig. 2, IP); this also served to determine whether the immune response was of the IgG type (for details, see Emini et al. 1983a). As can be seen, a lasting IgG response of more than 8.5 $\log_{10}$ plaque-titer reduction was observed after three inoculations (column 1) or after a single inoculation (column 2) with peptide 1. The extent of plaque reduction is the same as that obtained with hyperimmune sera (column 7).

The priming of a neutralizing immune response with peptide 1 is specific for PV-1, although some cross-reactivity was observed toward poliovirus type 2 (PV-2). Of interest is column 4, which shows that upon challenge with PV-3, antibodies specific for PV-3 were produced (IP +), but these antibodies did not neutralize PV-3. Thus, the priming with peptide 1, whose sequence is shared by both PV-1 and PV-3, yields antibodies specific for the configuration of epitopes of the challenging virus.

Very similar data were obtained with peptides 2–5 (Emini et al. 1983a). The priming with peptide 5 identified a new N-Ag. Moreover, peptide 9, which is specific for sequences of capsid polypeptide VP2, primed the immune response, although the final plaque reduction titer was only 4 $\log_{10}$ pfu/ml (E. Emini et al. unpubl.).

The phenomenon of priming has also been observed with the three larger capsid polypeptides VP1, VP2, and VP3 (van Wezel et al. 1983). Although the titers obtained were lower than those described here with peptides, some of the sera were found to interact with heterotypic virus.

Mechanism of Neutralization

The advent of N-mAbs that interact with specific surface structures of the poliovirion has led to new experiments aimed at the mechanism(s) by which neutralization of poliovirus occurs. We summarize here only the most recent results: (1) The binding of many different N-mAbs directed against N-Eps of VP1 all change the isoelectric point (pI) of the virus from approximately 7.0 to approximately 4.0 (Emini et al. 1983b,d), a phenomenon observed first by Mandel (1971), who used hyperimmune serum. Binding of nonneutralizing monoclonal antibodies to poliovirus does not change the pI, an observation that appeared to support a mechanism of neutralization that involves an apparent structural change of the virion. A change of the pI, however, does not occur upon neutralization with anti-VP4/VP3 (Emini et al. 1983b,c,d). (2) In a study with a single N-mAb, it was found that neutralization required a minimum of four antibody molecules per virion (Icenogle et al. 1983). It remains to be seen whether this ratio will be found for other N-mAbs also. (3) Under nonsaturating conditions, neutralization requires bivalent attachment of the antibody molecules (Emini et al. 1983b; Icenogle et al. 1983). Again, the neutralizing anti-VP4/VP3 antibodies do not appear to follow this requirement (Emini et al. 1983b).

These data suggest that the changes imposed upon a virion by antibody binding may differ from antigenic site to antigenic site. It remains to be seen whether neutralization follows a single multistep pathway or whether different mechanisms can interfere with the early steps in viral proliferation, adsorption, penetration, and uncoating.

CONCLUSION

We have identified by two different methods five different independent antigenic sites at the surface of the intact poliovirion (type 1, Mahoney) that are involved in neutralization: Three N-Ags are associated with VP1, one N-Ag with VP2, and one N-Ag with VP3. In the case of two of the N-Ags of VP1, we have found that each of these N-Ags harbors multiple N-Eps, since we isolated multiple genetic variants resistant to the corresponding N-mAbs. We consider it likely that the other three N-Ags consist of clusters of N-Eps, although this must await confirmation with additional N-mAbs.

Our results establish that the poliovirion contains multiple N-Ags. Any N-Ag can be expected to be more "immunopotent" than others, and the potency of an N-Ag may differ from one type of poliovirus to another. Our strategy for identifying N-Ags was based on peptides specifically selected according to hydrophilic regions of the large capsid proteins of poliovirus. Those peptides with a chain length of 6–12 amino acids were probed for their binding with N-mAb; they were used as antigens to elicit neutralizing antibodies directly; and, finally, they were used to prime a neutralizing immune response. Clearly, more work must be carried out before the proper size or the "perfect" sequence of a peptide for maximal biological activity can be established.

Priming with synthetic peptides could be used to activate an immune response directed against N-Ags that are less immunogenic than others. This may be of great advantage in viral or bacterial systems where the immunopotent N-Ags undergo rapid genetic changes leading to antigenic drifts or shifts. In any case, as has been discussed elsewhere (Emini et al. 1983a), synthetic peptides, even though their ability to elicit neutralizing antibodies may be weak or absent, may be potent components of new vaccination programs against infectious disease.

ACKNOWLEDGMENTS

We thank Akio Nomoto for making available to us the sequences of the Sabin strains of PV-1, PV-2, and PV-3 prior to publication; Bruce Erickson and Bruce Merrifield for instructing us in peptide synthesis; and Jean Leibowitz for the synthesis of peptide 9. This work was supported by U.S. Public Health Service grants AI-15122 and CA-28146. E.A.E. was recipient of a U.S. Public Health Service postdoctoral fellowship (AI-06485).

REFERENCES

Blondel, B., R. Crainic, and F. Horodniceanu. 1982. Le polypeptide structural VP1 du poliovirus type 1 induit des anticorps neutralisants. *C. R. Acad. Sci.* **294:** 91.

Chow, M. and D. Baltimore. 1982. Isolated poliovirus capsid protein VP1 induces a neutralizing response in rats. *Proc. Natl. Acad. Sci.* **79:** 7518.

Dernick, R., J. Heukeshoven, and M. Higbrig. 1983. Induction of neutralizing antibodies by all three structural poliovirus polypeptides. *Virology* **130:** 243.

Dorner, A.J., L.F. Dorner, G.R. Larsen, E. Wimmer, and C.W. Anderson. 1982. Identification of the initiation site for translation of poliovirus polyprotein synthesis. *J. Virol.* **42:** 1017.

Emini, E.A., M. Elzinga, and E. Wimmer. 1982a. Carboxy-terminal analysis of poliovirus proteins: The termination of poliovirus RNA translation and the location of unique poliovirus polyprotein cleavage sites. *J. Virol.* **42**: 194.

Emini, E.A., B.A. Jameson, and E. Wimmer. 1983a. Priming for and induction of anti-poliovirus neutralizing antibodies by synthetic peptides. *Nature* **304**: 699.

Emini, E.A., P. Ostapchuk, and E. Wimmer. 1983b. Bivalent attachment of antibody onto poliovirus leads to conformational alteration and neutralization. *J. Virol.* **48**: 547.

Emini, E.A., A.J. Dorner, L.F. Dorner, B.A. Jameson, and E. Wimmer. 1983c. Identification of a poliovirus neutralization epitope through use of neutralizing antiserum raised against a purified viral structural protein. *Virology* **124**: 144.

Emini, E.A., B.A. Jameson, A.J. Lewis, G.R. Larsen, and E. Wimmer. 1982b. Poliovirus neutralization epitopes: Analysis and localization with neutralizing monoclonal antibodies. *J. Virol.* **43**: 997.

Emini, E.A., S.-Y. Kao, A.J. Lewis, R. Crainic, and E. Wimmer. 1983d. Functional basis of poliovirus neutralization determined with monospecific neutralizing antibodies. *J. Virol.* **46**: 466.

Erickson, B.W. and R.B. Merrifield. 1976. In *The proteins* (ed. H. Neurath and R.L. Hill), p. 255. Academic Press, New York.

Hopp, T.P. and K.R. Woods. 1981. Prediction of protein antigenic determinants from amino acid sequences. *Proc. Natl. Acad. Sci.* **78**: 3824.

Icenogle, J., H. Shiwen, G. Duke, S. Gilbert, R. Rueckert, and J. Anderegg. 1983. Neutralization of poliovirus by a monoclonal antibody: Kinetics and stoichiometry. *Virology* **127**: 412.

Kitamura, N., B.L. Semler, P.G. Rothberg, G.R. Larsen, C.J. Adler, A.J. Dorner, E.A. Emini, R. Hanecak, J.J. Lee, S. van der Werf, C.W. Anderson, and E. Wimmer. 1981. Primary structure, gene organization, and polypeptide expression of poliovirus RNA. *Nature* **291**: 547.

Larsen, G.R., C.W. Anderson, A.J. Dorner, B.L. Semler, and E. Wimmer. 1982. Cleavage sites within the poliovirus capsid protein precursors. *J. Virol.* **41**: 340.

Lee, Y.F. and E. Wimmer. 1976. "Fingerprinting" high molecular weight RNA by two-dimensional gel electrophoresis: Application to poliovirus RNA. *Nucleic Acids Res.* **3**: 1647.

Lerner, R.A. 1982. Tapping the immunological repertoire to produce antibodies of predetermined specificity. *Nature* **299**: 592.

Mandel, B. 1971. Characterization of type 1 poliovirus by electrophoretic analysis. *Virology* **44**: 554.

―――. 1979. Interaction of viruses with neutralizing antibodies. In *Comprehensive virology* (ed. H. Fraenkel-Conrat and R.R. Wagner), vol. 15, p. 37. Plenum Press, New York.

Minor, P.D., G.C. Schild, J. Bootman, D.M.A. Evans, M. Ferguson, P. Reeve, and M. Spitz. 1983. Location and priming structure of the antigenic site for poliovirus neutralization. *Nature* **301**: 674.

Nomoto, A., T. Omata, H. Toyoda, S. Kuge, H. Horie, Y. Kataoka, Y. Genba, Y. Nakano, and N. Imura. 1982. Complete nucleotide sequence of the attenuated poliovirus Sabin 1 strain genome. *Proc. Natl. Acad. Sci.* **79**: 5793.

Racaniello, V.R. and D. Baltimore. 1981. Molecular cloning of poliovirus cDNA and determination of the complete nucleotide sequence of the viral genome. *Proc. Natl. Acad. Sci.* **78**: 4887.

Semler, B.L., R. Hanecak, C.W. Anderson, and E. Wimmer. 1981a. Cleavage sites in the polypeptide precursors of poliovirus protein P2-X. *Virology* **114**: 589.

Semler, B.L., C.W. Anderson, R. Hanecak, L.F. Dorner, and E. Wimmer. 1982. A membrane-associated precursor to poliovirus VPg identified by immunoprecipitation with antibodies directed against a synthetic heptapeptide. *Cell* **28**: 405.

Semler, B.L., C.W. Anderson, N. Kitamura, P.G. Rothberg, W.L. Wishart, and E. Wimmer. 1981b. Poliovirus replication proteins: RNA sequence encoding P3-1b and the sites of proteolytic processing. *Proc. Natl. Acad. Sci.* **78**: 3464.

Toyoda, H., K. Michinori, Y. Kataoka, T. Suganama, T. Omata, N. Imura, and A. Nomoto. 1984. Complete nucleotide sequence of all three poliovirus serotype genomes: Implications for genetic relationship, gene function, and antigenic determinants. *J. Mol. Biol.* (in press).

van Wezel, A.L., P. van der Marel, T.G. Hazendonk, V. Boer-Bak, and M.A.C. Henneke. 1983. Antigenicity and immunogenicity of poliovirus capsid proteins. *Dev. Biol. Stand.* (in press).

Walter, G. and R.F. Doolittle. 1983. Antibodies against synthetic peptides. In *Genetic engineering* (ed. J.K. Setlow and A. Hollaender), vol. 5, p. 61. Plenum Press, New York.

Wimmer, E., E.A. Emini, and B.A. Jameson. 1983. Peptide priming of an anti-poliovirus neutralizing antibody response. *Rev. Infect. Dis.* (in press).

Molecular Basis of Antivirus Serotype Specificity

**Thomas M. Shinnick, J. Gregor Sutcliffe,
Nicola Green, James L. Bittle,
Hannah Alexander, and Richard A. Lerner**
*Department of Molecular Biology
Research Institute of Scripps Clinic
La Jolla, California 92037*

John L. Gerin
*Division of Molecular Virology and Immunology
Georgetown University Medical Center
Rockville, Maryland 20852*

David J. Rowlands and Fred Brown
*Biochemistry Department, Animal Virus
Research Institute, Pirbright, Surrey, England*

Vaccination to prevent virus infection has been practiced for over 200 years, yet the process has changed relatively little since the time of Jenner. The immunogen of choice is still a killed or attenuated virus, although attention has recently turned toward designing and producing subunit vaccines consisting of nonviable and noninfectious portions of the pathogenic agent that are capable of eliciting a protective immune response. The use of subunit vaccines is attractive in part because it enables us to circumvent some of the concerns often associated with intact viral immunogens, such as incomplete inactivation or attenuation of the virus stock and possible biological contamination of the inoculum that may be introduced during large-scale growth of the virus. Subunit immunogens might be produced by purifying individual proteins from virions, by recombinant DNA technology, or by chemical synthesis. However, before we can rationally design a subunit vaccine, we need to learn more about the details of a protective immune response to virus infection. In particular, what are the essential characteristics of the components (or subunits) of the virus that elicit the neutralizing antibodies, and how can one produce a subunit vaccine that immunologically mimics such a key component? We have chosen to study this by analyzing the precise chemical nature of synthetic oligopeptides that can mimic known seroepidemiological markers, the thought being that if serotypic markers are a direct reflection of the specificity of neutralizing antibodies, then we should be able to learn how to mimic the viral immunogenic sites that elicit the protective antibodies.

The serotype of a virus is usually defined on the basis of the specificity of the antibody-virus reaction. In one procedure, serotypes are defined by the pattern of reactivity of the purified virus with known typing sera or by the pattern of reactivity of the antisera elicited by the new virus with known typing viruses, the typing reagents having been defined in a broad-range seroepidemiological study. In this manner, the hepatitis-B viruses (HBVs) have been classified into four serotypes (LeBouvier 1971; Gold et al. 1976; Peterson et al. 1977; Shih et al. 1978). Alternatively, viruses can be classified into serotypes on the basis of cross-neutralization behavior. A virus is assigned to a given serotype if antibodies elicited by it are capable of neutralizing known members of a serotype or if antibodies elicited by viruses of a particular serotype could cross-neutralize the new virus. In this way, for example, the strains of foot-and-mouth disease virus (FMDV) have been classified into seven serotypes, A, O, C, SAT1, SAT2, SAT3, and Asia 1 (Della-Porta 1983). Such serotyping is conceptually much like complementation grouping in genetics. The serotypes can often be divided into subtypes by quantitative analysis of the neutralizing activity, since antibodies often neutralize the homologous virus more efficiently than a heterologous virus of the same serotype. The A serotype of FMDV, for example, has been divided into about 30 subtypes in this manner (Della-Porta 1983).

Such antibody specificity must be caused by a variation in the immunogenic and antigenic determinants of the viruses. Furthermore, since for many viruses most of the neutralizing immune response is directed at one particular protein on the surface of the virus, the serotypic variation should be reflected in variation of the structure of this particular protein. The problem we address here is the precise chemical nature of the variation in protein sequence that leads to the serological differences. In particular, we review our studies on the chemical nature of the *d/y* serotype variation in HBV strains and serotypic variation in FMDV.

Hepatitis-B Virus

In the course of an immune response to infection by HBV, neutralizing antibodies are elicited that are primarily directed against the hepatitis-B surface antigen (HBsAg) (Peterson et al. 1977). The HBsAg protein carries the three serotypic markers that define the four possible serotypes of the HBVs (LeBouvier 1971; Gold et al. 1976; Peterson et al. 1977; Shih et al. 1978). Seroepidemiological studies have shown that the several strains of HBV have one serological marker in common, which is designated the *a* determinant, as well as two other serologically defined determinants. At one of the loci the strain displays either the *d* or *y* serotype, and at the other locus it has either the *w* or *r* serotype (LeBouvier 1971; Holland et al. 1972). Thus, the four serotypes are *ayw, ayr, adw,* and *adr.*

Since all three serotypic markers map to the HBsAg polypeptide, we compared the amino acid sequences of the HBsAg proteins from three strains of HBV in order to get an idea of which portions of this polypeptide might be responsible for the serotypic variation. (The amino acid sequences had been deduced from the published nucleotide sequences of the *S* genes of HBV [Galibert et al. 1979; Pasek et al. 1979; Valenzuela et al. 1979].) Most of the 19 positions that varied among the three strains were scattered throughout the 226-residue sequence, but six changes were clustered in a 21-residue region (amino acids 114–134), thereby suggesting that this region might be a candidate for encoding at least one of the serotypic determinants.

To identify or to prove which of these variable six residues are critical for the determination of serotype, one needs a set of proteins that vary at the different residues such that a comparison of reactivities would identify the key residues. If one were lucky, sequencing of additional virus strains might identify such a set. Two observations suggest an alternative approach in which the investigator can design and synthesize such a set of reagents. First, short synthetic oligopeptides can immunogenically mimic portions of a protein in that the peptides often elicit antibodies that react with the native, full-length protein. Second, oligopeptides can sometimes antigenically mimic portions of a protein in that, occasionally, antibodies elicited by native proteins can react with appropriate oligopeptides (for review, see Arnon 1980; Lerner 1982; Shinnick et al. 1983; Sutcliffe et al. 1983). Hence, we initiated a study of the chemical nature of the hepatitis-B serotypes by chemically synthesizing peptides corresponding to the above-identified variable region of the HBsAg.

Initially, we used as a blueprint the amino acid sequence of a surface antigen deduced from the nucleotide sequence of a virus displaying the *ayw* serotype and synthesized a peptide corresponding to residues 110–137, designated peptide 49 (Gerin et al. 1983). To determine whether the peptide carried one of the hepatitis-B serotypic determinants, the peptide was iodinated and then analyzed with antisera monospecific for the *a, d,* or *y* determinants. ^{125}I-labeled peptide 49 was immunoprecipitated by the antisera monospecific for the *a* and *y* determinants but not by the antiserum monospecific for the *d* determinant. These results suggest that the region encompassing residues 110–137 contains an *a* and a *y* determinant.

To investigate further the role of this region in the determination of serotype, we raised antibodies to peptide 49 and assayed for the ability of the antipeptide antibodies to react with purified ^{125}I-labeled HBsAg by immunoprecipitation. The anti-peptide-49 antibodies reacted with HBsAg of serotypes *ayw* and *adw* but showed a clear preference for the *ayw* serotypes (Alexander and Lerner 1983; Gerin et al. 1983). To quantitate the reaction, competitive immunoprecipitation experiments were done in which anti-peptide-49 antibodies were premixed with varying amounts of purified surface antigen of the *ayw* or *adw* serotype and then assayed for the ability to immunoprecipitate ^{125}I-labeled surface antigen of the *ayw* serotype. Whereas native HBsAg of serotype *ayw* completely inhibited the immunoprecipitation of ^{125}I-labeled HBsAg (*ayw*) by antibodies to peptide 49, native HBsAg of serotype *adw* was able to compete out only 15–20% of the reactivity, thus indicating that the predominant immune response to peptide 49 displays the *y* serotype specificity.

To define further the region involved in the *y* serotype specificity, we next synthesized a 13-amino-acid peptide (designated peptide 49a) corresponding to residues 125–137 of the HBsAg of the serotype *ayw* (Gerin et al. 1983). Antibodies elicited by this peptide react only with HBsAg carrying the *y*-serotype marker (Alexander and Lerner 1983; Gerin et al. 1983). In a competitive inhibition experiment, pretreatment of the anti-peptide-49a antibodies with the *ayw* surface antigen efficiently inhibited the immunoprecipitation of the labeled *ayw* surface antigen, whereas pretreatment with the *adw* surface antigen had little or no effect. This suggests that at least a portion of the *y* determinant and its alternative, the *d* determinant, lies within this 13-amino-acid sequence. Thus, one should be able to synthesize a peptide corresponding to the *d* determinant by using the predicted amino acid sequence of this region of a serotype *adw* surface antigen as a blueprint. The sequence we chose next (peptide 72a, residues 125–137 of serotype *adw*) differs from peptide 49a (residues 125–137 of serotype *ayw*) at only four positions (Alexander and Lerner 1983). Antibodies elicited by peptide 72a display strict *d* serotype specificity (Alexander and Lerner 1983). Therefore, we can conclude that the region between positions 125 and 137 plays an important role in the expression of the two mutually exclusive serotype determinants *d* and *y* and that at least a portion of the difference between the *d* and *y* serotypes is reflected in the four amino acid differences found in this region. Perhaps the *d/y* variation is brought about by fewer than four amino acid substitutions. We are now in the position where we can make a battery of peptides that differ at the various residues and analyze the role of each residue in determining the *d/y* serotypes. Recent evidence (Peterson et al. 1982) suggests that only two of these residues are crucial for the *d/y* serotype determinant, since an analysis of the amino acid sequence of protein fragments derived from *ayw* or *adw* surface antigen revealed that amino acid differences in the peptides at positions 131 and 134 were consistent with the serotype specificity of the donor protein. Clearly, very subtle changes in the amino acid sequence of a protein—a threonine for an asparagine at position 131 and a tyrosine for a phenylalanine at position 134 in the case of the *d/y* serotype—can have profound effects on the serology of the virus. We should note here that the studies with the antipeptide antibodies help define the crucial residues for determining the *d/y* serotype specificities in the region corresponding to amino acid residues 125–137. Possibly, other amino acid residues outside this region play a role in determining the *d/y* serotype of the entire surface antigen. In this regard, other investigators have reported a role for regions corresponding to residues 138–149 (Prince et al. 1982) and 4–121 (Mackay et al. 1982) in determining *d/y* serotype specificity. Further studies with chemically synthesized peptides should clarify any role of these regions in the *d/y* serotype specificity.

In toto, our studies with the HBsAg have revealed that only a small region of a protein may be involved in serotypic variation and that synthetic peptides can immunogenically mimic such a small region. Furthermore, if the *d/y* serotype variation in the immune response to HBV infection (defined on the basis of in vitro binding assays) is a consequence of a variation in the reactivities of neutralizing antibodies, then we have also identified a region of the HBsAg that interacts with the biologically important, neutralizing antibodies. If so, then we have produced synthetic peptide reagents that can immunologically mimic a key immunogenic site of the virus, i.e., a key site in eliciting neutralizing antibodies. One might expect that such synthetic peptides could form the basis of a chemically defined vaccine against HBV. Moreover, since there appear to be only two possible serotypes at this locus (*d* and *y*), a vaccine that provides protection against all of the known serotypes of HBV might be made by combining a synthetic peptide immunogen that elicits an anti-*y* response with one that elicits an anti-*d* response. Indeed, such a peptide mixture does elicit sera that react equally well with HBsAg isolated from either serotype. Unfortunately, no nonprimate host for HBV exists, so that a detailed investigation of the molecular basis of serotypic variation with respect to virus neutralization would be quite difficult. Therefore, to look directly at virus neutralization, we have studied serotypic variation in FMDV, since the serotypes of this virus are defined on the basis of neutralization assays and hence serotypic variation is a direct reflection of variation in the neutralizing immune response.

Foot-and-Mouth Disease Virus

FMDV occurs naturally as seven distinct serotypes that are defined on the basis of cross-neutralization behavior. The neutralizing immune response to FMDV infection appears to be primarily directed against VP1 (one of the four capsid proteins of this picornavirus) in part because treatment of this virus with trypsin cleaves only VP1 yet abolishes the protective immunogenicity of the viral particle (Wild et al. 1969; Kaaden et al. 1977; Meloen et al. 1979). Thus, this protein should carry the serotypic determinants. Furthermore, two lines of evidence suggested that the key immunogenic regions of the VP1 polypeptide involve approximately amino acid residues 130–160 and 190–213. First, an analysis of the immunogenicity of protein fragments derived from VP1 by chemical or enzymatic cleavage showed that fragments containing residues from regions 145–154 and 200–213 elicited neutralizing antibodies (Strohmaier et al. 1982). Second, a comparison of several VP1 amino acid sequences revealed that sequence variation among the VP1s from viruses of different serotypes clustered in the regions of residues 130–160 and 190–213 (Kleid et al. 1981; Kurz et al. 1981; Bittle et al. 1982; Boothroyd et al. 1982). Therefore, we chose to synthesize peptides corresponding to these presumptive immunogenic regions and used as a blueprint the amino acid sequence of VP1 of the serotype O, subtype 1, strain Kaufbeuren FMDV.

Antisera elicited by peptides corresponding to residues 141–160 and 200–213 were capable of neutralizing the Kaufbeuren strain of FMDV (Bittle et al. 1982). However, the neutralizing activity of the antisera elicited by residues 141–160 was much greater than that of the antisera to residues 200–213. The serotype specificity of the antibodies elicited by these peptides was determined in a bioassay using the homologous virus and heterologous viruses of serotypes A and C. As expected, the antisera elicited by either peptide efficiently neutralized the O serotype strain but displayed little or no cross-neutralization of the A and C strains. Similarly, antisera elicited by peptides corresponding to residues 141–160 of the VP1 sequence of a virus of the A serotype and one of the C serotype displayed the appropriate serotype-specific neutralization behavior in that the antisera could efficiently neutralize only the virus from which the sequence of the peptide immunogen had been derived (F. Brown et al. unpubl.). Overall, these results indicate that the serotype specificity of the antisera elicited by the peptide immunogens mimics that found with antisera elicited by whole virus, thereby suggesting that at least a portion of the A, O, and C serotype differences is due to amino-acid-sequence variation in these regions.

The FMDV serotypes have been divided into many subtypes based on the quantitation of the neutralizing activity. These subtype differences also appear to be located within residues 141–160 of VP1. In this region, the amino acid sequence of the serotype A, subtype 10, strain A61, differs by 10 of the 20 residues from the sequence of the serotype A, subtype 12, strain 119, and cross-neutralization by antivirion sera is 10^3- to 10^4-fold less efficient than neutralization of the homologous virus (Kleid et al. 1981; Boothroyd et al. 1982; Rowlands et al. 1983). As expected, a peptide corresponding to the subtype-10 sequence elicited antibodies that efficiently neutralized the subtype-10 virus but not the subtype-12 virus. Conversely, antibodies to a peptide corresponding to the subtype-12 sequence could efficiently neutralize the subtype-12 virus but not the subtype-10 virus. However, both antipeptide sera could very weakly cross-neutralize the other subtype. Possibly, this reactivity is due to the limited sequence homology between the two strains. Nonetheless, the antipeptide sera do mimic the subtype specificity of antivirus sera and this suggests that at least a portion of the key immunogenic determinants for subtype specificity must lie within residues 141–160 of VP1.

We have not yet investigated the key amino acid differences between the serotypes or subtypes because of the large number of residues in the region of 141–160 that vary among the strains. We have, however, been able to identify key residues that are involved in strain-specific neutralization behavior (Rowlands et al. 1983). (These studies are presented in detail elsewhere in this volume [Rowlands et al.] and are only summarized here.) It appears that variation at residues 148 and 153 of the VP1 amino acid sequence is responsible for certain observed differences in strain neutralization; i.e., one strain of serotype A subtype 12 differs from another strain of serotype A subtype 12 only at positions 148 and 153, yet antivirion sera can easily distinguish between the two strains (Rowlands et al. 1983). An antiserum to a peptide corresponding to the sequence of residues 141–160 of one of the strains displays a neutralization titer against the homologous virus roughly 100–1000-fold higher than that against the heterologous strain. Moreover, a third strain that differs by only one of the two residues is neutralized about 10–30-fold less well than the homologous virus. Similar analyses with a series of peptides that vary at one or both positions have revealed that both residues are important in the strain-specific neutralization by antipeptide sera. A change at either position appears to reduce the neutralization titer by about 10-fold, and changes at both positions lead to roughly 100-fold less neutralization. Once again, the peptides can mimic the serotypic differences between virus strains, and the results suggest that rather subtle changes in the amino acid sequence of a protein can have profound effects on its immunogenicity and antigenicity and on the ability of a virus to escape a neutralizing immune response.

Immune Response to Serological Determinants

It seems reasonable to expect that two amino acid changes in a short oligopeptide should have a profound effect on the specificity of the elicited antibodies, but why should a rather subtle change in a large protein (e.g., 2 out of 213 amino acids for the VP1 of subtype-12 strains) dramatically alter antibody binding in such a way that might allow the entire virus to escape a neutralizing immune response? Clues to understanding this may come from a consideration of the nature of the immunogenic sites that can elicit neutralizing antibodies. Not all portions of a protein are equally immunogenic in that proteins display immunologically dominant, recessive, and silent regions. One might expect that in order to get a strong neutralizing immune response, the sites that elicit neutralizing antibodies should correspond to or overlap an immunodominant region. If so, then sites that elicit neutralizing antibodies may be relatively rare on proteins, since immunodominant regions appear to be relatively rare. For example, more than 95% of the antibodies elicited by the globular protein myoglobin bind to five discrete regions of the protein that comprise less than 25% of the protein sequence. Immunodominant sites that elicit virus-neutralizing antibodies may be less frequent than the immunodominant sites of a soluble protein such as myoglobin, since large portions of a viral surface protein are often inaccessible to serum antibodies or cell-surface receptors when that protein is part of a virion. Furthermore, although antibody binding to the virus surface appears to be required for neutralization, it is not sufficient. Rather, neutralizing antibodies affect a domain of the protein that is functionally or structurally important in virus infection. For example, neutralizing antibodies might sterically block infection by binding to the viral protein that binds to the cell receptor. Such functional regions appear to be a subset of the protein's immunogenic sites, since only a fraction of a battery of monoclonal antibodies elicited by the surface glycoprotein of a murine retrovirus was capable of neutralizing the virus (H.L. Niman and J. Gautsch, unpubl.), perhaps suggesting that only a portion of the surface-accessible immunodominant sites might elicit antibodies capable of neutralizing virus. In toto, these considerations and observations suggest that the sites capable of eliciting neutralizing antibodies may be relatively rare, small, and functionally or structurally important regions of a protein exposed on the surface of the virus. Perhaps, as suggested by our results, only one or two sites are important in eliciting neutralizing antibodies. If so, then it would not be surprising that only a few amino acids need to be changed in order to alter serotype specificity.

In FMDV, two amino acid substitutions in the region of residues 141–160 of VP1 are sufficient to reduce neutralization titer by about three orders of magnitude. How might these substitutions alter the secondary or tertiary structure of this region in such a way as to dramatically reduce antibody binding? On the basis of a computer model of protein folding, Pfaff et al. (1982) have suggested that residues 144–159 of the VP1 of serotype O subtype-1 virus form an *a*-helical segment that is exposed on the surface of the protein. Rowlands et al. (1983) have similarly predicted the structure of the two VP1s that display amino acid differences at residues 148 and 153 and whose cross-neutralization titers are about 1/1000 the neutralization titer against the homologous virus. Both viruses are predicted to form *a*-helices in the region of 141–160 of VP1, but of different lengths. For the VP1 of the serotype A, subtype 12, strain 119-A, residues 150–159 are predicted to form an *a*-helix (about one helical turn shorter than the corresponding region of the serotype-O VP1), whereas only residues 154–159 of the VP1 of the serotype A, subtype 12, strain 119-USA are predicted to form an *a*-helix due to the presence of a helix-disrupting proline at residue 153. Perhaps it is this rather major variation in secondary structure that is at least partly responsible for the dramatic differences in neutralization titers between these strains and possibly even between serotypes.

Local secondary structure could also be dramatically altered by other changes in sequence. For example, the substitution of a polar residue for a hydrophobic residue may lead to the exposure of previously buried residues. This appears to be the case when the phenylalanine at position 148 of strain 119-USA is replaced with a serine in strain 119-A (Rowlands et al. 1983). Additional serotype specificity might be related to the exact amino acid sequence of this region. For example, the substitution of a charged residue such as lysine for a polar residue such as threonine could greatly alter antibody affinity. Other minor changes such as a leucine for a phenylalanine may also account for a portion of the strain specificity of neutralization.

Overall, the considerations presented here suggest that virus neutralization may be mediated by antibody binding to one or a few key portions of a viral surface protein. Such regions have in common the ability to elicit antibodies, to react with antibodies in solution when present in intact virus, and to block a required step in virus infection when bound by antibody. The serotype specificity of virus neutralization is reflected in the amino acid sequence of the key neutralizing sites. Therefore, alterations in the amino acid sequence of a key neutralizing site (which may appear quite minor when the protein sequence is viewed as a whole) could dramatically affect antibody binding to the site and hence alter serotype specificity. The key then to designing synthetic vaccines may lie in identifying these sites. As we learn more about these sites and how they vary between serotypes or subtypes, we may be able to design a synthetic vaccine that incorporates the important structural features of such sites from more than one serotype and thereby generate a vaccine that may provide broad-range protection.

ACKNOWLEDGMENTS

Portions of this work were supported by grants from the American Cancer Society (NP-359), the National Institutes of Health (1P01-CA-27489), and Johnson & Johnson Industries. This is Publication No. 3275-MB from the Research Institute of Scripps Clinic.

REFERENCES

Alexander, H. and R.A. Lerner. 1983. Chemically synthesized peptide analogs of the hepatitis B surface antigen. In *Advances in hepatitis research* (ed. F. Chisari). (In press.)

Arnon, R. 1980. Chemically defined antiviral vaccines. *Annu. Rev. Microbiol.* **34:** 593.

Bittle, J.L., R.A. Houghten, H. Alexander, T.M. Shinnick, J.G. Sutcliffe, R.A. Lerner, D.J. Rowlands, and F. Brown. 1982. Protection against foot-and-mouth disease by immunization with a chemically synthesized peptide predicted from the viral nucleotide sequence. *Nature* **298:** 30.

Boothroyd, J.C., T.J.R. Harris, D.J. Rowlands, and P.A. Lowe. 1982. The nucleotide sequence of cDNA coding for the structural proteins of foot-and-mouth disease virus. *Gene* **17:** 153.

Della-Porta, A.J. 1983. Serotype variation in foot-and-mouth disease virus. *Aust. Vet. J.* **60:** 129.

Galibert, F., E. Mandart, F. Fitoussi, P. Tiollais, and P. Charney. 1979. Nucleotide sequence of the hepatitis B virus genome (subtype ayw) cloned in *E. coli. Nature* **281:** 646.

Gerin, J.L., H. Alexander, J.W.-K. Shih, R.H. Purcell, G. Dapolito, R. Engle, N. Green, J.G. Sutcliffe, T.M. Shinnick, and R.A. Lerner. 1983. Chemically synthesized peptides of hepatitis B surface antigen duplicate the d/y specificities and induce subtype-specific antibodies in chimpanzees. *Proc. Natl. Acad. Sci.* **80:** 2365.

Gold, J.W.M., J.W.-K. Shih, R.H. Purcell, and J.L. Gerin. 1976. Characterization of antibodies to the structural polypeptides of HBsAg: Evidence for subtype-specific determinants. *J. Immunol.* **117:** 1404.

Holland, P.V., R.H. Purcell, H. Smith, and H.J. Alter. 1972. Subtyping of hepatitis-associated antigen (HBAg): Simplified technique with counter electrophoresis. *J. Immunol.* **109:** 420.

Kaaden, O.R., K.-H. Adam, and K. Strohmaier. 1977. Introduction of neutralizing antibodies and immunity in vaccinated guinea pigs by cyanogen bromide-peptides of VP of foot-and-mouth disease virus. *J. Gen. Virol.* **34:** 397.

Kleid, D.G., D. Yansura, B. Small, D. Dowbenko, D.M. Moore, M.J. Grubman, P.D. McKercher, D.O. Morgan, B.H. Robertson, and H.L. Bachrach. 1981. Cloned viral protein vaccine for foot-and-mouth disease: Response in cattle and swine. *Science* **214:** 1125.

Kurz, C., S. Forss, H. Kupper, K. Strohmaier, and H. Schaller. 1981. Nucleotide sequence and corresponding amino acid sequence of the gene for the major antigen of foot-and-mouth disease virus. *Nucleic Acids Res.* **9:** 1919.

LeBouvier, G.L. 1971. The heterogeneity of Australia antigen. *J. Infect. Dis.* **123:** 671.

Lerner, R.A. 1982. Tapping the immunological repertoire to produce antibodies of predetermined specificity. *Nature* **299:** 592.

Mackay, P., M. Pasek, M. Magzin, R.I. Kovacic, B. Allet, S. Stahl, W. Gilbert, H. Schaller, S.A. Bruce, and K. Murray. 1982. Production of immunologically active surface antigens of hepatitis B virus by *Escherichia coli. Proc. Natl. Acad. Sci.* **78:** 4510.

Meloen, R.H., D.J. Rowlands, and F. Brown. 1979. Comparison of the antibodies elicited by the individual structural polypeptides of foot-and-mouth disease and polio viruses. *J. Gen. Virol.* **45:** 761.

Pasek, M., T. Goto, W. Gilbert, B. Zink, H. Schaller, P. Mackay, G. Leadbetter, and K. Murray. 1979. Hepatitis B virus genes and their expression in *E. coli. Nature* **282:** 575.

Peterson, D.L., N. Nath, and S.F. Gavilanes. 1982. Structure of hepatitis B surface antigen. *J. Biol. Chem.* **257:** 10414.

Peterson, D.L., I.M. Roberts, and G.N. Vyas. 1977. Partial amino acid sequence of two major component polypeptides of hepatitis B surface antigen. *Proc. Natl. Acad. Sci.* **74:** 1530.

Pfaff, E., M. Massgay, H.O. Bohm, G.E. Schulz, and H. Schaller. 1982. Antibodies against a preselected peptide recognize and neutralize foot and mouth disease virus. *EMBO J.* **1:** 869.

Prince, A.M., H. Ikram, and T.P. Hopp. 1982. Hepatitis B virus vaccine: Identification of HBsAg/a and HBsAg/d but not HBsAg/y subtype antigenic determinants on a synthetic immunogenic peptide. *Proc. Natl. Acad. Sci.* **79:** 579.

Rowlands, D.J., B.E. Clarke, A.R. Carroll, F. Brown, B.H. Nicholson, J.L. Bittle, R.A. Houghten, and R.A. Lerner. 1983. The chemical basis for variation in the major antigenic site eliciting neutralizing antibodies in foot-and-mouth disease. *Nature* (in press).

Shih, J.W.-K., P.L. Tan, and J.L. Gerin. 1978. Antigenicity of the major polypeptides of hepatitis B surface antigen. *J. Immunol.* **120:** 520.

Shinnick, T.M., J.G. Sutcliffe, N. Green, and R.A. Lerner. 1983. Synthetic peptide immunogens as vaccines. *Annu. Rev. Microbiol.* **34:** 425.

Strohmaier, K., R. Franze, and J.-H. Adam. 1982. Location and characterization on the antigenic portion of the FMDV immunizing protein. *J. Gen. Virol.* **59:** 295.

Sutcliffe, J.G., T.M. Shinnick, N. Green, and R.A. Lerner. 1983. Antibodies that react with predetermined sites on proteins. *Science* **219:** 660.

Valenzuela, P., P. Gray, M. Quiroga, J. Zalvidar, H.M. Goodman, and W.J. Rutter. 1979. Nucleotide sequence of the gene coding for the major protein of hepatitis B surface antigen. *Nature* **280:** 815.

Wild, T.F., J.N. Burroughs, and F. Brown. 1969. Surface structure of foot-and-mouth disease virus. *J. Gen. Virol.* **4:** 313.

Synthetic Approaches to Vaccination against Cholera Toxin

**Michael Sela, Chaim O. Jacob,
and Ruth Arnon**
Department of Chemical Immunology, The Weizmann
Institute of Science, Rehovot, Israel

Our studies on synthetic polypeptide antigens led us many years ago (Arnon 1972) to suggest that synthetic vaccines might soon become a reality by making use of antigens containing unique synthetic determinants capable of provoking antibodies that neutralize efficiently a virus or a bacterial toxin. This hypothesis was strengthened by the evidence that antibodies produced against a synthetic peptide corresponding to the "loop" region of lysozyme reacted with a conformation-dependent region of the native protein. We later showed the synthetic approach to be successful for the RNA-containing coliphage MS2, where a totally synthetic antigen, composed of a synthetic peptide corresponding to sequence 89–108 of its coat protein and of the synthetic adjuvant N-acetylmuramyl-L-alanyl-D-isoglutamine (MDP), both attached covalently to multichain poly-DL-alanine, led to the production in rabbits of antibodies capable of neutralizing the virus (Arnon et al. 1980). Similarly, a successful synthetic approach in our laboratory to influenza hemagglutinin (see Arnon and Shapira, this volume) led to significant protection in mice.

The same approach may be used for bacterial toxins, and Audibert et al. (1981) have reported on a synthetic peptide analogous to a region of diphtheria toxin (188–201), which, after attachment to bovine serum albumin, led to the production in guinea pigs of antibodies capable of neutralizing the dermonecrotic activity of diphtheria toxin. This work was extended to additional peptides, and these were attached together with MDP to multichain poly-DL-alanine. The resulting totally synthetic immunogen, when administered in aqueous solution, provoked neutralizing antibodies in mice (Audibert et al. 1982).

We report here a synthetic approach to immunogens that provoke antibodies

87

cross-reactive with cholera toxin and that are capable of partially neutralizing its biological activity. The vaccines used in humans against cholera are prepared from killed bacteria and have a limited effectiveness. On the other hand, purified B subunit is a protecting antigen against experimental cholera in rabbits (Holmgren et al. 1977). The toxin of *Vibrio cholerae* is composed of two subunits, A and B. The A subunit activates adenylate cyclase, which triggers the biological activity, whereas the B subunit is responsible for binding to cell receptors and expresses most immunopotent determinants. Antibodies to the B subunit are capable of neutralizing the biological activity of the intact toxin. The B subunit (choleragenoid) is a pentamer, each of the chains containing 103 amino acid residues.

Synthetic Peptides of the B Subunit of Cholera Toxin

In view of its immunodominant role, the B subunit was the obvious candidate for our investigation (Fig. 1). To locate the regions relevant for antigenic determinants, the B subunit was cleaved by cyanogen bromide (CNBr) to yield three fragments with the following sequences: 1–37 and 69–101 (linked by a disulfide bridge between cysteines at positions 9 and 86), 38–68, and 102–103. The fragments were separated on a Sephadex G-50 column, and the two large peptides were tested for reactivity with antisera prepared against cholera toxin. The largest peptide was partially cross-reactive with anti-cholera-toxin sera, whereas peptide 38–68 did not bind directly to antisera but was capable of inhibiting binding of intact cholera toxin to homologous antisera. Considerations based on the results obtained with the CNBr fragments of the B subunit, as well as several previous studies on antigenically important regions of this protein, dictated the selection of peptides for chemical synthesis. In this context, a peptide surrounding the arginine at position 35, namely, residues 30–42 (CTP 2), was synthesized, since it was suggested, based on chemical modification experiments, that argi-


```
                                    10
Thr- Pro- Gln - Asn - Ile - Thr  - Asp - Leu - Cys - Ala - Glu - Tyr - His - Asn -
                                    20
Thr- Gln- Ile - His - Thr-Leu - Asn - Asn - Lys - Ile - Phe - Ser - Tyr - Thr -
       30                                             40
Glu- Ser - Leu - Ala - Gly - Lys - Arg - Glu - Met - Ala - Ile - Ile - Thr - Phe -
                                    50
Lys - Asn - Gly - Ala - Thr - Phe - Glu - Val - Glu - Val - Pro - Gly - Ser - Gln -
          60                                          70
His - Ile - Asp - Ser - Gln - Lys - Lys - Ala - Ile - Glu - Arg - Met - Lys - Asn -
                                    80
Thr - Leu - Arg - Ile - Ala - Tyr - Leu - Thr - Glu - Ala - Lys - Val - Glu - Lys -
                    90
Leu - Cys - Val - Trp - Asn - Asn - Lys - Thr - Pro - His - Ala - Ile - Ala - Ala -
   100      103
Ile - Ser - Met - Ala - Asn
```

Figure 1
Primary amino acid sequence of the B subunit of cholera toxin as quoted by Lai (1980). Regions of the protein chosen for synthesis are underlined.

nine 35 or the region surrounding it may be involved in antibody and receptor binding activity. Another peptide, residues 83–97 (CTP 6), consisting of the region surrounding tryptophan at position 88 was synthesized, since results based on chemical modification of this residue suggest that the tryptophan is near or in the binding site of the B subunit. Since it was claimed that the point of highest local average hydrophilicity is located in or immediately adjacent to an antigenic determinant, a peptide containing this area of the B subunit (residues 79–84) was chosen according to a statistical method of prediction. On the basis of the reported role of tyrosine residues for antigenicity, peptides containing tyrosine were included, namely, CTP 1 (residues 8–20) and CTP 5 (residues 75–85). Since the latter peptide contained only 11 residues, we prepared an additional peptide with a longer sequence (residues 69–85, CTP 4). Peptide 50–64 (CTP 3) is a part of the inhibitory CNBr fragment 38–68. The peptides were synthesized by solid-phase methodology, coupled to tetanus toxoid as carrier (Jacob et al. 1983) either via a water-soluble carbodiimide or via an azo bond, and injected into rabbits.

Immunological Cross-reactions

The conjugates of tetanus toxoid with all six peptides led to peptide-specific antibodies. To determine whether the antibodies raised against the various peptides could react with the B subunit and whole native cholera toxin, we assayed their ability to bind these proteins in solid-phase radioimmunoassay (Fig.2). The reactivity of the various antisera was further examined by immunoprecipitation, as well as by the immunoblotting technique, where the cholera toxin was separated into its subunits by SDS-polyacrylamide gel electrophoresis, transferred to nitrocellulose, and probed with antiserum. The reaction was visualized by autoradiography after binding ^{125}I-labeled goat anti-rabbit immunoglobulin. Both techniques showed similar results, which were in accord with those obtained by radioimmunoassay.

Taken together, these data indicate that four antisera out of the six that were raised against the appropriate peptides also reacted, to different extents, with the B subunit and the native cholera toxin, whereas two peptides, namely, CTP 2 and CTP 5, elicited antibodies with specificity limited to the respective peptides. The antisera against the peptides CTP 1 and CTP 6 showed a very high level of reactivity with the respective homologous peptides but reacted only slightly (several orders of magnitude difference) with the intact B subunit or cholera toxin. On the other hand, peptide CTP 3 induced antibodies that, although of lower absolute titer, gave a very strong cross-reactivity with the intact toxin, very similar in its level to that of the homologous peptide-antipeptide reaction. Furthermore, this peptide reacted also with antiserum against the native cholera toxin. The CTP 4 and CTP 5 peptides are of interest from another point of view: Antibodies to CTP 5 were incapable of cross-reacting with either the B subunit or whole toxin, although they showed an appreciable reactivity with the homologous peptide. Elongation of this peptide by six amino acid residues resulted in CTP 4, which elicited antibodies cross-reactive with the intact proteins, even though the homologous antipeptide titer was not significantly higher than in the case of CTP 5.

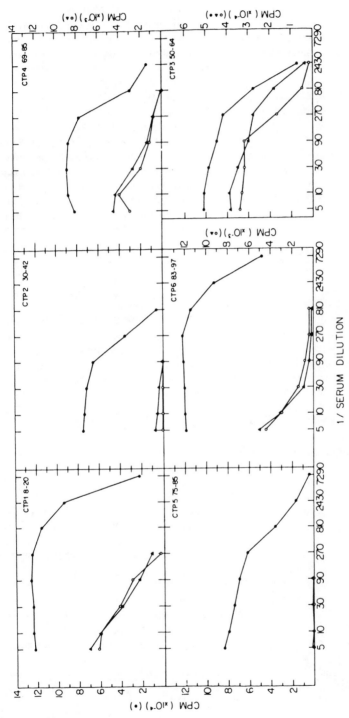

Figure 2

Antibody response of rabbits to different peptides of the B subunit of cholera toxin. Reactions were carried out with homologous peptides (●), the B subunit of cholera toxin (▲), and cholera toxin (○). Note the difference in the scales of the reactions with the peptide and the intact proteins in the case of all peptides except CTP 3.

90

Neutralization of Biological Activity

Antibodies to the various peptides were tested for their capacity to provide protection against the biological effects of cholera toxin. Antisera against CTP 3 were found effective, as demonstrated by two different assays.

One assay was a skin test in which the increased permeability in rabbit skin induced by cholera toxin is inhibited by antibodies (Lai 1980). We found that anti-CTP 3 at a 1:10 dilution was as effective as a 1:200 dilution of anti-cholera toxin in completely neutralizing 1 ng of the toxin. Under the same conditions, 0.5 ng of the toxin could be neutralized by a 20-fold dilution of anti-CTP 3.

In another in vivo assay, the antiserum against CTP 3 was capable of partially preventing the fluid accumulation induced by cholera toxin in ligated small intestinal loops of rabbits (Table 1). These results indicate that peptide CTP 3, which showed the strongest immunological cross-reaction with cholera toxin, has an appreciable ability to induce antibodies capable of neutralizing the biological activity of cholera toxin. Preliminary experiments indicate that the antiserum against CTP 3 is also capable of neutralizing the cholera-toxin-induced cAMP in an in vitro assay.

CONCLUSIONS

Antigenic determinants may be sequential or conformation-dependent. Even though the determinants of globular proteins belong in the great majority of cases

Table 1
Neutralization of Cholera Toxin by Antisera to Peptide CTP 3 (50–64)

Cholera toxin (μg)	Serum	Dilution	weight/cm loop (g)	reduced secretion (%)[a]
			Ligated ileal loop	
0.0	none (saline)		0.20	
1.5	none (saline)		1.30	
1.5	anti cholera toxin	1:20	0.45	
1.5	anti-CTP 3	1:2	1.02	40
1.5	normal rabbit serum	1:2	1.25	
3.0	none (saline)		1.36	
3.0	anti cholera toxin	1:20	0.51	
3.0	anti-CTP 3	1:2	1.08	33
5.0	none (saline)		1.42	
5.0	anti cholera toxin	1:20	0.58	
5.0	anti-CTP 3	1:2	1.32	12
7.5	none (saline)		1.42	
7.5	anti cholera toxin	1:20	0.60	
7.5	anti-CTP 3	1:2	1.32	12
10.0	none (saline)		1.50	
10.0	anti cholera toxin	1:20	0.69	
10.0	anti-CTP 3	1:2	1.50	0

[a]Assuming that the reduction effected by antiserum to cholera toxin is 100%.

to the second category, this does not mean that smaller peptides with sequences corresponding to various stretches of such globular proteins cannot give rise to antibodies capable of cross-reacting with the intact protein. This may be due to the fact that the peptide synthesized already possesses a three-dimensional structure similar to that characteristic of the same sequence within the protein or it may result from the ability of the particular protein segment of being transconformed upon reacting with the antibody against the peptide. The results discussed here show clearly that various peptides do not behave in a similar manner, some leading to antibodies cross-reacting strongly with the B subunit and the intact cholera toxin (CTP 3), others leading to a weaker cross-reaction (e.g., CTP 1), and still others being incapable of any cross-reaction (CTP 2 and CTP 5). It is of interest that antibodies to CTP 5 are not cross-reactive, whereas those to CTP 4 (in which an additional six residues were added to CTP 5) are definitely cross-reactive.

The results reported here suggest that the peptide with sequence 50–64 (CTP 3) may be a good candidate for the development of a synthetic vaccine against cholera, because it produced antibodies that not only cross-react immunologically very strongly with the cholera toxin, but also are capable of partially neutralizing the biological activity of the toxin, as tested by two independent methods. Finally, any realistic approach must necessarily include not only the ability to produce the right specific antigenic determinants, but also built-in adjuvanticity (e.g., our previous studies making use of MDP), as well as efforts to obtain a long-lasting immunity.

REFERENCES

Arnon, R. 1972. Synthetic vaccines—Dream or reality. In *Immunity of viral and rickettsial diseases* (ed. A. Kohn and A.M. Klinberg), p. 209. Plenum Press, New York.

Arnon, R., M. Sela, M. Parant, and L. Chedid. 1980. Antiviral response elicited by a completely synthetic antigen with built-in adjuvanticity. *Proc. Natl. Acad. Sci.* **77:** 6769.

Audibert, F., M. Jolivet, L. Chedid, R. Arnon, and M. Sela. 1982. Successful immunization with a totally synthetic diphtheria vaccine. *Proc. Natl. Acad. Sci.* **79:** 5042.

Audibert, F., M. Jolivet, L. Chedid, J.E. Alouf, P. Boquet, P. Rivaille, and O. Siffert. 1981. Active antitoxic immunization by a diphtheria toxin synthetic oligopeptide. *Nature* **289:** 593.

Holmgren, J., A.M. Svennerholm, I. Lonnroth, M. Fall-Persson, B. Markman, and H. Lundbeck. 1977. Development of improved cholera vaccine based on subunit toxoid. *Nature* **269:** 602.

Jacob, C.O., M. Sela, and R. Arnon. 1983. Antibodies against synthetic peptides of the B subunit of cholera toxin: Cross reaction and neutralization of the toxin. *Proc. Natl. Acad. Sci.* **80:** 7611.

Lai, C.Y. 1980. The chemistry and biology of cholera toxin. *CRC Crit. Rev. Biochem.* **9:** 171.

Chemical Basis for Variation in the Major Antigenic Site Eliciting Neutralizing Antibodies in Foot-and-Mouth Disease Virus

David J. Rowlands, Berwyn E. Clarke,
Anthony R. Carroll, and Fred Brown
Animal Virus Research Institute
Pirbright, Surrey, England

Bruce H. Nicholson
Biochemistry Department
The University
Reading, England

James L. Bittle, Richard A. Houghten,
and Richard A. Lerner
Research Institute of Scripps
Clinic, La Jolla, California 92037

Foot-and-mouth disease is probably the most important virus disease of farm animals. Control is by slaughter in those countries where the disease does not normally occur but by vaccination in endemic areas. The size of the problem can be measured by the fact that about 3×10^9 doses of vaccine are used each year.

Most of the vaccines are prepared by inactivating virus grown in tissue culture with formaldehyde or an imine. These vaccines, properly prepared and applied, are effective and have essentially allowed the eradication of the disease from western Europe. However, the disease is still widespread in many parts of Africa, Asia, and South America where efficient control is complicated by inherent deficiencies in the production and quality of currently available vaccines (Bittle et al., this volume) and by the extreme antigenic variability of the virus. The virus occurs as seven serotypes, many of which contain several subtypes that are sufficiently different to pose problems in the choice of vaccine strains. This variation, which complicates the control of the disease, has provided the opportunity to investigate the biochemical basis of antigenicity.

The observation that immunizing activity is associated only with VP1 of the four capsid proteins of the virus furnished the first step in these investigations (Wild et al. 1969). Cleavage of this protein in situ by proteolytic enzymes reduced the immunizing activity of the viral particles. It was subsequently shown that VP1 isolated from the viral particles had low but significant activity (Laporte et al. 1973).

Mapping of the viral genome established the position of VP1 on the RNA (Sangar et al. 1977), and this allowed the cDNA corresponding to the region of the RNA coding for the protein to be produced and expressed in *Escherichia coli* cells as part of a fusion protein. This expressed protein had the same low immunizing activity as VP1 isolated from viral particles (Kleid et al. 1981). The location of the antigenic site(s) on VP1 was predicted by Strohmaier and his colleagues (1982) from the activity of fragments of the protein obtained by chemical or enzymatic cleavage. By assigning the positions of the fragments on the amino acid sequence of VP1 derived from the corresponding nucleotide sequence (Kurz et al. 1981), these workers predicted that residues 146–154 and 201–213 of the 213-amino-acid chain would contain antigenic sites.

With additional information accruing from the sequence studies on viruses of different serotypes and subtypes, it became possible to compare the amino acid sequences of several VP1s. There was considerable sequence variation at residues 41–60 and 131–158 (Fig.1). From this, it was reasoned that these regions had been subjected to antibody pressure and were possible antigenic sites. However, the 41–60 region is largely hydrophobic, suggesting that it is unlikely to be on the surface of the viral particle. In contrast, the 131–158 region is largely hydrophilic and, moreover, is variable in length in the different viruses. Furthermore, preliminary experiments by Bittle and his colleagues (1982) showed that peptides corresponding to this region elicited neutralizing and protective antibodies. The present paper is an extension of these early observations.

DISCUSSION

Activity of Amino Acid Tracts in the 135–160 Region of VP1

It had been shown previously that a peptide corresponding to amino acids 141–160 elicited a level of neutralizing antibody in guinea pigs that protected the animals against experimental infection, whereas peptide 200–213, corresponding to the second predicted site, gave much lower levels of neutralizing antibody and did not afford protection. We have consequently concentrated our efforts on the region of VP1 containing amino acids from the variable hydrophilic region referred to above. The neutralizing antibody response of guinea pigs receiving a single injection and of rabbits given four injections of different tracts from this region is shown in Table 1. The results show that the 135–160 region contains an important immunogenic site. However, the precise location will require examination of synthetic peptides within this region. Our results so far indicate that the most important region lies within residues 141–155. Results with peptides from serotypes A and C confirm this observation (Bittle et al., this volume).

Mimicking of Subtype Specificity by Peptide 141–160

The problem of subtype specificity in foot-and-mouth disease is clearly demonstrated in a comparison of viruses belonging to subtypes 10 and 12 of serotype A. These viruses were chosen for this comparison because the derived se-

```
A-12 THR THR ALA THR GLY GLU SER ALA ASP PRO VAL THR THR THR VAL GLU ASN TYR GLY GLY
A-10         THR
0-1          SER ALA
C-3          THR                                                                  20

A-12 GLU THR GLN VAL GLN ARG ARG HIS HIS THR ASP VAL SER PHE ILE MET ASP ARG PHE VAL
A-10 ASP                                          GLY
0-1          ILE          GLN
C-3          ILE                        ALA          VAL LEU                       40

A-12 LYS ILE LYS SER LEU ASN PRO THR HIS VAL ILE ASP LEU MET GLN THR HIS GLN HIS GLY
A-10         ASN          SER                                            LYS
0-1  VAL THR PRO GLN      GLN ILE ASN ILE LEU              ILE PRO SER          THR
C-3  VAL HIS VAL SER GLY ASN GLN      THR LEU      VAL          VAL     LYS ASP SER  60

A-12 LEU VAL GLY ALA LEU LEU ARG ALA ALA THR TYR TYR PHE SER ASP LEU GLU ILE VAL VAL
A-10 ILE
0-1                                      SER                              ALA
C-3  ILE                                                                  ALA      80

A-12 ARG HIS ASP GLY ASN LEU THR TRP VAL PRO ASN GLY ALA PRO GLU ALA ALA LEU SER ASN
A-10
0-1  LYS     GLU     ASP                              LYS          ASP
C-3  THR     THR     LYS                          VAL SER          ASP            100

A-12 THR GLY ASN PRO THR ALA TYR ASN LYS ALA PRO PHE THR ARG LEU ALA LEU PRO TYR THR
A-10     SER
0-1      THR                                          LEU
C-3      ALA                      HIS         GLY     LEU                         120

A-12 ALA PRO HIS ARG VAL LEU ALA THR VAL TYR ASN GLY THR ASN LYS TYR SER ALA SER GLY
A-10                                          ASP                                  ASP
0-1                              GLU CYS ARG             ASN ARG ASN ALA
C-3              THR             THR                 THR ALA         THR         ALA 140

A-12 SER GLY  -  VAL ARG GLY ASP PHE GLY SER LEU ALA PRO ARG VAL ALA ARG GLN LEU PRO
A-10       -  ARG SER  -              LEU         ILE     ALA              THR
0-1  VAL PRO ASN LEU              LEU GLN VAL         GLN LYS         THR
C-3   -   -  ARG  -               LEU ALA HIS         ALA ALA HIS         HIS    160

A-12 ALA SER PHE ASN TYR GLY ALA ILE LYS ALA GLU THR ILE HIS GLU LEU LEU VAL ARG MET
A-10                              GLN     GLN ALA
0-1  THR                                 THR ARG VAL THR              TYR
C-3  THR         PHE     VAL              THR     THR                        180

A-12 LYS ARG ALA GLU LEU TYR CYS PRO ARG PRO LEU LEU ALA ILE GLU VAL SER SER GLN ASP
A-10                      LYS                              LYS     THR
0-1          THR                                      HIS PRO THR GLU  -  ALA
C-3                                      VAL         PRO VAL GLN PRO THR GLY  -    200

A-12 ARG HIS LYS GLN LYS ILE ILE ALA PRO GLY LYS GLN LEU  -
A-10     TYR                          ALA          LEU
0-1              VAL              VAL          THR LEU
C-3          PRO LEU              ALA          LEU
                    210
```

Figure 1
Comparative amino acid sequence of the VP1 protein of viruses of type A_{12} (Kleid et al. 1981), A_{10} (Boothroyd et al. 1982), O_1 (Kurz et al. 1981), and C_3 (Makoff et al. 1983). The sequence for the A_{12} VP1 is given in full, and only the amino acid residues of the other viruses that differ from this are shown. Alignment of the sequences results in the appearance of gaps, which are indicated by a dash.

quences of VP1 were available (Boothroyd et al. 1982; Kleid et al. 1981). The data in Table 2 show the neutralization of each virus by antisera produced by inoculation of either inactivated viral particles or peptides corresponding to the 141–160 sequences of each VP1. The results show that the difference between

Table 1

Neutralizing Antibody Response of Guinea Pigs and Rabbits to Injection of Peptides from Different Regions of VP1 of FMDV Serotype O_1

Antiserum to region	Log_{10} virus neutralized by 0.015 ml serum
1–41	
rabbit	nil
guinea pig	0.9
135–150	
rabbit	3.4
guinea pig	1.7
135–160	
rabbit	>6.3
guinea pig	2.9
141–155	
rabbit	3.7
guinea pig	2.9
141–160	
rabbit	6.0
guinea pig	2.7
136–144	
rabbit	2.1
guinea pig	1.7
146–155	
rabbit	1.3
guinea pig	0.7
200–213	
rabbit	3.7
guinea pig	1.1

Rabbits were immunized with peptide coupled via an added cysteine to keyhole limpet hemocyanin (KLH), inoculating 200 μg in complete Freund's adjuvant (1:2) subcutaneously in the footpad on day 0; 200 μg in incomplete Freund's adjuvant subcutaneously on day 14; and 200 μg with 4 mg of aluminum hydroxide intraperitoneally on days 21 and 50. The animals were bled on day 57. The guinea pigs were given one injection of 100 μg of the peptide, linked to KLH and adsorbed to aluminum hydroxide and bled 3 weeks later.

the subtypes is mimicked in the peptide sequences, thus indicating that the 141–160 region contains a major antigenic site of the virus.

Amino Acid Sequence of 130–160 of Different Serotypes

The importance of the 141–160 region of VP1 in eliciting neutralizing antibody prompted us to compare the sequences of this region from several serotypes in the virus. Three important features emerged from this comparison: (1) the highly variable nature of the region; (2) the presence of insertions and deletions, particularly between amino acids 140 and 145; and (3) differences in the helical content of this region between various viruses as deduced from the secondary structure predictions of Chou and Fasman (1978).

Table 2
Neutralizing Antibody Response of Guinea Pigs to Injection of
Inactivated Viral Particles and the 141–160 Region of VP1 of
the A_{10} and A_{12} Subtypes of FMDV

Antiserum	Log_{10} virus neutralized by 0.015 ml serum	
	A_{10}	A_{12}
A_{10} antivirus particle	2.5	0.9
A_{10} antipeptide	2.7	0.5
A_{12} antivirus particle	0.7	3.5
A_{12} antipeptide	0.5	2.5

Antivirus particle sera were 1:100 dilution. Antipeptide sera were
undiluted.

We have used another method to predict the side chains that are in contact
with the hydrophobic core of VP1 (Nicholson 1982). Examples of the use of this
method are shown in Figure 2, in which we depict models of the antigenic site of
viruses of the same and different serotypes. The models of two subtypes O_1 and
O_6 of serotype O show the effects of relatively small sequence changes. Thus, in
O_1, eight residues are in contact with the core of VP1, firmly embedding it in the
surface. Of the six polar residues on the hydrophilic side of the helix, four are
present as a prominent band. In O_6, there are three amino acid differences that
substitute the hydrophilic threonine and serine for three of the four core-predicted residues shown in the top half of O_1 (Fig. 2). The alteration in sequence is
such that the fourth, unaltered, residue is no longer predicted in core. The effect
of these changes is that the O_6 helix is higher on the protein surface and rotated
slightly. The band of four polar residues in O_1 is also present in O_6 and, in addition, extra, potentially antigenic, hydrophilic side chains are present on the surface.

Virus C_3, a member of a distinct serotype, but still belonging to the Eurasian
group of viruses (O, A, C, and Asia 1), has a different amino acid sequence but
nevertheless has a basically a-helical structure in the 144–159 region. Core-predicted residues are absent from one side, but new core-predicted residues are
found on the other side so that the axis of the helix is in much the same position
as in O_1, but the entire helix has been rotated through approximately 80°, with
the consequent exposure of a new hydrophilic side.

In all three viruses, the integrity of the helix has been preserved. However, in
virus SAT2, we see the insertion of a tripeptide that could have lengthened the
helix by one turn. Instead, the presence of a tyrosine at position 152 breaks the
helix after 2.5 turns. The shorter helix is bound on the carboxyterminal side by a
sequence lacking defined secondary structure and on the aminoterminal side by
a sequence predicted to be a β-sheet (Fig. 2). These changes have the effect of
elongating this region, since an a-helix is the most compact form of an amino
acid tract. In addition, only two residues are predicted in core. All of these predictions suggest that the amino acid tract may loop out from the protein surface.

Pfaff et al. (1982) argued that the maintenance of the important antigenic features of the protein in a synthesized peptide would require a rigid secondary
structure such as is provided by an a-helix. Such a structure is present in the

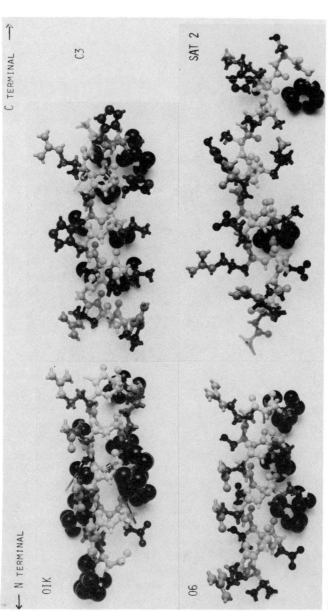

← N TERMINAL

C TERMINAL →

OIK

C3

O6

SAT 2

Figure 2

Structure proposed for the sequence 144-159 of four viruses by predictive methods (Chou and Fasman 1978; Nicholson 1982). The side chains predicted to form part of the protein core are shown with space-filling shells; the skeletal side chains (uppermost) are exposed on the protein surface. Residues 141–143 (not shown) are always nonhelical. The increased length of SAT2 is due to the insertion of a tripeptide and a reduction in the α-helical content (2.5 turns), compared to the other viruses, which allows the sequence on either side to adopt a less-compact structure. In all four structures, various amino acid substitutions have taken place, with effects on the positioning and length of the helix.

Table 3
Neutralizing Antibody Response of Guinea Pigs to Injection of the 141–160 Region of VP1 of Four Different Strains of FMDV

Virus	Log_{10} virus neutralized by 0.015 ml serum at 21 days
O_1 (Kaufbeuren)	2.7
A_{12}	3.1
A_{10}	2.7
C_3 (Indaial)	2.1

Peptide (100 μg) linked to keyhole limpet hemocyanin and adsorbed to aluminum hydroxide gel was injected subcutaneously into groups of four guinea pigs. The lower level of neutralizing activity in the animals that received the C_3 peptide was found in sera taken at intervals ranging from 1 to 51 weeks (Bittle et al., this volume).

141–160 region of type-O and type-C viruses. Nevertheless, peptides 141–160 in which the a-helix is shorter, e.g., A_{10} and A_{12}, are as active as the O_1 peptide (Table 3). These observations suggest that the more rigid structure of an a-helix compared with other types of secondary structures is not necessary for a synthetic peptide to mimic the antigenic site of a protein. The surface features defining an antigenic determinant can apparently be reproduced with peptides corresponding to regions of a nonhelical nature. Whether the interaction with the carrier protein or with cellular receptors constrains the predicted random orientation that such small peptides would assume in free solution and induces in them a more stable secondary structure related to that of the antigenic site on the complete virus remains to be determined.

Importance of Single Amino Acid Substitutions in Determining Serological Activity

During our studies on the antigenic activity of the 141–160 region of the VP1 of several viruses, we found that the antibody elicited by the peptide corresponding to this region of the A_{12} virus neutralized only poorly our stock of the virus. However, the serum did neutralize the virus that had been used for producing the clones from which the nucleotide sequence had been determined (Kleid et al. 1981). Closer examination of our stock virus, which had been passaged only once in tissue-culture cells, compared with the multiple passaging in different cell systems referred to by Kleid et al. (1981), revealed the presence of three viruses with VP1 sequences that differed at positions 148 and 153 from each other and from the virus used by the American workers (see Table 4) (Rowlands et al. 1983). Antisera against the intact viral particles and peptides corresponding to the 141–160 region of VP1 revealed marked antigenic differences between these viruses. The good correlation between the antigenic specificity displayed by the antivirus and antipeptide sera further supports the contention that the 141–160 region of VP1 contains the dominant site on the virus responsible for eliciting neutralizing antibodies. The lack of discrimination we have observed in

Table 4
Neutralizing Antibody Response of Guinea Pigs to Injection of Inactivated Viral Particles and the 141–160 Region of VP1 of Different Plaque Isolates of FMDV A_{12}

		Log_{10} virus neutralized by 0.015 ml serum			
Antiserum		A 148 Ser 153 Leu	B Leu Pro	C Ser Ser	D Phe Pro
148 Ser	antivirus particle	3.3	1.3	1.7	0.7
153 Leu	antipeptide	—	—	—	—
148 Leu	antivirus particle	0.9	3.7	0.9	2.1
153 Pro	antipeptide	0.0	3.2	0.5	2.2
148 Ser	antivirus particle	3.5	2.9	4.1	2.5
153 Ser	antipeptide	1.5	0.1	2.6	1.5
148 Phe	antivirus particle	1.3	2.5	1.1	3.7
153 Pro	antipeptide	0.0	2.0	0.0	2.7

Antivirus particle sera were 1:200 dilution. Antipeptide sera were undiluted.

immunoprecipitation tests with antivirus sera indicates that there are antigenic sites on the viral particle that are of minor importance in neutralization. In contrast, the antipeptide sera are very discriminating in this test (Rowlands et al. 1983). The influence of these amino acid changes on the folding of the 141–160 region of VP1 is discussed in detail by Rowlands et al. (1983).

Practical Implications

There would be several advantages in using a peptide vaccine compared with a conventional vaccine based on the inactivation of viral particles. (1) There would be no problems regarding residual infectivity. (2) The product would be defined precisely in chemical terms. (3) There would be no storage problems; indeed, the shelf life should be infinite. (4) It would be possible to match exactly the sequence of the peptide with that of the corresponding tract of VP1 of the virus causing the outbreak.

The primer extension method (Ghosh et al. 1980) would allow the sequencing of the RNA of a field strain within a few days and ensure that the virus (or peptide) used for production matched exactly in the antigenic site.

CONCLUSIONS

Our work has shown the potential of peptides as vaccines in foot-and-mouth disease. Not only would they have considerable practical advantages over the conventional vaccines, but they would bring to their formulation a precision that cannot be attained with current methods. In addition to these immediate practical advantages, they also bring an understanding of the structural features, in the most fundamental terms, that are required for antigenicity. Probably the most significant feature of the work, however, lies in the fact that it has shown the potential of peptide vaccines for those diseases such as hepatitis A and B where the causative agent cannot be grown in sufficient quantity to allow the production of conventional vaccines.

REFERENCES

Bittle, J.L., R.A. Houghten, H. Alexander, T.M. Shinnick, J.G. Sutcliffe, R.A. Lerner, D.J. Rowlands, and F. Brown. 1982. Protection against foot-and-mouth disease by immunization with a chemically synthesized peptide predicted from the viral nucleotide sequence. *Nature* **298:** 30.

Boothroyd, J.C., T.J.R. Harris, D.J. Rowlands, and P.A. Lowe. 1982. Nucleotide sequence of cDNA coding for the structural proteins of foot-and-mouth disease virus. *Gene* **17:** 153.

Chou, P.Y. and G.D. Fasman. 1978. Prediction of the secondary structure of proteins from their amino acid sequence. *Adv. Enzymol.* **47:** 45.

Ghosh, P.K., V.B. Reddy, M. Piatak, P. Lebowitz, and S. Weissman. 1980. Determination of RNA sequences by primer directed synthesis and sequencing of their cDNA transcripts. *Methods Enzymol.* **65:** 580.

Kleid, D.G., D. Yansura, B. Small, D. Dowbenko, D.M. Moore, M.J. Grubman, P.D. McKercher, D.O. Morgan, B.H. Robertson, and H.L. Bachrach. 1981. Cloned viral protein vaccine for foot and mouth disease: Responses in cattle and swine. *Science* **214:** 1125.

Kurz, C., S. Forss, H. Kupper, K. Strohmaier, and H. Schaller. 1981. Nucleotide sequence and corresponding amino acid sequence of the gene for the major antigen of foot-and-mouth disease virus. *Nucleic Acids Res.* **9:** 1919.

Laporte, J., J. Grosclaude, J. Wantyghem, S. Bernard, and P. Rouze. 1973. Neutralization en culture cellulaire du pouvoir infectieux du virus de la fievre aphteuse par les serums provenant de porcs immunisee a l'aide dune proteine viral purifee. *C. R. Seances Hebd. Acad. Sci. Ser. D.* **276:** 3399.

Makoff, A.J., C.A. Paynter, D.J. Rowlands, and J.C. Boothroyd. 1982. Comparison of the amino acid sequence of the major immunogen from three serotypes of foot and mouth disease virus. *Nucleic Acids Res.* **10:** 8285.

Nicholson, B.H. 1982. Correlation of sequence and spatial position in globular proteins. *Biochem. Soc. Trans.* **10:** 387.

Pfaff, E., M. Mussgay, H.O. Bohm, G.E. Schulz, and H. Schaller. 1982. Antibodies against a preselected peptide recognize and neutralize foot and mouth disease virus. *EMBO J.* **1:** 869.

Rowlands, D.J., B.E. Clarke, A.R. Carroll, F. Brown, B.H. Nicholson, J.L. Bittle, R.A. Houghten, and R.A. Lerner. 1983. The chemical basis for neutralization of foot-and-mouth disease virus. *Nature* **306:** 694.

Sangar, D.V., D.N. Black, D.J. Rowlands, and F. Brown. 1977. Biochemical mapping of the foot and mouth disease virus genome. *J. Gen. Virol.* **35:** 281.

Strohmaier, K., R. Franze, and K.H. Adam. 1982. Location and characterization of the antigenic portion of the FMDV immunizing protein. *J. Gen. Virol.* **59:** 295.

Wild, T.F., J.N. Burroughs, and F. Brown. 1969. Surface structure of foot and mouth disease virus. *J. Gen. Virol.* **4:** 313.

Immunization against Foot-and-Mouth Disease with a Chemically Synthesized Peptide

James L. Bittle, Patricia Worrell,
Richard A. Houghten, and Richard A. Lerner
Research Institute of Scripps
Clinic, La Jolla, California 92037

David J. Rowlands and Fred Brown
Animal Virus Research Institute
Pirbright, Surrey, England

Foot-and-mouth disease is one of the most serious livestock diseases, causing severe economic losses, not only in loss of productivity, but also in the disruption it causes to trading between countries. The disease is controlled either by eradication programs or by vaccination. Despite the widespread use of vaccines, only the continents of North America and Australia are free from the disease.

By far the greatest number of vaccines are prepared by chemically inactivating virus grown in tissue-culture cell systems. In general, these are effective in preventing the disease, but there are some problems connected with their manufacture and application: (1) Special containment facilities are required for growing and handling the large amounts of virus required for vaccine production. (2) It is difficult to ensure that complete inactivation of infectivity has been achieved. (3) The vaccines have a limited shelf life because of the instability of the viral particle. (4) The necessary storage at refrigerator temperatures presents difficulties under field conditions.

A radically new approach to the problem has been developed during the last few years. On the basis of the observation that the major immunizing site is located on only one (VP1) of the four capsid proteins of the virus (Wild et al. 1969) and the location of this protein on the viral RNA by biochemical mapping (Sangar et al. 1977), it became possible to express the protein in *Escherichia coli* cells by recombinant DNA technology (Kleid et al. 1981). This antigen has been shown to elicit neutralizing antibody in cattle and swine and to protect them against experimental infection.

Dissection of VP1 into immunogenic fragments by either cyanogen bromide cleavage of the isolated protein or enzymatic cleavage in situ allowed Strohmaier

103

et al. (1982) to predict that two amino acid sequences, 146–154 and 201–213 of the 213-amino-acid-long protein from virus of serotype O, contained antigenic sites. This was followed shortly afterward by our demonstration (Bittle et al. 1982) that a chemically synthesized peptide corresponding to residues 141–160 of the polypeptide, when coupled to keyhole limpet hemocyanin (KLH), elicited by one injection a level of neutralizing antibody that protected guinea pigs against experimental challenge with the homologous virus. The level of the antibody response was sufficient to encourage us to investigate whether peptides corresponding to the same region of the VP1 polypeptide of other strains of the virus would give a similar response and to determine whether the response could be enhanced by (1) linking the peptide to different carrier proteins, (2) varying the method of coupling, and (3) using different adjuvants. As a result of these studies, a vaccine formulation effective in inducing levels of antibody in cattle compatible with protection has been derived.

DISCUSSION

Antibody Response to the 141–160 Region of Different Viruses

A single injection of the 141–160 region from three different viruses, A_{10}, A_{12}, and C_3 linked to KLH via an added cysteine residue, gave a significant neutralizing antibody response in guinea pigs. There was little or no response at 6 days, but the level of neutralizing antibody at 14 days for type A and 21 days for type C would be expected to protect the animals against experimental infection. The response to the C peptide was lower than that to the other peptides. The antibody titer against the A viruses was maintained at a high level over several months and was still significant after 1 year (Table 1).

The long duration of the antibody response was also found in rabbits. In one experiment in which two rabbits were injected with the type-O peptide on days 0, 14, and 21, the serum antibody levels at 35, 70, and 365 days were 4.5, 5.8, and 4.8 logs, respectively.

Table 1
Response of Guinea Pigs to Injection of the 141–160 Region of VP1 of Three Viruses

Virus	Weight of peptide (μg)	Log_{10} virus neutralized by 0.015 ml serum (weeks after injection)							
		1	2	3	6	22	41	46	51
A_{10}	40	0.9	3.5	≥4.1	2.9	2.9	1.9		1.7
	200	0.1	2.7	2.7	2.7	2.7	2.1		2.3
	1000	1.4	≥3.9	3.3	3.1	≥3.5	2.3		2.1
A_{12}	40	0.7	3.1	3.3	3.1	≥3.7	2.5		2.1
	200	1.1	3.1	≥4.1	3.1	≥3.7	4.1		3.1
	1000	2.5	≥3.3	2.5	3.5	3.9	4.1		3.1
C_3	40	0.3	1.5	2.1	1.5	0.9	0.3		0.1
	200	0.1	1.9	2.1	1.7	0.9	1.1		1.1
	1000	0.3	2.1	2.9	1.9	2.1	1.9		1.7

Peptides were linked to KLH via a cysteine residue and adsorbed onto aluminum hydroxide before subcutaneous injection.

Effect of Different Carriers, Method of Coupling, and Adjuvants on the Antibody Response in Guinea Pigs

Much of our early work was done with peptides that had been attached to KLH via an added cysteine residue at the carboxyl terminus. However, it was appreciated that this carrier was unlikely to be used on a large scale because of its cost and availability, so other carriers were examined. The method of coupling was also varied.The results in Table 2 show that bovine serum albumin and tetanus toxoid were as good as KLH as carriers. Moreover, coupling with glutaraldehyde gave preparations that were as active as those obtained by attaching with *N*-maleimidobenzoyl-*N*-hydroxysuccinimide (MBS) via an added cysteine.

We also found that preparations obtained by polymerizing the peptide with glutaraldehyde or air-oxidizing a peptide containing an added cysteine at each end of the chain were also active. Such preparations would have clear advantages over those in which a carrier protein is used. The response to the monomeric form of the peptide was much lower. The neutralizing antibody levels at 4 weeks were similar for any particular preparation regardless of whether saponin or incomplete Freund's was used as an adjuvant. However, the response was longer lasting when incomplete Freund's adjuvant was used, and high levels were maintained for at least as long as 36 weeks (Table 3).

The possible value of immunostimulants other than conventional adjuvants has also been explored. We have found that the addition of muramyl dipeptide to incomplete Freund's adjuvant before emulsifying with the peptide gave a preparation that elicited a high level of antibody. However, the high cost of this compound persuaded us to investigate other immunostimulants. Preliminary results indicate that preparations containing sodium selenite enhance the neutralizing antibody response.

Table 2
Effect of Carrier, Method of Coupling, and Adjuvant on the Antibody Response in Guinea Pigs to Peptide 141–160 of VP1 of Serotype O_1

Carrier	Linking agent	Adjuvant	Log_{10} virus neutralization by 0.015 ml serum (at four weeks)
KLH	MBS	incomplete Freund's	3.1
KLH	MBS	saponin	2.9
KLH	glutaraldehyde	incomplete Freund's	2.8
KLH	glutaraldehyde	saponin	2.5
BSA	MBS	incomplete Freund's	3.1
BSA	MBS	saponin	3.7
Tetanus toxoid	MBS	incomplete Freund's	2.5
Tetanus toxoid	glutaraldehyde	incomplete Freund's	2.9
Polylysine	MBS	incomplete Freund's	2.6
Polymerized with glutaraldehyde	none	incomplete Freund's	3.3
Polymerized via cysteine	none	incomplete Freund's	2.3
None	none	incomplete Freund's	0.9

Peptide (100 µg) injected subcutaneously into each of five guinea pigs.

Table 3
Duration of Neutralizing Antibody Response in Guinea Pigs to Various Formulations of the O_1 141–160 Peptide

Carrier protein	Adjuvant	Log_{10} virus neutralized by 0.015 ml serum (weeks after injection)				
		4	8	12	24	36
None	incomplete Freund's	0.7	2.3	1.1	2.1	1.7
KLH	incomplete Freund's	2.7	3.4	3.3	3.5	3.3
KLH[a]	incomplete Freund's	2.9	3.6	3.8	3.8	4.7
Tetanus toxoid	incomplete Freund's	2.9	2.3	2.9	3.5	3.5
Tetanus toxoid[a]	incomplete Freund's	2.7	4.3	3.9		
Tetanus toxoid	saponin	2.1	2.1	2.7		

Each guinea pig received 100 μg of peptide emulsified with incomplete Freund's adjuvant.
[a]The incomplete Freund's adjuvant contained 10 μg muramyl dipeptide.

Response of Cattle to Peptide 141–160

In foot-and-mouth disease, the acceptability of a vaccine for use in cattle is dependent on whether animals will withstand infection when injected in the tongue with 10,000 ID_{50} of challenge virus. The degree of protection is correlated with the level of neutralizing antibody in the serum at the time of challenge. It has been shown with many vaccines that a level of neutralizing antibody in the serum of about 2.5 logs will afford protection. Our aim has been to achieve this level with one injection of the peptide. We have found that the peptide coupled to tetanus toxoid and injected with Freund's adjuvant containing muramyl dipeptide elicited levels of neutralizing antibody that would be expected to afford protection (Table 4). However, a better and longer lasting response was obtained when the Freund's adjuvant contained sodium selenite. Challenge experiments with cattle that have received this formulation are in progress.

Table 4
Neutralizing Antibody Response in Cattle to the 141–160 Peptide of VP1 Serotype O_1 Coupled to Tetanus Toxoid

Adjuvant	Log_{10} virus neutralized by 0.015 ml serum (weeks after injection)		
	4	8	10
Incomplete Freund's	1.9	2.3	1.8
Incomplete Freund's/MDP	2.3	2.8	2.3
Saponin/aluminum hydroxide	1.5	1.2	1.5
Saponin/aluminum hydroxide/MDP	2.4	2.1	1.6
Incomplete Freund's/ sodium selenite	2.4	3.2	3.0

Titers are averages of three animals.

CONCLUSIONS

Our results show that a neutralizing antibody response can be elicited in guinea pigs and in cattle with a chemically synthesized peptide corresponding to the major antigenic site of the virus that is sufficiently high to protect the animals against experimental infection. This demonstration thus foreshadows a stage in the development of foot-and-mouth disease vaccines in which a safe and stable, chemically synthesized product will be available.

REFERENCES

Bittle, J.L., R.A. Houghten, H. Alexander, T.M. Shinnick, J.G. Sutcliffe, R.A. Lerner, D.J. Rowlands, and F. Brown. 1982. Protection against foot-and-mouth disease by immunization with a chemically synthesized peptide predicted from the viral nucleotide sequence. *Nature* **298**: 30.

Kleid, D.G., D. Yansura, B. Small, D. Dowbenko, D.M. Moore, M.J. Grubman, P.D. McKercher, D.O. Morgan, B.H. Robertson, and H.L. Bachrach. 1981. Cloned viral protein vaccines for foot and mouth disease: Responses in cattle and swine. *Science* **214**: 1125.

Sangar, D.V., D.N. Black, D.J. Rowlands, and F. Brown. 1977. Biochemical mapping of the foot and mouth disease virus genome. *J. Gen. Virol.* **35**: 281.

Strohmaier, K., R. Franze, and K.H. Adam. 1982. Location and characterization of the antigenic portion of the FMDV immunizing protein. *J. Gen. Virol.* **59**: 295.

Wild, T.F., J.N. Burroughs, and F. Brown. 1969. Surface structure of foot and mouth disease virus. *J. Gen. Virol.* **4**: 313.

Anti-influenza Synthetic Vaccine

Ruth Arnon and Michal Shapira
Department of Chemical Immunology
The Weizmann Institute of Science
Rehovot 76100, Israel

Early studies in our laboratory have demonstrated that synthetic antigens containing an immunoreactive region of a protein molecule can give rise to an immune response toward the intact native protein. Often, the specificity of the response is toward a conformation-dependent antigenic determinant (Arnon et al. 1971). When the protein in question was a component of a virus, e.g., the coat protein of MS2 coliphage, the resultant antibodies toward a synthetic fragment were capable of neutralizing the viability of the phage (Langbeheim et al. 1976). These findings paved the way for the study of synthetic virus vaccines. We have subsequently employed the synthetic approach to the influenza virus system. This virus provides a suitable model, since detailed information is available on the structure, function, and antigenic properties of its surface protein components, to allow the synthesis of peptides with potential immune reactivity. Moreover, since this is an animal virus infectious for mice, the immune response against the synthetic peptides can be evaluated not only for the in vitro reactivity, but also for its protective effect in vivo. In the following, we report on the synthesis of peptides from two regions in the influenza hemagglutinin (HA) molecule, which induce anti-influenza immune response, as well as partial protection of mice against virus infection.

The first peptide we synthesized, before the three-dimensional structure was known, contained 18 amino acid residues corresponding to the sequence 91–108 of the influenza HA molecule. This region, which is common to at least 12 H3 strains, is a part of a larger cyanogen bromide (CNBr) fragment previously shown by Jackson and his colleagues (1979) to be immunologically active. According to our computer-predicted folded structure of the HA polypeptide chain, this peptide segment should have comprised a folded region with a short a-helical segment, and hence an exposed area in the molecular structure. It also contains three tyrosine and two proline residues that had been demonstrated in our previous studies to play a dominant role in antigenicity of several proteins or synthetic antigens. The 91–108 peptide that contains these "ingredients" was anticipated to be immunologically reactive.

Indeed, a conjugate of this peptide with tetanus toxoid elicited in both rabbits and mice antibodies that reacted immunochemically with the synthetic peptide, as well as with the intact influenza virus of several strains of type A. These antibodies were capable of inhibiting the capacity of the HA of the relevant strains to agglutinate chicken red blood cells. They also interfered with the in vitro growth of the virus in tissue culture. But, most importantly, mice immunized with the peptide-toxoid conjugate were partially protected against further challenge infection with the virus (Müller et al. 1982).

One of the crucial factors concerning the influenza vaccine is the tremendous genetic variations among the various virus strains—shifts and drifts—and their reflection on the serological specificities. Detailed studies of amino acid sequences and X-ray diffraction (Wiley et al. 1981) resulted in the location of four antigenic sites, designated A through D, on the HA molecule. Amino acid substitutions at these sites caused by mutation led to the development of new virus strains with changed immunogenic properties, whereas other regions were shown to be "constant." The peptide 91–108 was deliberately chosen to be part of a conserved sequence; although it does not overlap with any of the four proposed antigenic determinants of the native HA (Fig. 1), it is adjacent in the three-dimensional structure to the antigenic site D. This could provide an explanation for the partial protective effect achieved by immunization with this peptide. Furthermore, since the same sequence is present in the HA of several influenza strains, it was of interest to determine whether immunization with the same conjugate will elicit protection against more than one H3 strain. The finding that this is indeed the case (Table 1) is an indication that the synthetic approach might lead to multivalent vaccines for cross-strain protection.

As evident from the three-dimensional structure of the influenza HA (Wiley et al. 1981), the region 140–146, which forms antigenic site A, is a "loop" of seven amino acids unusually protruding from the surface of the molecule (Fig. 1). It is also exposed in the trimeric structure assumed by the HA on the virus surface. One would expect that peptides corresponding to this region, where "natural" immunogenic determinants of the HA molecule are located, would elicit a better and more specific immune response against the virus. It was of interest, therefore, to synthesize peptides covering the loop region for immunization purposes. Jackson et al. (1982) have used a synthetic peptide representing the sequence 123–151 that includes the loop region for immunization of rabbits. They did not find significant binding between the antipeptide antibodies and the X-31 virus. However, antibodies raised against the intact X-31 virus did exhibit some binding to the synthetic peptide.

In our studies, four peptides have been synthesized. Two of them corresponded to the sequence 139–146, with either Gly or Asp at position 144. The third peptide corresponded to the sequence 147–164, and the fourth included both regions and corresponded to the sequence 138–164. The location of these peptides is shown in Figure 1. Conjugates of these four peptides to tetanus toxoid were used for immunization of rabbits and mice.

All four conjugates elicited high antibody titer against the respective homologous peptides, with a significant extent of cross-reactivity among them. Of particular interest is the high cross-reactivity between the two octapeptides differing at residue 144 (Gly for Asp exchange), a finding that is contrasted by the significant effect of the same exchange on the serological specificity of the intact HA, which

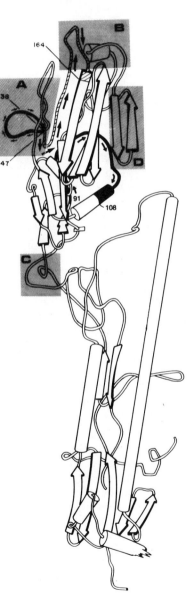

Figure 1
Schematic diagram of the folding of the influenza HA polypeptide chain (according to Wiley et al. 1981). The proposed antigenic sites A to D are shaded. Peptides 91–108, 139–146, 147–164, and 138–164 are designated.

Table 1
Protection of Mice against Challenge Infection with Influenza Virus

Immunizing conjugate	Infectious strain	Group	Incidence of infection at 10^{-2} dilution into egg	Mouse lung virus titer
(91-108)-TT	A/Tex/77	immunized[a]	19/36 (52%)	$10^{-1.98}$
		control[b]	21/23 (91%)	$10^{-3.56}$
(91-108)-TT	A/PC/75	immunized	4/18 (22%)	$10^{-0.61}$
		control	8/19 (42%)	$10^{-1.53}$
(91-108)-TT	A/Eng/42/72	immunized	8/18 (44%)	$10^{-1.61}$
		control	15/21 (71%)	$10^{-2.9}$
(91-108)-TT	A/PR/81/34	immunized	18/19 (95%)	$10^{-3.47}$
	(H1)	control	20/21 (95%)	$10^{-3.95}$
(138-164)-TT	A/Eng/42/72	immunized	4/11 (36%)	$10^{-1.18}$
		control	7/10 (70%)	$10^{-2.6}$
(147-164)-TT	A/Eng/42/72	immunized	6/11 (55%)	10^{-2}
		control	7/10 (70%)	$10^{-2.6}$

[a]Immunized with the respective conjugate in complete Freund's adjuvant.
[b]Control groups were injected with tetanus toxoid alone in complete Freund's adjuvant.

is manifested by the existence of monoclonal-antibody-selected variants that escape neutralization due to this single amino acid substitution.

The four synthetic peptides differed in their cross-reactivities with the intact H3 influenza virus. Thus, antibodies against the two loop octapeptides showed very low binding capacity to the virus, whereas antibodies against the two longer peptides, namely, 147–164 or 138–164, recognized the intact virus and showed considerable binding to it (Table 2).

In interfering with the biological functions of the virus, we found that the only peptide that showed activity was fragment 138–164. Its reactivity was manifested first in the capacity of its antiserum to inhibit the hemagglutination activity of the intact virus; moreover, immunization of mice with the tetanus toxoid conjugate of this peptide resulted in their partial protection against infection with the A/Eng/ 42/72 strain, with which the sequence of the synthetic peptide corresponds. It is of interest that antibodies raised against the intact virus were capable of recog-

Table 2
Characterization of the Various Conjugates

Conjugate	Peptide to carrier ratio		Reactivity of antiserum with homologous peptide	Reactivity of antiserum with virus	Protective capacity
	W/W	M/M			
(139-146[144-Gly])-TT	10%	20:1	+	−	n.d.[a]
(139-146[144-Asp])-TT	19%	37:1	+	±	n.d.
(147-164)-TT	60%	40:1	+	+	−
(138-164)-TT	40–84%	19–40:1	+	+	+

[a]n.d. indicates not determined.

nizing the synthetic loop octapeptides and reacted partially with peptide 138–164, probably due to their recognition of the loop region, but did not react at all with peptide 147–164. These findings are indicative of the importance of the length and conformation of the synthetic peptide for its immunological reactivity. The short loop peptide is recognized by the antivirus antibodies but cannot elicit antiviral response, whereas the longer peptide 138–164 provides protective immunity against the virus.

CONCLUSIONS

The results presented here demonstrate that synthetic peptides corresponding to regions of relevance in the viral protein can indeed serve as a basis for a synthetic vaccine leading to protective immunity. These should not necessarily consist of the naturally occurring antigenic determinants. It is possible that a segment, which is immunosilent in the intact virus, when presented in an isolated form might induce antibodies that recognize the virus. As in the case of peptide 91–108, this may result in cross-strain reactivity. On the other hand, the short loop segment containing an antigenic site of the virus, when presented as an isolated peptide, does not necessarily fold into the native conformation. In such cases, use of a longer peptide might result in enforcing the right folding that is required for mimicking the native structure. Hence, a detailed study of each individual virus system is essential for elucidating this point and for achieving the optimal results.

ACKNOWLEDGMENT

We wish to thank Ms. Ziva Misulovin for excellent technical assistance.

REFERENCES

Arnon, R., E. Maron, M. Sela, and C.E. Anfinsen. 1971. Antibodies reactive with native lysozyme elicited by a completely synthetic antigen. *Proc. Natl. Acad. Sci.* **68:** 1450.

Jackson, D.C., L.E. Brown, D.O. White, T.A.A. Dopheide, and C.W. Ward. 1979. Antigenic determinants of influenza virus hemagglutinin. IV. Immunogenicity of fragments isolated from the hemagglutinin of A/Memphis/102/72. *J. Immunol.* **123:** 2610.

Jackson, D.C., J.M. Murray, D.O. White, C.N. Fagan, and G.W. Tregear. 1982. Antigenic activity of a synthetic peptide corresponding to the "loop" region of influenza virus hemagglutinin. *Virology* **120:** 273.

Langbeheim, H., R. Arnon, and M. Sela. 1976. Antiviral effect on MS-2 coliphage obtained with a synthetic antigen. *Proc. Natl. Acad. Sci.* **73:** 4636.

Müller, G., M. Shapira, and R. Arnon. 1982. Anti-influenza response achieved by immunization with a synthetic conjugate. *Proc. Natl. Acad. Sci.* **79:** 569.

Wiley, D.C., I.A. Wilson, and J.J. Skehel. 1981. Structural identification of the antibody-binding sites of Hong-Kong influenza hemagglutinin and their involvement in antigenic variation. *Nature* **289:** 373.

Immunogenic and Antigenic Activities of a Cyclic Synthetic HBsAg Peptide

Gordon R. Dreesman, James T. Sparrow, Ronald C. Kennedy, and Joseph L. Melnick
Department of Virology and Epidemiology and Department of Medicine, Baylor College of Medicine, Houston, Texas 77030

Antibody produced against hepatitis-B surface antigen (HBsAg), the lipoprotein envelope of hepatitis-B virus (HBV), provides protection from infection with this virus. Serological examination of HBsAg has revealed several distinct antigenic determinants that include an *a* cross-reactive group determinant and two sets of mutually exclusive subtype determinants referred to as *d* or *y* and *w* or *r* (for review, see Tiollais et al. 1981). Antibody against one of the four possible antigenic subtypes of HBV provides protection against infection or reinfection with a second subtype. These observations indicated that protective antibody is chiefly directed to the *a* determinant(s). Purified 22-nm particles associated with HBsAg derived from human plasma of HBV chronic carriers have proven to be a highly effective and safe vaccine in humans. However, the difficulty of obtaining source material and the high cost of the vaccine have prompted the investigation of an alternative source. The successful cloning of the entire DNA genome has provided the tools to develop two such alternatives. These include HBsAg produced by a vector containing the cloned gene for HBV surface antigen and a synthetic HBsAg peptide engineered from a computer analysis of the amino acid sequence of the major polypeptide of HBsAg (Tiollais et al. 1981). This study summarizes our recent experience with a synthetic peptide containing amino acid residues 122–137 of the 25,000-dalton polypeptide (p25) of HBsAg that was made cyclic by formation of a single disulfide bond between cysteine residues at positions 124 and 137.

DISCUSSION

Immunogenic Properties

The major task in the synthesis of an immunogenic peptide for possible use as an effective vaccine is the selection of the amino acid sequence containing the

115

required antigenic determinant (epitope) and the constraints that conformation may place on this epitope. On the basis of a computer analysis of the complete amino acid sequence of p25, we selected the amino acid residues 122–137, since this sequence represented a hydrophilic region with potential β turns (Dreesman et al. 1982). Earlier studies had demonstrated that intact disulfide bonds were critical for the maintenance of the native antigenic and/or immunogenic activity of HBsAg. Therefore, sequence 122–137 was especially attractive in that it contains two cysteine residues at positions 124 and 137 that could be utilized for the formation of an intrachain disulfide bond.

Peptide 122–137 was synthesized by the solid-phase Merrifield methodology and cyclized either by oxidation with potassium ferricyanide or by oxidation in the absence of reducing agents. After purification on ion exchange and gel-filtration columns, the peptide was incorporated into a series of adjuvant vehicles and used to immunize BALB/c mice. An immune response was noted 7–14 days after a single inoculation of liposome-incorporated peptide, as measured with a commercial solid-phase radioimmunoassay (Dreesman et al. 1982). A significant booster response was not observed after a second inoculation of liposome-entrapped peptide. Therefore, the cyclized peptide was aggregated into micelles by reaction with Triton X-100 or by reacting peptide with tetanus toxoid in the presence of carbodiimide. Two inoculations of alum-precipitated micelles or of peptide–tetanus toxoid conjugates elicited a significant booster response in BALB/c mice. Titers of antibodies against HBsAg (anti-HBs) recorded 30–35 days after the second dose of alum-precipitated, peptide–tetanus toxoid conjugate were similar to that noted in mice immunized with two doses of alum-precipitated, purified HBsAg 22-nm particles (Table 1). In contrast, the antibody response was markedly less in mice inoculated with a soluble pool of alum-adsorbed HBsAg-derived p25-gp30 subunits. The low antibody response was not unexpected, since the polypeptide-glycopeptide subunits were purified from solubilized 22-nm HBsAg particles by SDS-polyacrylamide gel electrophoresis in the presence of a reducing agent. The importance of the intrachain bond was substantiated in that injection of similar preparations of peptide 122–137, linearized by reduction and subsequent alkylation of the free thiol groups with iodoacetamide, failed to induce a detectable immune response.

Table 1
Mean Antibody Titers in Mice Immunized with Two Doses of Alum-adsorbed HBsAg Vaccine Candidates

HBsAg vaccines	Antibody titer 35 days after second inoculation
Intact 22-nm particle	6250
SDS-denatured p25-gp30	17
Peptide 122–137-tetanus toxoid	5500

For each alum-adjuvanted vaccine preparation, the antibody titer is expressed as the reciprocal of the geometric mean anti-HBs titers of sera from six individual mice, as measured by micro-solid-phase immunoradiometric assay. Mice were inoculated on days 0 and 35.

Major Epitopes Associated with Peptide 122–137

The next series of experiments was designed to define which epitopes were associated with this peptide using a panel of anti-HBs monoclonal antibodies developed in our laboratory. The peptide was analyzed by testing its potential capacity to inhibit the reaction of 14 different anti-*a* monoclonal antibodies with HBsAg (Ionescu-Matiu et al. 1983). Several points can be made from the results shown in Table 2. Preincubation of peptide 122–137 with six monoclonal antibody preparations with specificity for the group-*a* epitope inhibited the subsequent reaction of the antibody with intact HBsAg. However, the reactivity of the eight remaining anti-*a* monoclonal antibodies was unaltered in the presence of peptide 122–137. This demonstrates that the group-*a* specificity associated with HBsAg contains two or more distinct antigenic determinants and that the peptide contains one of these epitopes. In addition, we demonstrated that a sequential *y* epitope was associated with this peptide in that three anti-*y* monoclonal antibodies reacted with both the cyclic and linear peptides (Table 2). No *w* reactivity has been noted.

Reactivity of Human Anti-HBs with Cyclic Peptide 122–137

A tool that could aid in determining the ability of peptide 122–137 to elicit protective antibody resides with the idiotypic specificity of the anti-HBs antibodies produced by humans naturally infected with HBV. The region associated with the variable region of the immunoglobulin molecule and that contains the antigen-combining site has been defined as the idiotype of that immunoglobulin molecule. An anti-idiotype reagent was produced by inoculation of rabbits with specifically purified human anti-HBs. The subsequent rabbit antiserum was extensively adsorbed with normal human immunoglobulin negative for anti-HBs reactivity. The resultant antiserum thus recognized only that region of the immunoglobulin molecule that specifically reacted with HBsAg and is referred to as an anti-idiotype reagent. We demonstrated that humans infected with HBV generate anti-HBs that contains a common idiotype (CId). This conclusion was based on the

Table 2
Characterization of Synthetic Peptide 122–137 for HBsAg Group-*a* and Subgroup-*y* Epitopes by Using Monoclonal Antibodies

Monoclonal antibody specificity[a]	Inhibition of monoclonal antibody with			
	peptide 122–137		HBsAg	
	cyclic	linear	adw	ayw
Anti-*a* (6)	+	−	+	+
Anti-*a* (8)	−	−	+	+
Anti-*y* (3)	+	+	−	+

[a]Number in parentheses is the number of individual monoclonal preparations tested.

fact that preincubation of several different individual anti-HBs human sera with rabbit anti-Cld blocked reaction with ^{125}I-labeled idiotype.

The Cld was found to be associated with the a-group specificity in that purified 22-nm particles of adw, ayw, and adr specificities inhibited the Cld–anti-idiotype reaction to the same degree. Inhibition was also obtained with a nondenatured HBsAg polypeptide micelle preparation. Of particular importance to this study was that the cyclic peptide efficiently inhibited the reaction (Fig. 1). The major role of conformation was emphasized in that reduction of the intrachain disulfide bond (Cys 124–137) and alkylation of the free thiol groups destroyed the capacity of peptide to block the Cld–anti-idiotype reaction (Kennedy et al. 1983b). Similarly, SDS-denatured preparations of p25 and gp30 failed to inhibit the reaction significantly.

The relatedness of the epitope associated with peptide 122–137 to that of native HBsAg also has been shown in a preliminary experiment in which a chimpanzee with preexisting anti-HBs was inoculated with cyclic peptide. A heightened anti-HBs response was observed after a second inoculation of alum-precipitated, peptide–tetanus toxoid conjugate.

We have also studied the modulating effects of in vivo administration of anti-idiotype reagents that recognize the common anti-HBs idiotype prior to antigenic challenge with HBsAg at the cellular level. The injection of anti-idiotype antibodies prior to challenge with HBsAg resulted in an increased number of IgM anti-HBs-secreting cells. Anti-HBs-secreting cells were also induced by administration of anti-idiotype antibodies without antigen exposure (Kennedy et al. 1983a).

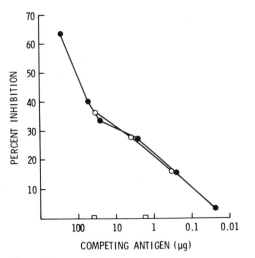

Figure 1
Inhibition of binding of ^{125}I-labeled common human idiotype (anti-HBs) to its respective rabbit anti-idiotypic antiserum by intact HBsAg/adw (○) and by cyclic (●) and linear (□) synthetic HBsAg peptide 122–137.

SUMMARY AND CONCLUSION

The above series of experiments clearly indicates that a vigorous immune response can be elicited in mice by two inoculations of alum-adsorbed preparations of cyclic peptide 122–137 aggregated into micelles or of the peptide covalently linked to a tetanus toxoid carrier. We have also demonstrated that our cyclic peptide contains an *a* determinant that reacts specifically with antibody produced by humans infected with HBV. In addition, the use of anti-idiotype reagents may represent valuable tools for priming the immune response of individuals prior to vaccination with either HBsAg or synthetic peptide. Continued investigations of the above and other defined HBsAg peptides with optimal adjuvant vehicles and administration schedules of various peptide formulations should form a foundation for the development of an economic and safe synthetic vaccine for HBV.

REFERENCES

Dreesman, G.R., Y. Sanchez, I. Ionescu-Matiu, J.T. Sparrow, H.R. Six, D.L. Peterson, F.B. Hollinger, and J.L. Melnick. 1982. Antibody to hepatitis B surface antigen after a single inoculation of uncoupled synthetic HBsAg peptides. *Nature* **295:** 158.

Ionescu-Matiu, I., R.C. Kennedy, J.T. Sparrow, A.R. Culwell, Y. Sanchez, J.L. Melnick, and G.R. Dreesman. 1983. Epitopes associated with a synthetic hepatitis B surface antigen peptide. *J. Immunol.* **130:** 1947.

Kennedy, R.C., K. Adler-Storthz, R.D. Henkel, Y. Sanchez, J.L. Melnick, and G.R. Dreesman. 1983a. Immune response to hepatitis B surface antigen: Enhancement by prior injection of antibodies to the idiotype. *Science* **221:** 853.

Kennedy, R.C., G.R. Dreesman, J.T. Sparrow, A.R. Culwell, Y. Sanchez, I. Ionescu-Matiu, F.B. Hollinger, and J.L. Melnick. 1983b. Inhibition of a common human anti-hepatitis B surface antigen idiotype by a cyclic synthetic peptide. *J. Virol.* **46:** 653.

Tiollais, P., P. Charnay, and G.N. Vyas. 1981. Biology of hepatitis B virus. *Science* **213:** 406.

Recombinant DNA and Synthetic Peptide Approaches to HBV Vaccine Development: Immunogenicity and Protective Efficacy in Chimpanzees

John L. Gerin
Division of Molecular Virology and
Immunology, Georgetown University Medical
Center, Rockville, Maryland 20852

Robert H. Purcell
Laboratory of Infectious Diseases, National
Institute of Allergy and Infectious Diseases
National Institutes of Health
Bethesda, Maryland 20205

Richard A. Lerner
Department of Molecular Biology,
Research Institute of Scripps Clinic
La Jolla, California 92037

Prospects for public health control of hepatitis-B virus (HBV) infection and disease sequelae depend on the availability of safe and effective vaccines (McAuliffe et al. 1980). Current vaccines consist of subviral particles of hepatitis-B surface antigen (HBsAg), which are isolated from the plasma of chronic HBV carriers, inactivated, and absorbed to alum. Clinical trials in high-risk populations established these vaccines to be safe and highly effective in the prevention of HBV infection and disease. However, the vaccines are limited in supply and relatively expensive for those populations of the world with the greatest burden of HBV-associated disease; also, certain risks may be associated with the plasma source material (e.g., the putative AIDS agent). These factors, coupled with recent advances in nucleic acid and peptide synthesis techniques, have stimulated an intense research effort to develop alternative HBV vaccines using modern approaches. Cloning of the HBV genome and determination of its sequence have identified a continuous nucleotide sequence (gene S) that encodes the surface antigen of HBV (see Tiollais et al. 1981), thereby providing opportunities for the production of HBsAg by either (1) S-gene expression using recombinant DNA methods or (2) chemical synthesis of peptides predicted from the S-gene nucleotide sequence.

DISCUSSION

HBsAg Produced by Recombinant DNA Methods

Gene-*S* expression in mammalian cell cultures is marked by the synthesis, assembly, and release of 22-nm forms of HBsAg to the culture medium. These particles have the same biophysical, biochemical, and antigenic properties as those isolated from human HBV carriers for use in current HBV vaccines. The immunogenicity and protective efficacy of a 22-nm HBsAg vaccine, derived by recombinant DNA methods (Moriarty et al. 1981), were evaluated in the chimpanzee model of response to HBV infection. HBsAg was purified from cell culture media by density gradient centrifugation, inactivated by formalin, and absorbed to alum by conventional methods. Each of two HBV-susceptible chimpanzees was inoculated intramuscularly with a 5-μg dose of HBsAg at 0 and 4 weeks. Both animals developed a brisk response in which antibodies to HBsAg (anti-HBs) rose to high levels following the 4-week booster dose. One chimpanzee was experimentally challenged at week 10 with $10^{3.5}$ chimpanzee infectious doses of HBV and monitored at weekly intervals for evidence of HBV infection and disease. The animal maintained a high level of anti-HBs activity for the 6-month follow-up period with no evidence of HBV infection (HBsAg or anti-HBc) or liver disease (elevated alanine aminotransferase, ALT). A relatively small dose of vaccine consisting of recombinant-DNA-derived HBsAg was therefore highly immunogenic and effective in the prevention of experimental HBV infection and disease, thereby establishing the potential application of this approach for new generations of HBV vaccines.

Chemically Synthesized Peptides of HBsAg

Chemically synthesized peptides, predicted from selected regions of the continuous nucleotide sequence of the *S* gene, stimulate antibodies that react with native HBsAg (Lerner et al. 1981). These peptides represent extremely useful reagents for the analysis of HBsAg and the effective host response to HBV vaccination, and, in turn, such chemically defined preparations have great potential for the production of safe and inexpensive HBV vaccines.

Specificities of Synthetic Peptides

The analysis of the specificities of antisera to selected peptides in terms of established HBsAg determinants indicates that the group-specific (*a*) determinant is derived from at least three nonoverlapping sequences (Gerin et al. 1983); HBsAg/*a* therefore appears to represent a collection of determinants, at least some of which depend on the local conformation of relatively short amino acid sequences. A protein region that encompasses amino acid residues 110–137 (numbered from the amino terminus of the *S*-gene product) and contains a high degree of sequence variation specifies the major *d/y*-subtype system; the *d* or *y* specificity appears to depend on one or more of four substitutions in the amino acid region 125–137.

The experience with conventional HBsAg vaccines indicates that antibody to the group-specific (*a*) determinant connotes protective efficacy. Since *a* represents a collection of determinants, the use of synthetic peptides in vaccination strategies could require combinations of peptides in order to obtain maximum protection. Alternatively, two similar peptides representing the *d* and *y* domains in combination may provide the broad protection required of alternative HBV vaccines. Accordingly, we have evaluated the immunogenicity and protective efficacy of one synthetic peptide (peptide 49; the *y*-subtype sequence encompassing amino acid residues 110–137) in the chimpanzee model of response.

Immunogenicity of Peptide 49 in Chimpanzees

Peptide 49 coupled to keyhole limpet hemocyanin (KLH) stimulated a brisk anti-HBs response in chimpanzees (Table 1). Depending on the adjuvant (FIA or alum) and dose (0.2–1.0 mg of coupled peptide 49), the first appearance of anti-HBs varied from 1 week to 5 weeks after primary inoculation of previously seronegative animals; maximum anti-HBs response for all animals ranged from 4 to 6 weeks. A major feature of the response in all animals was a passive decay of anti-HBs after maximum response. This transient anti-HBs activity could not be boosted by further inoculation, at least for chimpanzees 1–3. Sedimentation analysis of the anti-HBs response of chimpanzees 1 and 6 (Fig. 1) revealed that the anti-HBs activity was entirely IgM; therefore, immunization of chimpanzees with synthetic peptide 49 failed to result in the production of long-lasting IgG regardless of choice of adjuvant. Animals 4–7, however, are still on study, and their response to subsequent inoculations has not been determined.

Subtype analysis of the anti-HBs response to the linear form of peptide 49 (Table 2) revealed that the activity was entirely anti-*y*, consistent with the antigenic analysis of this peptide. Interestingly, the cyclic form of peptide 49 (intrapeptide disulfide bond between residues 137 and 124 or 122) stimulated a predominant anti-*a* response, indicating that conformational foldings within this peptide are involved in certain HBsAg specificities.

Table 1
Synthetic Peptide 49–KLH Complex: Anti-HBs Response in Chimpanzees

Animal no.	Peptide	Adjuvant[a]	Dose (μg)[b]	Anti-HBs response weeks to 1st	max.	max. (S/N)[c]
1	49	FIA	1000	1	6	77.1
2	49	alum	1000	2	6	6.4
3	49	alum	1000	2	6	5.2
4	49	alum	200	4	4	5.1
5	49	alum	200	4	4	2.8
6	49 cyclic	alum	200	5	5	51.5
7	49 cyclic	alum	200	4	5	9.2

[a]FIA indicates Freund's incomplete adjuvant.
[b]Dose (μg) of peptide at 0 and 4 weeks (intramuscular).
[c]Ratio of cpm of test sample (S) and negative (N) control in Ausab assay (Abbott); values ≥2.1 are considered positive.

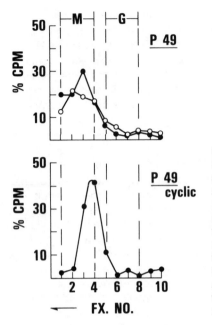

Figure 1
Sucrose gradient analysis of the anti-HBs response to synthetic peptide 49 in chimpanzees. Sera from the primary (O) and maximum (●) anti-HBs response to the linear peptide 49 (*top*) and the maximum response to cyclic peptide 49 (bottom; ●) were sedimented on a 7–30% (w/w) sucrose gradient for 7.5 hr at 45,000 rpm and 4°C in an SW 50.1 rotor. Gradient fractions were assayed by Ausab for anti-HBs activity. The relative positions of standard IgM and IgG are indicated by zones M and G, respectively.

Protective Efficacy of Peptide 49 in Chimpanzees

Late in the course of immunization, chimpanzees 1–3 (Table 1) were experimentally challenged by intravenous inoculation of $10^{3.5}$ infectious doses of HBV/*ayw*. One animal (no. 3) was totally protected against HBV infection, a second chimpanzee (no. 2) developed an attenuated infection without disease, and the third (no. 1) demonstrated a typical pattern of acute hepatitis when compared with response patterns of eight controls. Immunization with peptide 49 therefore provided at least partial protection against homologous virus despite low

Table 2
Synthetic Peptide 49: Specificity of Anti-HBs Response in Chimpanzees

Antiserum	% Inhibition: blocking HBsAg[a]		
	ay	ad	
Monotypic antibody Ctls.			
anti-HBs/*y*	100	7	
anti-HBs/*d*	3	100	
Chimpanzee serum[b]			
anti-peptide 49	88	12	anti-*y*
anti-peptide 49 cyclic	93	62	anti-*a* (anti-*y*)

[a]Percentage of inhibition of cpm in Ausab compared with FBS control.
[b]Two weeks after booster dose.

or undetectable levels of humoral anti-HBs activity at the time of challenge. These data indicate that synthetic peptides have potential in HBV vaccine strategies and also may provide a means of dissecting the effective immune response.

SUMMARY

Modern approaches to HBV vaccines involve the production of protective antigens by recombinant DNA techniques and chemical synthesis of selected peptides. Experimental evaluation of these approaches in the chimpanzee model of human response indicates that both approaches are effective and warrant continued development.

ACKNOWLEDGMENT

This work was supported, in part, by the National Institute of Allergy and Infectious Diseases under contract N01-AI-22665 with Georgetown University.

REFERENCES

Gerin, J.L., J.W.-K. Shih, R.H. Purcell, G. Dapolito, R. Engle, N. Green, H. Alexander, J.G. Sutcliffe, T.M. Shinnick, and R.A. Lerner. 1983. Chemically synthesized peptides of hepatitis B surface antigen duplicate the *d/y* specificities and induce subtype-specific antibodies in chimpanzees. *Proc. Natl. Acad. Sci.* **80:** 2365.

Lerner, R.A., N. Green, H. Alexander, F.-T. Liu, J.G. Sutcliffe, and T.M. Shinnick. 1981. Chemically synthesized peptides predicted from the nucleotide sequence of the hepatitis B virus genome elicit antibodies reactive with the native envelope protein of Dane particles. *Proc. Natl. Acad. Sci.* **78:** 3403.

McAuliffe, V.J., R.H. Purcell, and J.L. Gerin. 1980. Type B hepatitis: A review of current prospects for a safe and effective vaccine. *Rev. Infect. Dis.* **2:** 470.

Moriarty, A.M., B.H. Hoyer, J.W.-K. Shih, J.L. Gerin, and D.H. Hamer. 1981. Expression of the hepatitis B virus surface antigen gene in cell culture using a simian virus 40 vector. *Proc. Natl. Acad. Sci.* **78:** 2606.

Tiollais, P., P. Charnay, and G.N. Vyas. 1981. Biology of hepatitis B virus. *Science* **213:** 406.

Immunogenicity of the Unconjugated Synthetic Polypeptides of Hepatitis-B Surface Antigen

J.Wai-Kuo Shih, Robert J. Gerety, and D.Teh-Yung Liu
Office of Biologics, National Center of Drugs and Biologics, Bethesda, Maryland 20205

Haruaki Yajima, Nobutaka Fujii, Motoyoshi Nomizu, Yoshio Hayashi, and Shinichi Katakura
Kyoto University, Kyoto, Japan

Hepatitis-B virus surface antigen (HBsAg) polypeptides of residues between 1 and 20, 21 and 47, 48 and 81, and 156 and 185 were synthesized by the solid-phase procedures of Merrifield (1963; Merrifield et al. 1982). The sequences synthesized were based on the information obtained from the nucleotide sequence of cloned hepatitis-B virus (HBV) DNA of subtype *ayw* (Tiollais et al. 1981). Amino acid analysis confirmed the composition of the synthesized sequences; residues between 1 and 20, 21 and 47, and 156 and 185 were insoluble in the aqueous medium. Each of the four unconjugated polypeptide fragments emulsified in complete Freund's adjuvant was administered subcutaneously to a group of three rabbits at multiple sites. All polypeptide fragments were shown to be immunogenic by the induction of antibodies against HBsAg (anti-HBs). The rapid appearance of anti-HBs activity was observed after one booster inoculation in rabbits immunized with fragments of residues 1–20 and 48–81 (Fig. 1A,C). Anti-HBs titers were maintained in responders at 1:625 (measured by radioimmunoassay) for a period of at least 5 weeks (Fig. 2A,B). Antibody levels equivalent to 9375 and 6250 mIU/ml were observed 9 weeks postimmunization in some of the rabbits that received peptides 1–20 and 48–81, respectively. Lower antibody responses were seen in rabbits immunized with peptides 21–47 and 156–185 (Fig. 1B,D). With the exception of one animal that received peptide 21–47, all rabbits produced specific antibodies to HBsAg. Thus, short peptide fragments without coupling to a carrier protein were able to induce antibodies that reacted with the intact HBsAg. The insolubility in aqueous medium of three of the four polypep-

127

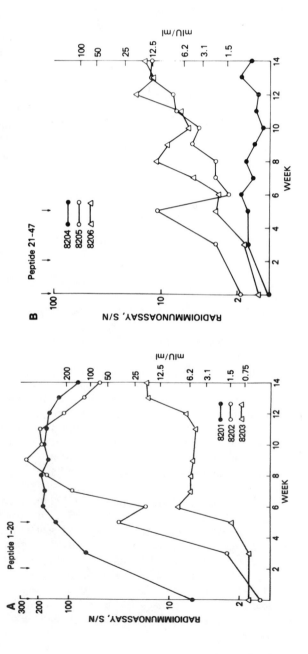

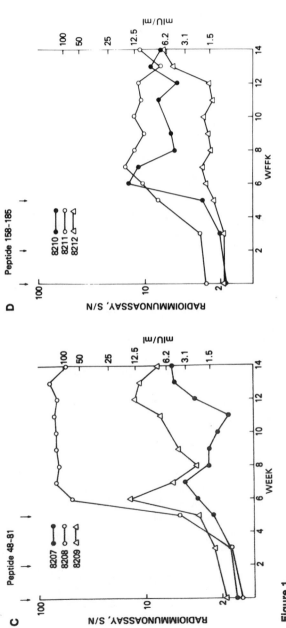

Figure 1

Immune response of rabbits to synthetic HBsAg polypeptide fragments of residues 1–20 (A), 21–47 (B), 48–81 (C), and 156–185 (D). Arrows indicate where first immunization or subsequent booster exposures to peptide fragments were administered.

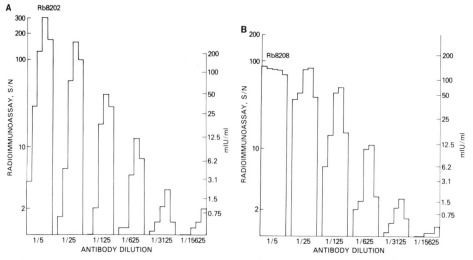

Figure 2
Anti-HBs titer of antibodies against peptide fragment 1–20 (A) and 48–81 (B). Serial bleedings from week 6, 7, 8, 9, and 12 from rabbit 8202 (peptide 1–20) and 8208 (peptide 48–81) were diluted and tested for anti-HBs activity against the WHO anti-HBs International Reference Preparation.

tides might have facilitated the immune response; each of the polypeptides was administered with adjuvant.

The anti-HBs fragments were analyzed for their subtype specificity by a modification of the procedure of Hoofnagle et al. (1977), using the HBsAg subtyping panel of the 1975 Paris Workshop (Courouce et al. 1976), as well as predetermined antigen subtypes characterized in our laboratory. All antibodies used behaved as monospecific antibodies. This result was not unexpected since each polypeptide immunogen contained a small fraction of the antigenic determinants of native HBsAg. Antibodies induced by fragment 21–47 reacted with all presubtyped antigens used in the blocking radioimmunoassay. This antibody activity appeared to represent anti-group-specific determinant activity, designated *a* according to the conventional serological identification scheme. The specificities of antibodies against other polypeptide fragments were undefinable by this procedure. The blocking assay showed clear-cut reactivity, either inhibition or no reaction with the testing antigens of known subtypes, but without a definite reaction pattern with respect to the subtype determinants. The complexity of the reaction patterns is illustrated in Table 1 and probably represents heterogeneity among the epitopes on the synthetic peptides and on the testing antigen and/or the quantitative and qualitative differences of the epitopes present on the different competing antigens. In either case, these data suggest that the conventional concept of a group-specific determinant, *a,* representing only one single common site requires revision.

Since antibody activity to the common group determinant is believed to be the only required protective antibody against the infection by different subtypes of

Table 1
Specificity of Rabbit Antibodies Elicited by Synthetic HBsAg Fragments

Rabbit no.	Residues	Blocking HBsAg subtype (% inhibition)[a]									
		ayw1	ayw2	ayw3	ayr	adw	adw4	adr	adw	ayw	adr
8202	1–20	93.8(+)	102(+)	0(−)	15.0(−)	100(+)	0.7(−)	0(−)	101(+)	100(+)	14.8(−)
8206	21–47	72.3(+)	76.1(+)	63.3(+)	71.1(+)	90.2(+)	51.9(+)	59.4(+)	98.2(+)	80.2(+)	75.5(+)
8208	48–81	97.9(+)	98.3(+)	4.0(−)	15.0(−)	94.4(+)	27.8(−)	8.4(−)	99.3(+)	18.9(−)	4.2(−)
8211	156–185	97.6(+)	11.2(−)	0(−)	2.3(−)	100(+)	2.3(−)	75.8(+)	100(+)	0.5(−)	0(−)

[a]First seven columns are HBsAg-positive sera subtyped at the First International Workshop, Paris, 1975. The last three columns are HBsAg-positive sera subtyped in our laboratory.

HBV (Murphy et al. 1974), the ability to identify the "neutralizing" antibody and its association with specific antigenic determinant(s) would be essential in designing a synthetic vaccine. The presence of more than one of the common group-specific determinants and their heterogeneity in distribution on the HBsAg particles could pose difficulty in identifying the biological functions of the selected synthetic peptide fragments.

REFERENCES

Courouce, A.M., P.V. Holland, J.Y. Muller, and J.P. Soulier, eds. 1976. *HBs antigen subtypes.* Karger, Basel.

Hoofnagle, J.H., R.J. Gerety, L.A. Smallwood, and L.F. Barker. 1977. Subtyping of hepatitis B surface antigen and antibody by radioimmunoassay. *Gastroenterology* **72:** 290.

Merrifield, R.B. 1963. Solid phase peptide synthesis. I. The synthesis of a tetrapeptide. *J. Am. Chem. Soc.* **85:** 2149.

Merrifield, R.B., L.D. Vizioli, and G.H. Boman. 1982. Synthesis of the antibacterial peptide Cecropin A (1-33). *Biochemistry* **21:** 5020.

Murphy, B.L., J.E. Maynard, and G.L. LeBouvier. 1974. Viral subtypes and cross-protection in hepatitis B virus infections of chimpanzees. *Intervirology* **3:** 378.

Tiollais, P., P. Charnay, and G.N. Vyas. 1981. Biology of hepatitis B virus. *Science* **213:** 406.

A General Method to Prepare Synthetic Peptide Conjugates

J.M. Robert Parker, Smita Bhargava, and Robert S. Hodges

*Department of Biochemistry, and the
Medical Research Council of Canada Group in
Protein Structure and Function
University of Alberta, Edmonton, Canada T6G 2H7*

Antibodies of selected specificity derived from synthetic peptide conjugates are utilized in various ways. These antibodies can be used to detect proteins predicted on the basis of nucleic acid sequences, to localize functionally active regions, and to follow the fate of protein domains both in studying exon usage during gene expression and in protein maturation. Synthetic peptide conjugates, which have been shown to induce neutralization antibodies to virus infections, are currently being studied to produce synthetic vaccines (Lerner 1982).

Several methods to prepare peptide conjugates, including carbodiimides, glutaraldehyde and bis-derivatized imidates, diazotized benzidines, N-hydroxysuccinimides, and maleimides, are employed to couple peptides to protein carriers. Of the many problems inherent with these reagents, perhaps the most outstanding is that they require a specific reactive group in the peptide. This can result in modification of functional groups such as amino, carboxyl, or sulfhydryl in the antigenic site itself. It is possible to incorporate at the carboxyl or amino terminus of the synthetic peptide an amino acid residue with a reactive functional group that does not occur in the antigenic site. However, this route would require a variety of coupling reagents and reaction conditions for every peptide sequence examined. Moreover, many bifunctional cross-linking reagents that require specific functional groups on the carrier for coupling restrict one's choice of a carrier molecule.

To avoid these problems, we are presenting a universal method using photoaffinity cross-linking reagents that are incorporated directly on the peptide during synthesis. It is important to note that no modification of any amino acid on the antigenic site will occur with this strategy. These reagents are stable under the

133

strong acidic conditions used in peptide synthesis, which are required to remove benzyl-type protecting groups as well as cleave the peptide from the resin. The photoprobes are inert until photolysis and are nonspecific for cross-linking so that carriers other than protein can be used.

EXPERIMENTAL PROCEDURES

Peptide Synthesis and Purification

Peptides were synthesized on a Beckman synthesizer (Model 990) with standard solid-phase methodology. The a-amino groups were protected by the Boc group, and the functional side chains were protected by benzyl-type protecting groups. Deprotection of Boc groups was carried out with 50% trifluoroacetic acid (TFA)/ methylene chloride, neutralization was carried out with 5% diisopropylethyl amine (DIEA)/methylene chloride, and two couplings of Boc-amino acids were performed for each amino acid residue, with diisopropyl carbodiimide (DIC) in trifluoroethanol/methylene chloride. The peptide was cleaved from the solid support (co-poly [styrene, 1% divinyl-benzene] benzhydrylamine•HCl resin or co-poly [styrene, 1% divinyl-benzene] chloromethyl resin) with hydrofluoric acid (HF)-anisole (10%) at 4°C. The crude probe peptides were purified on a reverse-phase high-performance liquid chromatography (HPLC) column (4.6 mm × 7.5 cm, Beckman Ultrapore C3; solvent A = 0.1% TFA/H_2O, solvent B = 0.05% TFA/ acetonitrile, gradient 1% B/min, flow = 1 ml/min).

Synthesis of Cross-linker

N^ϵ-(4-Benzoylbenzoyl)-N^α-t-butyloxycarbonyl-lysine. A solution of N^α-t-butyloxycarbonyl-lysine (246 mg, 1 mmole) in 1 M sodium bicarbonate (3 ml) was added to a suspension of N-hydroxysuccinimide ester of 4-benzoylbenzoic acid (300 mg, 0.9 mmole) in p-dioxane (8 ml) and stirred at room temperature overnight. The clear solution was diluted with H_2O (5 ml) and adjusted to pH 3.5 with citric acid. The solution was extracted with methylene chloride (3 times, 20 ml). The organic extracts were dried with sodium sulfate and concentrated to a white powder. This residue can be used directly or purified by reverse-phase HPLC on Synchropak RP-C18 preparative column (250 × 10 mm, flow = 4 ml/min, solvent A = H_2O, solvent B = acetonitrile, gradient 1% B/min).

Preparation of Peptide Conjugates

A five-to-one molar ratio of peptide to bovine serum albumin Fraction V (BSA) (1–2 mg of lyophilized probe peptide was dissolved in 75–150 μl of BSA stock solution prepared by dissolving 600 mg of BSA in 0.1 M KH_2PO_4 [5 ml] at pH 6.8) was photolyzed at 4°C for 1 hour in a RPR-208 preparative reactor equipped with RPR 3500-Å lamps (Rayonet, The Southern New England Ultraviolet Co.). The peptide conjugates were purified by reverse-phase HPLC on Synchropak RP-C18 column (250 × 10 mm, flow = 4 ml/min, solvent A = 0.1% TFA/H_2O, solvent B = 0.05% TFA/acetonitrile, gradient 2% B/min).

RESULTS

The four photoprobes studied are listed in Figure 1. The synthesis of (4-benzoyl-benzoyl)-glycine (BBGly) was first reported by Galardy et al. (1974). Escher et al. (1982) reported the use of p-NO$_2$-Phe as a photoprobe. N^ϵ-(4-Benzoylbenzoyl)-N^α-t-butyloxycarbonyl-lysine (Boc-BBLys) was synthesized from N^α-Boc-Lys as described in Experimental Procedures. Hodges and co-workers described the synthesis and applications of the N-hydroxysuccinimide ester of 4-azidobenzoic acid (ABOSu) (Chong and Hodges 1981; Worobec et al. 1983; Watts et al. 1983). Each of the photoprobes BBGly, BBLys, and pNO$_2$Phe was coupled directly on the resin after the peptide sequence had been synthesized by standard solid-phase methodology. These products were cleaved from the resin with HF and purified by HPLC. The azide photoprobe cannot be coupled directly to the peptide resin, since it is not stable under HF cleavage conditions. The peptide was synthesized, cleaved with HF, derivatized with ABOSu, and purified by HPLC.

A solution of probe peptide and BSA in 0.1 M KH$_2$PO$_4$ buffer (pH 6.8) was photolyzed for periods of 1/2, 1, and 3 hours. The peptide conjugates were purified by reverse-phase HPLC. The results are shown in Figure 2. BBGly and BBLys gave the best incorporation. This allows us to report a general strategy for synthetic peptide conjugates containing the protein aminoterminal amino acid residue, the protein carboxyterminal amino acid residue, or internal regions of the protein (Fig. 3). This is important since the amino- or carboxyterminal amino acid residue could be involved in the antigenic site.

The BBGly probe is added to the amino terminus of a synthetic peptide. We propose the incorporation of ^{14}C-labeled glycine preceding BBGly. This results in a two-residue spacer between the cross-linker attached to the carrier and the antigenic site. The radioactive label allows one to determine the degree of peptide incorporation onto carrier after photolysis. Similarly, we are recommending

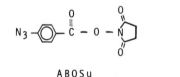

Figure 1
Structure of photoaffinity probes used in the preparation of synthetic peptide conjugates. (BBGly) N-(4-Benzoylbenzoyl)-glycine; (Boc-BBLys) N^ϵ-(4-benzoylbenzoyl)-N^α-t-butyloxy-carbonyl-lysine; (ABOSu) N-hydroxysuccinimide ester of 4-azidobenzoic acid; (Boc-p-NO$_2$-Phe) N^α-t-butyloxycarbonyl-p-nitrophenylalanine.

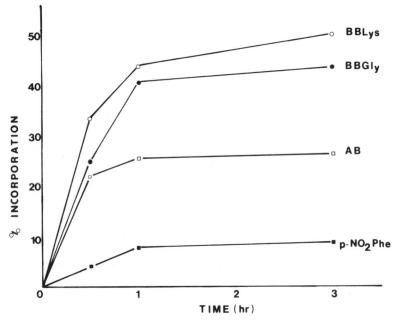

Figure 2
Incorporation of photoaffinity-labeled peptides to protein carrier (BSA, Fraction V). The photoprobes, BBGly (●), BBLys (○), and p-NO₂-Phe (■), were coupled to the aminoterminal residue to the peptide resin during solid-phase synthesis. 4-Azidobenzoyl (AB, □) was coupled to the free peptide. The sequence of the peptide is Glu-Leu-Ala-Pro-Glu-Asp-Pro-Glu-Asp-Ser, herpes simplex virus (type I)-glycoprotein D (292–301).

the coupling of BBLys to the resin, followed by ^{14}C-labeled glycine before the antigenic sequence, for synthetic peptides containing the aminoterminal residue of a protein. In this case, lysine and glycine act as a spacer. One may suggest that BBLys be used at either end of the antigenic sequence and serve as a universal cross-linker. However, for economical reasons as well as ease in chemical synthesis, we suggest that BBGly is suitable for most approaches.

The incorporation of BBGly or BBLys during peptide synthesis is readily verified where amino acid analysis indicates the addition of glycine for BBGly or lysine for BBLys. The benzophenone moiety offers another unique advantage during purification by HPLC. This group is detected by its strong absorption at 260 nm and is easily distinguished from peptides not coupled to the probe. Since the extinction of BBGly and BBLys ($\varepsilon_{260} = 26,000$) is greater than that for tyrosine or phenylalanine, the absorption of the photoprobes is unaffected if these other chromophores are present in the antigenic sequence. In addition, the hydrophobic character of benzophenone will add to the binding property of a hydrophilic peptide sequence in reverse-phase HPLC. It then offers unique photochemical properties for cross-linking the peptide to carrier. The free radical generated on photolysis is stable in aqueous solution until proton abstraction occurs. This results in a higher cross-linking efficiency when compared with the relatively unstable intermediates generated in azide photolysis. This is demonstrated in Figure

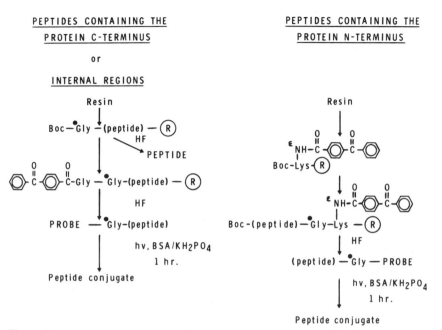

Figure 3

Strategy to prepare synthetic peptide conjugates. Standard solid-phase methodology is used for chemical synthesis of peptides. BBGly is used as the photoaffinity cross-linker when the synthetic peptide represents internal regions or contains the carboxyterminal residue of the protein. BBLys is used when the synthetic peptides contain the aminoterminal residue of a protein. Gly (●) represents the ^{14}C-labeled glycine residue used to determine the degree of incorporation of peptide into carrier. HF is used to cleave the peptide or peptide probe from the solid support. BSA, Fraction V, was used as the carrier.

2, where BBLys and BBGly peptides were incorporated at significantly higher levels than the *p*-azidobenzoyl peptide.

In these experiments, we used BSA as the carrier molecule. However, since photolysis requires no specific functional group on the carrier other than carbon-hydrogen bonds, different proteins or carriers other than proteins can be used.

CONCLUSIONS

Using the photoaffinity approach to prepare peptide conjugates, these studies have led to the following conclusions:

1. We have developed a universal strategy to prepare synthetic peptide conjugates.

2. BBGly or BBLys can be synthesized directly onto the peptide at the carboxyl or amino terminus and is stable to strong acids used to cleave the synthetic peptide from the resin and remove protecting groups in solid-phase peptide synthesis.

3. The use of benzophenone as a cross-linker is independent of the antigenic sequence. For example, BBLys could be used for all sequences.

4. The benzophenone moiety is carrier-independent.

This methodology is currently being used in our laboratory to study the antigenic determinants of herpes simplex virus (types I and II) glycoproteins with the eventual goal of studying their function and preparing a synthetic vaccine.

REFERENCES

Chong, P.C.S. and R.S. Hodges. 1981. A new heterobifunctional cross-linking reagent for the study of biological interactions between proteins. I. Design, synthesis and characterization. *J. Biol. Chem.* **256:** 5064.

Escher, E., R. Couture, G. Champagne, J. Mizrah, and D. Regoli. 1982. Synthesis and biological activities of photoaffinity labelling analogues of substance P. *J. Med. Chem.* **25:** 470.

Galardy, R.E., L.C. Craig, J.D. Jamieson, and M.P. Printz. 1974. Photoaffinity labelling of peptide hormone binding sites. *J. Biol. Chem.* **249:** 3510.

Lerner, R.A. 1982. Tapping the immunological repertoire to produce antibodies of predetermined specificity. *Nature* **299:** 592.

Watts, T.H., P.A. Sastry, R.S. Hodges, and W. Paranchych. 1983. Mapping of the antigenic determinants of *Pseudomonas aeruginosa* PAK polar pili. *Infect. Immun.* **42:** 113.

Worobec, E.A., A.K. Taneja, R.S. Hodges, and W. Paranchych. 1983. Localization of the major antigenic determinant of EDP208 pili at the N-terminus of the pilus protein. *J. Bacteriol.* **153:** 955.

Localization of the Immunodominant Domains of Rabies Virus Glycoprotein

Roderick I. Macfarlan, Bernhard Dietzschold,
and Hilary Koprowski
The Wistar Institute of Anatomy and Biology
Philadelphia, Pennsylvania 19104

Mary Kiel, Richard Houghten,
Richard A. Lerner, and J. Gregor Sutcliffe
The Scripps Clinic and Research Foundation
La Jolla, California 92037

The glycoprotein of rabies virus is the only virion component that induces the production of and reacts with neutralizing antibody and that protects animals from challenge (Wiktor et al. 1973). The next generation of rabies vaccines could therefore consist of either the glycoprotein (perhaps produced using recombinant methods) or chemically synthesized peptides representing immunogenic segments of the glycoprotein. With this in mind, a number of approaches have been used to define which segments possess immunoreactivity.

Biological Activities of Cyanogen Bromide Cleavage Peptides

Glycoprotein was isolated from the ERA strain of rabies virus by means of a monoclonal antibody affinity column and then subjected to cyanogen bromide (CNBr) cleavage. The fragments were reduced and carboxymethylated and then separated by SDS gel electrophoresis. The aminoterminal sequence of each of seven large peptides was determined and compared with the deduced amino acid sequence of the glycoprotein (Anilionis et al. 1981). Peptides designated Cr1, Cr2, Cr2A, Cr3, Cr4, Cr5, Cr6, and Cr7 corresponded to residues 1–44, 244–291, 386–452, 292–323, 103–178, 324–376, 188–236, and 57–102, respectively. Peptides Cr2 and Cr2A resolved as a single band and were differentiated only after sequencing (Dietzschold et al. 1982).

To determine whether these peptides could induce antibody responses, mice were inoculated with individual peptides emulsified in Freund's adjuvant. After two boosts, serum antibody titers were determined. It was found that although all peptides induced glycoprotein-binding antibody, the highest titers were obtained with sera against Cr1, Cr2 + Cr2A, Cr3, and Cr4. Furthermore, these were the only peptides that induced neutralizing antibody. In the rapid fluorescent focus inhibition test, titers were 180 (Cr1), 60 (Cr2 + Cr2A), 270 (Cr3), and 510 (Cr4), expressed as the reciprocal dilution of serum resulting in 50% reduction of infection (Dietzschold et al. 1982).

Because rabies glycoprotein is a T-dependent antigen, these reduced CNBr peptides were tested for their capacity to stimulate proliferation of virus-primed splenic T lymphocytes from A/J mice, using a modification of the assay described by Walker et al. (1981). Figure 1 shows that viral glycoprotein stimulated a strong in vitro proliferative response, as measured by [³H]thymidine incorporation on day 5 of culture; a mixture of reduced CNBr peptides also stimulated a response. Of the isolated peptides, significant proliferation was seen with Cr1, Cr2 + Cr2A, and Cr3; Cr4, Cr5, Cr6, and Cr7 did not stimulate. Not shown are results demonstrating that prior immunization of the mice was necessary for a proliferative response to any of these antigens. It is interesting that Cr4 gave rise to a strong antibody response, yet failed to stimulate T cells in vitro. The proliferation assay will measure only T-cell specificities that have been expanded following priming of mice with virus. If Cr4 had acquired new T-cell-stimulating structures as a result of partial unfolding, then it might be expected that this peptide could stim-

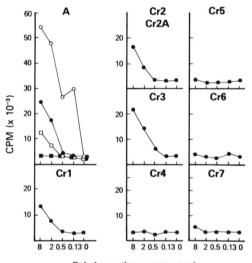

Relative antigen concentration
(based on μg/ml of glycoprotein)

Figure 1
Stimulation of rabies-specific lymphocytes by glycoprotein antigens. Spleen cells from rabies-immune A/J mice were passed through nylon wool columns. The resulting T lymphocytes were cultured (2.5 × 10⁶/ml) with irradiated spleen cells from nonimmunized A/J mice (2.5 × 10⁶/ml) plus various antigens. Proliferation was evaluated on day 5 of culture by measuring incorporation of [³H]thymidine added 16 hr previously. (A) Native glycoprotein (○); CNBr-cleaved glycoprotein (●); trypsin-cleaved glycoprotein (□); chymotrypsin-cleaved glycoprotein (■). Other panels show stimulation with isolated reduced CNBr fragments as indicated.

ulate a primary T-dependent antibody response in vivo, yet fail to stimulate a secondary proliferative response by virus-primed lymphocytes in vitro. It should also be noted that although the data in Figure 1 indicate that three T-cell determinants are shared between native glycoprotein and reduced CNBr fragments, this figure is a minimum estimate.

Biological Activities of Synthetic Peptides

On the basis of hydrophilicity and partial homology with biologically active CNBr peptides, 26 peptides were synthesized. These ranged in size from 6 to 36 residues and covered most of the glycoprotein sequence. These peptides were used to stimulate virus-primed T lymphocytes. Figure 2 shows the positive results obtained. Synthetic peptide R21, and to a lesser extent R20, stimulated proliferation. R21 was as potent as glycoprotein; however, there was a large shift in the dose-response curve, particularly when considered in molar concentrations. Conjugation of peptide R21 with keyhole limpet hemocyanin (KLH) did not change its activity. The lack of stimulation seen with peptide R23 is representative of results obtained with all other synthetic peptides tested, including those sharing sequences with Cr2 and Cr3. Both R21 (residues 9–44) and R20 (residues 32–44) share amino acid sequences with Cr1 (residues 1–44). Other peptides from this region that did not stimulate were R1 (residues 1–25), R2 (residues 23–35), and R25 (residues 10–31). Thus, the data are consistent with a major T-cell determi-

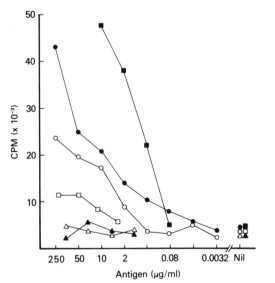

Figure 2
Stimulation of rabies-specific T lymphocytes by synthetic peptides. (●) Peptide R21; (○) peptide R21-KLH; (□) peptide R20; (△) peptide R23; (▲) peptide R23-KLH; (■) glycoprotein. See Fig. 1 for methodology. Vertical axis is incorporation of [³H]thymidine on day 5 of culture.

nant located toward the carboxyl terminus of Cr1 and the amino terminus of the glycoprotein molecule.

Following inoculation of mice with R21 conjugated with KLH, very low titers of virus-neutralizing antibody were obtained. However, most of the response was to KLH determinants. These immunization experiments are being repeated using unconjugated peptide R21, which is of sufficient size (36 residues) to act as its own carrier and has been shown to have T-cell reactivity.

Subpopulations of Lymphocytes Stimulated by Peptides

Monoclonal antibodies toward lymphocyte differentiation antigens were used to examine the phenotype of lymphocytes responding to stimulation. Table 1 shows that glycoprotein R21 and R20 stimulated exclusively T lymphocytes (Thy-1-positive, Iak-negative). There was a significant difference between glycoprotein and the peptides, however, in that only the latter stimulated proliferation of Lyt-2-positive lymphocytes. In some experiments, Lyt-2 antigen could be detected on 40% of lymphocytes responding to peptide R21. Lyt-2 is expressed by both cytotoxic and suppressor T lymphocytes. Experiments are being carried out to determine the function of these Lyt-2-positive cells and whether they play a role in immunization. Preliminary results indicate that culture supernatants from R21-stimulated cultures contain interleukin 2, demonstrating that at least some of the T lymphocytes have helper function.

DISCUSSION

There are two main problems in designing a synthetic vaccine. The first is to define a peptide sufficiently similar to a structure in the native molecule to enable

Table 1
Cell-surface Phenotype of Proliferating Cells

Antigen	Complement	Monoclonal antibody			
		a-Thy-1	a-Lyt-1	a-Lyt-2	a-Iak
Glycoprotein	—	0.8[a]	0	3.4	0
(2 µg/ml)	1/30	77.6	37.6	1.8	0
R20	—	0[a]	0	0	0
(125 µg/ml)	1/30	76.0	30.5	8.6	0
R21	—	0.8[a]	0	0	0
(125 µg/ml)	1/30	79.4	41.3	14.7	0
	1/10	96.2	89.7	37.5	1.1
Glycoprotein	—	2.0[b]	14.1	6.1	n.t.
(2 µg/ml)	1/10	55.3	58.1	5.5	n.t.

Lymphocytes were cultured with antigen as indicated for Fig. 1, except that the viable cells were recovered from culture and subjected to treatment with monoclonal antibody plus rabbit complement. n.t. indicates not tested.
[a]Percentage of cells killed measured by dye exclusion.
[b]Percentage of inhibition of [^{3}H]thymidine incorporation after treatment.

immunological cross-reaction, and the second is to find conditions under which the peptide is immunogenic. Our contention is that these two steps are best evaluated independently. In other words, tests of immunogenicity (such as production of neutralizing antibody) should not be used to search for immunoreactive peptides. The approach used here has been to examine the reactivity of peptides with virus-primed lymphocytes. A rabies-immunoreactive peptide (R21) has been identified, and the next task is to enhance its immunogenicity. At this stage in the development of synthetic peptide technology, some generalizations are applicable: (1) The use of strong carriers (such as KLH) may result in a primarily anticarrier immune response. (2) The kinetics of antipeptide immune responses may be markedly different from those of anti-large-protein responses. (3) In some systems, it may not be necessary to achieve high levels of neutralizing antibody, but rather to prime animals to make a rapid secondary response upon challenge.

ACKNOWLEDGMENT

This work was supported by grant AI-09706 from the National Institute of Allergy and Infectious Diseases.

REFERENCES

Anilionis, A., W.H. Wunner, and P.J. Curtis. 1981. Structure of the glycoprotein gene in rabies virus. *Nature* **284:** 275.

Dietzschold, B., T.J. Wiktor, R. Macfarlan, and A. Varrichio. 1982. Antigenic structure of rabies virus glycoprotein. Ordering and immunological characterization of the large CNBr cleavage fragments. *J. Virol.* **44:** 595.

Walker, S.M., E.L. Morgan, and W.O. Weigle. 1981. Regulation of the in vitro secondary antibody response. II. Antigen-induced murine splenic T cell proliferation. *J. Immunol.* **126:** 766.

Wiktor, T.J., E. Gyorgy, M.D. Schlumberger, F. Sokol, and H. Koprowski. 1973. Antigenic properties of rabies virus components. *J. Immunol.* **110:** 269.

Synthesis of an Antigenic Determinant of the HSV gD That Stimulates the Induction of Virus-neutralizing Antibodies and Confers Protection against a Lethal Challenge of HSV

Bernhard Dietzschold and Angela Varrichio
The Wistar Institute of Anatomy and Biology
Philadelphia, Pennsylvania 19104

Gary Cohen
Department of Microbiology and Center for
Oral Health Research, School of Dental
Medicine, University of Pennsylvania
Philadelphia, Pennsylvania 19104

Roselyn Eisenberg
Department of Microbiology, School of
Veterinary Medicine, University of Pennsylvania
Philadelphia, Pennsylvania 19104

One new approach in modern vaccine production utilizes short synthetic peptides selected from immunogenic proteins. For a given viral antigen, the strategy employed for the design of a synthetic peptide vaccine includes the prediction of immunogenic domains of the antigen and their chemical synthesis and attachment to suitable carriers. We have used this approach to produce a synthetic herpes vaccine.

Localization of an Antigenic Determinant of HSV Glycoprotein D

Herpes simplex virus glycoprotein D (HSV gD) appears to be the major structural antigen of the virus responsible for the induction of humoral and cellular immunity. Using a panel of gD-specific monoclonal antibodies, eight separate antigenic determinants were delineated on the gD molecule (Eisenberg et al. 1982). The group VII monoclonal antibody (no. 170), which has neutralizing activity, rec-

145

ognized gD that had been reduced and alkylated, indicating that the determinants specified by this monoclonal antibody appear to be continuous or sequential in nature. The determinant was then localized employing chemical and immunological analysis of gD-1 cleavage fragments.

After V8-protease digestion of gD-1, a 12,000-dalton fragment was isolated that bound to the group VII monoclonal antibody. This fragment contained a type-common, arginine-containing, tryptic fragment designated f (Cohen et al. 1983). The sequence of this peptide (N-Met-Ala-Asp-Pro-Asn-Arg-C) matched residues 11–16 of the deduced amino acid sequence of gD (Cohen et al. 1983), indicating that the determinant recognized by the group VII monoclonal antibody is localized near the amino terminus of the gD molecule.

The secondary structure of gD was predicted from the rules established by Chou and Fasman (1974). Using stringent criteria (the probability of a β-turn is $\geq 5 \times 10^{-5}$), 17 β-turns were predicted for the gD sequence. The first predicted β-turn at the amino terminus is the most important because it includes the sequence of f, the type-common peptide. As predicted by the Hopp and Woods analysis (1981), the sequence of this first β-turn is highly hydrophilic.

Peptide Synthesis

Chemical and immunological information obtained from cleavage fragments, together with the computer analysis, which predicted the secondary structure and hydrophilicity of gD, localized a major antigenic determinant of gD. To characterize the fine structure of this determinant, we synthesized overlapping peptides ranging from 7 to 23 amino acids in length, and covering positions 1–23 of the gD sequence.

Binding Properties of Peptides

The synthetic peptides were then tested for their ability to react with gD-specific polyclonal and monoclonal antibodies. An antigen spot test employing different antigens and antisera is shown in Figure 1. In the lower panel, monoclonal antibody 170 can be seen to react with gD-1, gD-2, and synthetic peptides ranging from amino acids 8 to 23, 3 to 23, and 1 to 23 of gD. Rabbit anti-gD-1 hyperimmune serum reacted exactly as the monoclonal antibody 170 did but also recognized the shorter peptides ranging from amino acid positions 17 to 23 and 13 to 23 of gD. In contrast, rabbit anti-gD-2 hyperimmune serum only recognized the largest peptide (1–23) as seen in panels 3 and 4.

The fact that the synthetic peptide ranging from amino acid 3 to 23 was not recognized by the anti-gD-2 immune serum implicated the lysine residues at positions 1 and 10 in the anti-gD-2 recognition process. To confirm this implication, peptide 1–23 was citraconylated, and the activity with the anti-gD-2 immune serum was abolished. Furthermore, after removal of the blocking group, the activity was restored, proving the importance of the lysine residues in the recognition process by anti-gD-2 immune serum.

To localize specifically the region of peptide 1–23 that reacts with gD-2, we then synthesized a series of peptides ranging from residues 1 to 16 with either

ANTIGEN

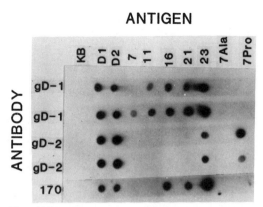

Figure 1
Dot-blot analysis of synthetic peptides, gD-1, and gD-2 with polyclonal and monoclonal anti-gD antibodies. Nitrocellulose strips were spotted with purified gD-1, gD-2, and synthetic peptides and treated as described recently (Cohen et al. 1983). The strips were then allowed to react with the antibodies. After incubation, the bound antibodies were visualized with ^{125}I-labeled ProA by autoradiography.

alanine (HSV-1-specific) or proline (HSV-2-specific) at position 7. In Figure 1, we show that the peptide with alanine at position 7 (7Ala) did not react with any of the antisera, whereas the same peptide with proline at position 7 (7Pro) was recognized only by the anti-gD-2 immune serum. This single amino acid substitution from alanine to proline at position 7 results in an additional β-turn at the amino terminus. This additional β-turn probably represents the binding site for anti-gD-2 immune sera.

Immunogenicity of Peptides

After coupling to either keyhole limpet hemocyanin (KLH) or ovalbumin (OVA), the immunogenicities of peptides 1–23 and 8–23 were assessed by injecting them into rabbits or mice. Immunoprecipitates from lysates of HSV-1-infected KB cells or HSV-2-infected BHK cells labeled with [^{35}S]methionine were analyzed by SDS-polyacrylamide gel electrophoresis (data not shown). Similarly to the anti-gD-1 and anti-gD-2 immune sera, antisera raised against peptide 8–23 specifically precipitated pgD-1 and pgD-2. The reactivity of the antipeptide sera was also tested in a dot-blot assay. The antisera raised against peptides 8–23 and 1–23 both recognized gD-1. However, only the sera raised against peptide 1–23 recognized gD-2, and the reactivity was significantly less than that obtained for gD-1.

Neutralizing Activity of Peptide Antisera

The group VII monoclonal antibody, which recognized peptides 1–23, 3–23, and 8–23, exhibited low titers of neutralizing antibodies. Therefore, antisera prepared against peptides 1–23, 3–23, and 8–23 were tested for their capability to neutralize HSV-1 or HSV-2. As demonstrated in Table 1, immune sera from mice prepared against peptide 1–23 or peptide 8–23 coupled to either KLH or OVA neutralized both HSV-1 and HSV-2. The neutralizing titer against HSV-1 was about four times higher than the neutralizing activity against HSV-2. The neutralizing activity of this antipeptide sera is comparable to that of the group VII monoclonal antibody 170.

Protection Experiments with Synthetic Peptides

To investigate whether peptides can confer protection against a lethal challenge infection with HSV-2, groups of mice were immunized with KLH, gD-1, or peptide 1–23 or peptide 8–23, both coupled to KLH. Complete Freund's adjuvant was used in each immunization. It can be depicted from Table 2 that 80% of animals immunized with either one of the conjugated peptides survived the challenge. The observation that only a partial protection against HSV-2 could be induced with a peptide vaccine can be attributed to the fact that most of the immunological activities of the peptides are directed against gD-1. Peptides with an identical sequence to gD-2 are currently being investigated for their immunizing capacity.

It should be mentioned in this context that recognition of these peptides by human T lymphocytes is being studied. Donor T lymphocytes, primed in vitro with peptide 1–23, give a unique response pattern for each individual tested upon restimulation with peptide 1–23 and its subsets. Furthermore, when the experiments were repeated at a later time, T lymphocytes donated from the same individual gave a response pattern identical with that obtained previously. These data suggest that the recognition of these peptides by T lymphocytes is genetically restricted (E. DeFrietas, unpubl.). The fact that human T lymphocytes can

Table 1
Serum Neutralization of HSV Infectivity

Antiserum	Neutralization titer (50% reduction)[a]	
	HSV-1 (HF)	HSV-2 (Savage)
gD-1	1024	800
gD-2	640	1600
Group VII mAb 170	64	32
8–23	0	0
8–23-KLH	64	8
8–23-OVA	8	8
1–23-KLH	80	20
1–23-OVA	120	30

BALB/c mice were immunized four times at biweekly intervals by intraperitoneal injection of 15 μg of peptide 8–23 or 1–23 alone or covalently bound to either KLH or OVA and emulsified in 50% complete Freund's adjuvant. Control mice were sham-immunized with complete Freund's adjuvant alone.
[a]HF and Savage are strains of HSV-1 and HSV-2, respectively.

Table 2
Protection of BALB/c Mice against Lethal
Challenge by HSV-2

Immunization group[a]	Survivors after challenge
KLH/CFA	0/10
gD-1/CFA	10/10
8–23-KLH/CFA	8/10
1–23-KLH/CFA	8/10

[a]Groups were challenged intraperitoneally with 10 LD_{50} of HSV-2 14 days after final immunization. Each mouse was immunized with a total of 6 μg of gD-1 or 200 μg of KLH peptide conjugate. Immunization procedure for mice is identical to the conditions described in Table 1, except that only peptides coupled to KLH were used for immunization. CFA indicates complete Freund's adjuvant.

be stimulated by synthetic peptides makes these peptides potentially useful for vaccination purposes. However, the genetic restriction of the T-cell stimulation by synthetic peptides should be taken into consideration.

ACKNOWLEDGMENT

This work was supported by U.S. Public Health Service grants AI-09768, AI-18289, and DE-02623 and by a grant to R.J.E. and G.H.C. from the American Cyanamid Company.

REFERENCES

Chou, P.W. and G.D. Fasman. 1974. Prediction of protein conformation. *Biochemistry* **13**: 222.

Cohen, G.H., B. Dietzschold, M. Ponce De Leon, D. Long, E. Golub, A. Varrichio, L. Pereira, and R.J. Eisenberg. 1983. Localization and synthesis of an antigenic determinant of herpes simplex virus glycoprotein D that stimulates the production of neutralizing antibody. *J. Virol.* **49**: 102.

Eisenberg, R.J., D. Long, L. Pereira, B. Hampar, M. Zweig, and G.H. Cohen. 1982. Effect of monoclonal antibodies on limited proteolysis of native glycoprotein gD of herpes simplex virus type 1. *J. Virol.* **41**: 478.

Hopp, T.P. and K.R. Woods. 1981. Prediction of protein antigenic determinants from amino acid sequences. *Proc. Natl. Acad. Sci.* **78**: 3824.

Structures in Influenza A/USSR/90/77 Hemagglutinin Associated with Epidemiologic and Antigenic Changes

Alan P. Kendal and Nancy J. Cox
WHO Collaborating Center for Influenza
Centers for Disease Control
Atlanta, Georgia 30333

Setsuko Nakajima and Katsuhisa Nakajima
Department of Microbiology
Institute of Public Health, Tokyo, Japan

**Lucy Raymond, Andy Caton,
and George Brownlee**
Department of Pathology
University of Oxford, Oxford, England

Robert G. Webster
Department of Virology, St. Jude
Children's Hospital for Research
Memphis, Tennessee 38101

Following the appearance of A/USSR/90/77 virus in 1977, several studies have been undertaken to investigate the properties of the antigenic sites in its hemagglutinin (HA). Such studies have involved the preparation of monoclonal antibodies specific for the A/USSR HA (by R.G.W.), the selection of variants in the presence of these monoclonal antibodies (by S.N. and K.N., who have now sequenced their HAs), and the sequencing of the HAs of several field strains that have evolved from A/USSR/77 in the period up to about mid-1980 (by A.C., G.B., and L.R.). In this paper, we summarize the findings of these studies using as a common theme the antigenic variation detected with monoclonal antibodies.

During the period from 1977 to 1980, a large number of H1N1 virus isolates were compared with a panel of monoclonal antibodies that had originally been shown by reaction with old, reference H1N1 strains from the 1950s to be directed at distinct epitopes. This analysis revealed first that considerable heterogeneity could be detected among the isolates, with about 20 different reaction types observed (Kendal et al. 1981) (Fig. 1), and second that, in 1978, a change in the HA appeared that resulted in lost reactivity with monoclonal antibody 264 (mAb

151

264). This change in the HA became conserved in all subsequent strains, and likewise a change resulting in lost reactivity with mAb 110 became conserved in strains appearing from 1980 to the present time (Webster et al. 1979; Cox et al. 1983).

In terms of epidemiologic properties, A/Brazil/11/78 was selected as the reference strain for variants bearing the single conserved change affecting reaction with mAb 264, and A/England/333/80 was selected as the reference strain for variants that, additionally, contained the conserved change affecting reaction with mAb 110. Thus, commencing in 1978, A/Brazil/11/78-like strains began to displace A/USSR/77-like strains, and commencing in 1980, A/England/333/80-like

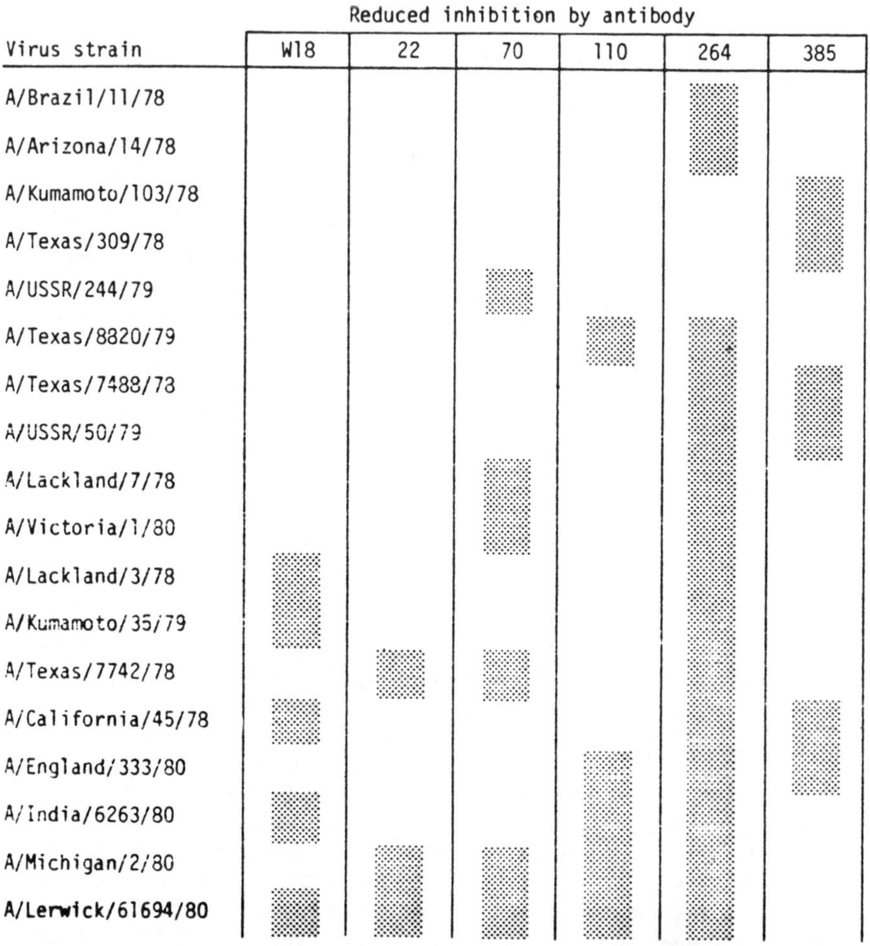

| | | Reduced inhibition by antibody | | | | |
Virus strain	W18	22	70	110	264	385
A/Brazil/11/78					▓	
A/Arizona/14/78					▓	
A/Kumamoto/103/78						▓
A/Texas/309/78						▓
A/USSR/244/79			▓			
A/Texas/8820/79				▓	▓	
A/Texas/7488/78					▓	▓
A/USSR/50/79					▓	
A/Lackland/7/78			▓		▓	
A/Victoria/1/80			▓		▓	
A/Lackland/3/78	▓				▓	
A/Kumamoto/35/79	▓				▓	
A/Texas/7742/78		▓	▓		▓	
A/California/45/78	▓				▓	▓
A/England/333/80				▓	▓	▓
A/India/6263/80	▓				▓	▓
A/Michigan/2/80		▓	▓		▓	
A/Lerwick/61694/80	▓	▓	▓		▓	

Figure 1
Monoclonal antibody reaction patterns of natural influenza A (H1N1) variants since 1977. Shaded area indicates significantly reduced HI reactivity with A/USSR/90/77 HA-specific monoclonal antibody.

Table 1
Monoclonal Antibody Reaction Patterns of Field Strains and Laboratory Variants
Whose HA$_1$ Sequence Has Been Determined

| | Selecting | HI titer with monoclonal antibody | | |
Antigen	antibody	264	W18	110
Field strains				
A/USSR/90/77	none	3200	1600	1600
A/Brazil/11/78	none	<100	800	1600
A/Lackland/3/78	none	<100	<100	1600
A/England/333/80	none	<100	1600	<100
A/India/6263/80	none	<100	200	<100
Laboratory mutants				
clone B-1	264	<100	3200	1200
clone C-2	W18	<100	≤100	1600
clone D-1	110	6400	3200	<100

strains displaced A/Brazil/11/78-like strains, and within each era all other variants shared the mutations detected with the monoclonal antibody panel, although, as shown in Figure 1, a proportion of the field strains had additional mutations in their HA.

It was of particular interest to determine the amino-acid-sequence changes responsible for loss of reactivity to those two monoclonal antibodies that were associated with evolution of successful new field strains. Mutants of A/USSR/77 were therefore prepared by growth in the presence of each monoclonal antibody (Nakajima and Kendal 1981). As shown in Table 1, laboratory variants were obtained that had lost the ability to react with the mAbs 264, 110, and W18. It was further shown that the epitope recognized by mAb W18 overlapped with that recognized by mAb 264, since variant C-2 selected with antibody W18 also failed to react with mAb 264, even though the reverse was not true for variant B-1 selected with mAb 264.

The amino acid changes detected in single clones of variants selected with mAbs W18, 264, and 110 are shown in Table 2. It can be seen that mAb 264 selected a variant with a single change at residue 190, and mAb 110 selected a variant with a single change at residue 125C. (The amino acid numbering system is based on that described by Winter et al. [1981], where sequence positions in H1 HA are maximally aligned with those in H3 HA; the suffix C after residue 125

Table 2
Sequence Mutations in Laboratory Variants Selected by mAbs W18,
264, and 110

Mutant	Selecting antibody	Amino acid sequence change
B-1	264	190: Asp to Asn
C-2	W18	125C: Arg to Gly; 189: Glu to Lys
D-1	110	125C: Arg to Lys

indicates that this is the last of a three-amino-acid insertion occurring in H1 HA compared with H3 HA after residue 125.)

The mutant selected with mAb W18, however, contained two amino acid changes; one was at residue 189. This is adjacent to the change at site 190 in the mutant B-1 selected with mAb 264, consistent with the existence of overlap between epitopes recognized by mAbs W18 and 264. However, the second mutation was at residue 125C, the same position where a mutation was selected by mAb 110, albeit resulting in a different amino acid substitution. Because the mutation in variant D-1 at site 125C had no effect on binding of mAb W18, the existence of a mutation at site 125C in variant C-2 selected by mAb W18 may have been quite coincidental. This is supported by sequence data of additional clones of variants selected with mAb W18 (unpubl.). These findings therefore suggested that residues 189 and 190 affected the binding of mAb W18 and/or mAb 264 and that an Arg to Lys mutation at residue 125C affected binding of mAb 110, although an Arg to Gly mutation at residue 125C did not.

The sequence analysis of field strains of H1N1 viruses is summarized in Figure 2. Because of the likelihood that a variety of mutations will occur in field strains of which only a proportion are biologically or antigenically significant (Both et al. 1983), it is highly desirable to sequence more than one field strain for each time point studied so as to identify which mutations are conserved. It can be seen that only six amino acid changes appear to have been conserved in HA₁ of viruses evolving up until A/Brazil/11/78.

None of these conserved mutations are in the same sequence (i.e., 189 and 190) found in the laboratory variants B-1 and C-2 that failed to react with mAb

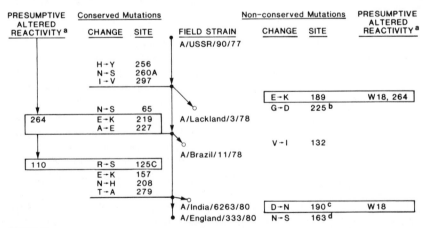

Figure 2
Evolution of influenza H1 HA, 1977-1980. (a) Lost reactivity with indicated monoclonal antibody. (b) Change at site 225 may also affect binding of mAb W18. (c) Change in reactivity with mAb W18 may result from the effect of mutation at site 190 in combination with the conserved change at sites 219 and/or 227. (d) Site 163 may affect binding of mAb 110, in addition to the conserved change at 125C. (●) Deduced evolutionary line containing mutations that are conserved in successive variants; (○) variants containing different (or additional) mutations that have not been conserved.

264, even though the 1978 field strains no longer reacted with this antibody. Examination of the three-dimensional structure of the HA, and assuming that a similar structure exists for H1 and H3 subtypes, reveals, however, that residues 219 and 227 (which have changed between 1977 and 1978 in field strains) are adjacent to each other and are adjacent to residues 189 and 190. The only reasonable explanation that can be found for the loss of reactivity by the field strains to mAb 264, therefore, is the conserved mutations Glu to Lys and Ala to Glu in residues 219 and/or 227, respectively. Thus, it can be concluded that the epitope in A/USSR/90/77 HA recognized by mAb 264 includes the Glu, Asp, Glu, and Ala of residues 189, 190, 219, and 227 on the outer surface of the HA. The site bounded by these residues is adjacent to the proposed receptor pocket (Wiley et al. 1981) and includes elements of the Sb and Ca_2 domains reported in A/PR/8/34 HA by Gerhard and co-workers (Caton et al. 1982).

Additional conserved mutations occurring from 1978 to 1980 are at residues 125C, 157, 208, and 279. The correspondence in position of a change (Arg to Ser) at residue 125C in field strains losing reactivity with mAb 110, and in the laboratory mutant D-1 selected with mAb 110 (albeit a different amino acid change Arg to Lys, in the mutant B-1), supports the view that residue 125C is indeed involved in the epitope recognized by mAb 110. Because of the three-amino-acid insertion after residue 125 in H1 HA compared with H3 HA, the exact three-dimensional location of residue 125C in H1 HA is not known. Almost certainly, however, the residue is on the outermost face of the protein on the opposite side to the receptor pocket, in an area likely to correspond to the Sa site of A/PR/8/34 HA (Caton et al. 1982). The mutation Asn to Ser at amino acid 163 in A/England/333/80 is believed to be in the Sa site (Caton et al. 1982) and may also affect the epitope recognized by mAb 110.

Finally, sequencing the field strains revealed that the variants A/Lackland/3/78 and A/India/6263/80 (each of which represented a minority of isolates compared with contemporary strains A/Brazil/78 and A/England/333/80, respectively) contained amino acid substitutions at residues 189 and 225 or 190 and 225, respectively. The failure of A/Lackland/3/78 to react with mAbs W18 and 264 is consistent with the existence of a Glu to Lys change at residue 189 in this variant. This change is identical with that found in the laboratory mutant C-2, which also fails to react with mAbs W18 and 264. The change at residue 225 in A/Lackland/3/78 also might affect the mAb W18/264 epitopes, particularly taking into account the reduced reactivity of A/India/6263/80 with mAb W18. Thus, the Asp to Asn change uniquely seen at residue 190 in the A/India/6263/80 field strain has been seen in the laboratory mutant B-1, which still reacts well with mAb W18. Our interpretation of these data is that the epitope recognized by mAb W18 in A/USSR/90/77 virus includes site 225 as well as 189, and it is this additional change at site 225 in A/India/6263/80 that finally results in an alteration of the mAb W18 epitope of sufficient magnitude to affect binding of this antibody.

Although further analysis of the sequence results is desirable in the future, looking in more detail at the orientation of amino acid side chains in the three-dimensional structure of the H1 HA as this information becomes available, the following summary can be made.

1. Those monoclonal antibodies (110, 264) that have detected conserved antigenic changes evolving in H1 HA since 1977 select laboratory variants with

mutations in regions of the molecule similar to those detected in naturally occurring field variants.

2. The epitope recognized by mAb 264 is in a region of the HA molecule along the outer edge of the proposed receptor binding pocket. Residues 189, 190, 219, and/or 227 are included in this epitope, and this knowledge approximately defines the epitope as an area incorporating the lower region of the Sb site and the upper region of the Ca_2 site defined by Gerhard and co-workers on H1 HA (Caton et al. 1982). Changes at three of the four residues described that appear to affect binding of mAb 264 involve increased basicity (Glu to Lys at residue 189, Asp to Asn at 190, and Glu to Lys at 219), indicating the likely importance of electrical charge in determining the antigenic specificity of this region of the HA molecule. The changes in binding patterns of another monoclonal antibody (W18) with laboratory variants or field strains appear to depend slightly on the particular combination of amino acid substitutions that take place, but clearly include the same general area of the HA molecule that forms the epitope for mAb 264. Loss of binding of mAb W18 also is associated with changes in charge of amino acids in the region (Glu to Lys at 189 and Gly to Asp at residue 225 in A/Lackland/3/78 and mutant C-2; Gly to Asn at residue 225 in A/India/6263/80).

3. The epitope recognized by mAb 110 includes amino acid 125C, on an opposite face of the HA to the region recognized by mAb 264. This residue is likely to be in the domain identified as the Sa site of H1 HA by Gerhard and collaborators (Caton et al. 1982). Because mutation in this site appears to have minimal effect on binding of A/USSR/90/77-specific antibodies, as judged by hemagglutination-inhibiting tests with ferret sera, the evolution and conservation of a change at site 125C may result from biological, rather than immunological, factors.

ACKNOWLEDGMENTS

Monoclonal antibodies to A/USSR/77 hemagglutinin were prepared with the support of National Institutes of Health grant AI-08831 to R.G.W.

REFERENCES

Both, G.W., M.J. Sleigh, N.J. Cox, and A.P. Kendal. 1983. Antigenic drift in influenza virus H3 hemagglutinin from 1968 to 1980: Multiple evolutionary pathways and sequential amino acid changes at key antigenic sites. *J. Virol.* **48:** 52.

Caton, A.J., G.G. Brownlee, J.W. Yewdell, and W. Gerhard. 1982. The antigenic structure of the influenza virus A/PR/8/34 hemagglutinin (H1 subtype). *Cell* **31:** 417.

Cox, N.J., Z.S. Bai, and A.P. Kendal. 1983. Laboratory-based surveillance of influenza A (H1N1) and A (H3N2) viruses in 1980–81: Antigenic and genomic analysis. *Bull. WHO* **61:** 143.

Kendal, A.P., N.J. Cox, S. Nakajima, R.G. Webster, W. Bean, and A.S. Beare. 1981. Natural and unnatural variation in influenza A (H1N1) viruses since 1977. *ICN-UCLA Symp. Mol. Biol.* **22:** 489.

Nakajima, S. and A.P. Kendal. 1981. Antigenic drift in influenza A/USSR/90/77(H1N1) variants selected in vitro with monoclonal antibodies. *Virology* **113:** 656.

Webster, R.G., A.P. Kendal, and W. Gerhard. 1979. Analysis of antigenic drift in recently isolated influenza A (H1N1) viruses using monoclonal antibody preparations. *Virology* **96:** 258.

Wiley, D.C., I.A. Wilson, and J.J. Skehel. 1981. Structural identification of the antibody-binding sites of Hong Kong influenza hemagglutinin and their involvement in antigenic variation. *Nature* **289:** 373.

Winter, G., S. Fields, and G.G. Brownlee. 1981. Nucleotide sequence of the hemagglutinin gene of a human influenza virus H1 subtype. *Nature* **292:** 72.

Molecular Cloning of Rotaviral Genes: Implications for Immunoprophylaxis

Jorge Flores, Mitzi Sereno,
Anthony Kalica, Jerry Keith,
Albert Kapikian, and Robert M. Chanock
Laboratory of Infectious Diseases
National Institutes of Health
Bethesda, Maryland 20205

The etiological importance of rotavirus as a common cause of diarrhea in infants and young children has been well documented in studies from developed and developing countries. Some of these studies have pointed out that the severity of the diarrheal syndrome produced by rotavirus may be greater than that caused by other common agents. Thus, it is likely that a high proportion of the more than 5 million fatal cases of infantile diarrhea occurring in the world every year is due to rotavirus. In consequence, the development of immunizing agents against rotavirus diarrhea deserves high priority as they would have a sizable impact on the high infant mortality rates observed in developing countries. Rotavirus diarrhea is also commonly associated with mortality in newborn animals, and a vaccine against the syndrome is likely to be of economic importance.

Traditional approaches to vaccine development, such as the production of mutants by serial passage or chemical mutagenesis, or the use of naturally occurring host-restricted viruses, have now been joined by more direct approaches such as the in vitro production of subunit viral antigens. In the case of rotavirus, synthesis of the relevant protective antigens in bacteria or yeast directed by expression vectors containing cloned DNA copies of the appropriate rotaviral genes may provide abundant amounts of antigen for use in a vaccine. Expression of such antigens as fusion proteins on the surface of bacteria, which could transiently colonize the small intestine, may stimulate local immunity and provide protection. Alternatively, synthetic peptides representing the major antigenic determinants responsible for the induction of neutralizing antibody could be used for immunoprophylaxis.

159

DISCUSSION

Rotaviruses are nonenveloped viruses with a double capsid structure whose genetic material consists of 11 segments of double-stranded RNA that can be easily resolved by gel electrophoresis. Analysis of the individually isolated segments in in vitro translation systems (Dyall-Smith and Holmes 1981; McCrae and Mc-Corquodale 1982) indicates that each segment codes for a protein. To establish coding assignments for some of the rotaviral genes that express recognizable phenotypes, reassortants obtained by coinfection of cells with different rotavirus strains were analyzed (Greenberg et al. 1981; Kalica et al. 1981; Flores et al. 1982a). These studies led to the identification of the gene (sixth in order of migration during gel electrophoresis) that codes for the major structural component of the virus, the gene (eighth or ninth, depending on the rotavirus strain) that codes for the major neutralization antigen, and the gene (fourth) that codes for the protease-sensitive outer capsid protein.

We have directed our efforts to the cloning and characterization of these three genes. Sequencing of the sixth gene may provide information on the structure of the 42,000-dalton inner capsid protein and the nature of the antigenic determinants present on it. Although this protein comprises the major antigenic component that defines human and animal rotaviruses as a group, certain epitopes on the same molecule are responsible for an antigenic specificity that distinguishes two major rotavirus subgroups (Kapikian et al. 1981). It will be of interest to compare the amino acid sequence of this protein of the two rotavirus subgroups and that of the recently described "antigenically distinct rotaviruses," which do not share a common group antigen with conventional rotaviruses.

Cloning of the rotaviral eighth or ninth gene, which codes for the 34,000–38,000-dalton outer capsid glycoprotein, may allow the expression of antigens that have a potential use in immunization. Sequencing of this gene, which codes for the major protective antigen, may reveal the molecular basis of serotype differences that exist among rotavirus strains. This information may also allow us to deduce the amino acid sequences of the major antigenic sites present on this protective antigen.

Cloning, sequencing, and expression of the fourth gene should allow us to understand the molecular basis of several properties of the 88,000-dalton protein coded by this gene: (1) Trypsin cleavage of this protein is required for rotavirus cultivation and probably for infectivity in vivo; (2) this protein is responsible for the hemagglutination of red blood cells exhibited by some animal rotavirus strains; (3) this protein is responsible for the restriction of human rotaviruses in tissue culture; and (4) antibodies against this protein neutralize the virus, but not as well as antibodies against the 34,000–38,000-dalton protein.

Cloning and sequencing of other rotaviral genes may provide important information concerning their genetic structure and organization and may allow the identification of factors relevant to virulence, host range, genetic stability, and evolution of rotaviruses. In addition, probes obtained from rotaviral cloned DNA may have practical uses in the diagnosis of rotaviruses and in studies of their molecular epidemiology.

Synthesis of rotaviral cDNA for cloning in *Escherichia coli* was achieved by reverse transcription of either single-stranded or double-stranded rotaviral RNA;

single-stranded mRNA was obtained by in vitro transcription of rotaviral single-shelled particles (Flores et al. 1982b), whereas genomic double-stranded RNA was extracted from purified viral particles.

Neither the mRNAs nor the genomic RNAs of rotavirus are polyadenylated; thus, in order to create priming regions for reverse transcription, the RNAs were tailed (oligo[A]) with E. *coli* poly(A) polymerase and transcribed by priming with oligo(dT). Once cDNA was obtained, the RNA templates were eliminated by alkali digestion. To synthesize complementary strands to the DNA transcripts obtained from single-stranded RNAs, these transcripts were tailed at their 3' ends with oligo(dC), primed with oligo(dG), and transcribed by the action of reverse transcriptase. When double-stranded RNAs were used as a template, complementary DNA strands were allowed to hybridize and were then completed using reverse transcriptase. After second-strand synthesis, the double-stranded cDNAs were tailed with oligo(dC) and hybridized to plasmid pBR322 that had been linearized previously by digestion with *Pst*I and tailed with oligo(dG). The hybrids were then used to transform E. *coli* HB101, and the transformed colonies were probed by standard techniques using either ^{32}P-labeled single-stranded RNA synthesized in vitro or DNA probes obtained by nick translation of rotaviral cDNA of known gene origin.

The gene origin of the cDNA inserts in the recombinant clones was determined by screening the transformed bacterial colonies with individually isolated single-stranded RNA transcripts, by Northern blot analyses (Fig. 1A) or by a dot hybridization technique; in this latter procedure, individually isolated double-stranded RNA segments were extracted from acrylamide gels, heat-denatured, and dotted onto nitrocellulose membranes that were later incubated with nick-translation probes prepared from cDNA inserts (Fig. 1B). Although acrylamide gel electrophoresis allows high resolution of most rotaviral double-stranded RNA segments, it was not possible to separate segments 7-8-9 of any of three animal rotavirus strains studied. However, those segments were easily resolved with the human Wa rotavirus strain. By performing heterologous hybridization, it was possible to identify the gene origin of clones derived from the animal strains employed. In this case, probes derived from the animal rotaviral cDNA inserts were hybridized at low stringency to membranes on which the 11 individual genes of Wa virus had been dotted. In this manner, recombinant clones were obtained from several rotavirus strains including (1) the human Wa strain, which represents the most common human rotavirus serotype (serotype 1); (2) the simian Rh2 strain, which was originally isolated from an asymptomatic monkey and which has a neutralization specificity identical to human rotavirus serotype 3; and (3) the bovine UK and NCDV (Nebraska calf diarrhea virus) strains, which were originally isolated in England and the United States, respectively, and which belong to a serotype that is distinct from the known human rotavirus serotypes. Recombinant DNA clones representing each of the genes of these viruses were identified, except for genes *10* and *11*, which have not yet been sought. In each instance, the *Pst*I restriction sites initially used for insertion have been reconstructed, allowing the retrieval of the rotaviral cDNA with that enzyme.

More than 50 clones representing copies of the sixth gene of Wa have been identified, and the sizes of their cDNA inserts were determined after *Pst*I diges-

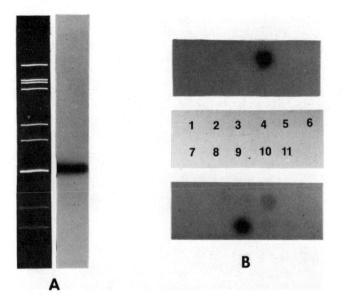

Figure 1
(A) Genomic RNA from the NCDV bovine rotavirus strain was electrophoresed in a 7.5% acrylamide gel (*left*), denatured, and then blotted onto DBM paper. A nick-translation probe prepared from the NCDV clone N-681 was hybridized to the blotted RNA; the probe reacted specifically with the band representing RNA segments 7-8-9 (*right*). (B) The 11 double-stranded RNA segments of Wa were individually extracted from acrylamide gels, dena-tured, and spotted onto nitrocellulose membranes according to the scheme shown (*mid-dle*). Nick-translation probes prepared from two Wa clones were hybridized to the individ-ually dotted segments and were found to hybridize specifically to the fourth (*top*, Wa clone 45A) or ninth (*bottom*, Wa clone 21b) Wa gene.

tion; 17 of these clones contained inserts of identical size and restriction pattern. Although their length suggests that they may represent entire copies of the gene, sequencing of the cDNA is required to establish this.

Clones representing genes coding for the major neutralization antigen (34,000–38,000-dalton glycoprotein) of the four strains studied have also been identified. Inserts from such clones that apparently represent full-size copies of the gene obtained from the Wa, Rh2, and NCDV strains have been mapped by restriction endonuclease analysis. Interestingly, 21 of the clones representing the Wa gene have a similar size, identical restriction maps, and the same orientation in the plasmid (Fig. 2).

The presence of two unevenly spaced *Hin*fI sites on the gene-9 cDNA has allowed the 5' labeling of three fragments of this gene for its initial sequencing. Preliminary comparisons have been made to sequences recently published for the corresponding genes of simian rotavirus strain SA11 (Both et al. 1983) and bovine strain UK (Elleman et al. 1983), which represent serotypes different from each other and from Wa. The strong degree of homology between these se-quences in the SA11 and UK glycoprotein genes is also shared by the areas

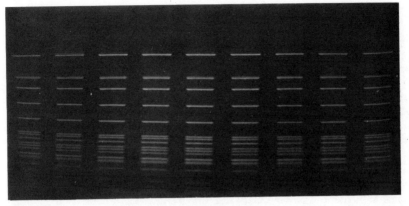

Figure 2
Electrophoretic analysis of plasmids prepared from nine separate Wa gene-*9* clones digested with *Hpa*II. The top band represents in each case the rotaviral cDNA insert flanked by 100 bases of pBR322. The other bands represent restriction fragments generated by *Hpa*II digestion of pBR322.

already sequenced in the Wa virus (about 60% of the gene). When the amino acid sequences are deduced from the DNA sequences, long stretches of homology are detected among the three viruses interrupted only by isolated variant amino acids and, in a few instances, by clusters of amino acid changes. One such cluster of amino acid replacements is encountered at amino acid positions 39–49; this area is, however, strongly hydrophobic, and hence should not represent an antigenic determinant. The strong hydrophilic area near the carboxyl end of the molecule, postulated by Elleman et al. (1983) as a strong antigenic determinant, may not be responsible for serotypic differences, since the amino acid sequences in that area are similar for the three strains. Other highly hydrophilic regions in the protein do not exhibit major differences among the three genes (or between the SA11 and UK genes in areas for which the Wa sequences have not yet been determined). It is possible that only a few amino acid replacements may produce major conformational changes in the molecule that could account for the serotypic differences. Recognition of such sites requires the completion of our sequencing, the examination of sequences of similar genes from viruses of other serotypes, or, alternatively, the expression of the protein (or portions of it) in a eukaryotic system followed by analysis with monoclonal antibodies that exhibit neutralizing activity.

We have also identified 55 Rh2 and 87 Wa gene-*4* clones in our library. Most of them contain rotaviral cDNA inserts of the same size (about 1400 bp or approximately two thirds of the entire gene); we have not yet identified a gene-*4* clone with a larger insert; this may be due to the presence of strong stop sequences for reverse transcription, the presence of potential self-priming sites for reverse transcription within the gene, or the deletion of a portion of the gene once it is introduced into bacteria.

The Wa gene-*9* cDNA has been useful as a probe in studying the genetic relatedness among different rotavirus strains. We have used such probes in a recently described dot hybridization assay (Flores et al. 1983). In this assay, stool specimens or tissue-culture samples containing rotavirus are heat-denatured, dotted on nitrocellulose membranes, and then incubated with the gene-9 probe. When hybridization is carried out at high stringency, it is possible to distinguish rotaviruses belonging to serotype 2 (such as the DS-1 strain), serotype 4 (such as the St. Thomas 4 strain), and many serotype-3 strains from the Wa strain and other type-1 rotaviruses. Application of this assay may prove useful in epidemiological studies, since it could allow identification of rotavirus serotype, obviating the need for cultivation of the virus.

The identification of Wa gene-4 clones has also been useful in studies of the molecular epidemiology of rotavirus. Nick-translation probes from such clones were used in the dot hybridization assay to detect homologies among several human and animal rotavirus strains and the Wa virus. Preliminary results have shown that the gene-4 probe recognized similar sequences in most of the human strains but did not react significantly with most of the animal rotavirus strains tested, suggesting that the product of this gene may be involved in host-range restriction. Differences in the sequence of this gene may be responsible for the known host specificity of different viral strains.

REFERENCES

Both, G.W., J.S. Mattick, and A.R. Bellamy. 1983. The serotype-specific glycoprotein of simian 11 rotavirus: Coding assignment and gene sequence. *Proc. Natl. Acad. Sci.* **80:** 3091.

Dyall-Smith, M.L. and I.H. Holmes. 1981. Gene-coding assignments of rotavirus double-stranded RNA segments 10 and 11. *J. Virol.* **38:** 1099.

Elleman, T.C., P.A. Hoyne, M.L. Dyall-Smith, I.H. Holmes, and A.A. Azad. 1983. Nucleotide sequence of the gene encoding the serotype-specific glycoprotein of UK bovine rotavirus. *Nucleic Acids Res.* **11:** 4689.

Flores, J., H.B. Greenberg, J. Myslinski, A.R. Kalica, R.G. Wyatt, A.Z. Kapikian, and R.M. Chanock. 1982a. Use of transcription probes for genotyping rotavirus reassortants. *Virology* **121:** 288.

Flores, J., J. Myslinski, A.R. Kalica, H.B. Greenberg, R.G. Wyatt, A.Z. Kapikian, and R.M. Chanock. 1982b. In vitro transcription of two human rotaviruses. *J. Virol.* **43:** 1032.

Flores, J., R.H. Purcell, I. Perez, R.G. Wyatt, E. Boeggeman, M. Sereno, L. White, R.M. Chanock, and A.Z. Kapikian. 1983. A dot hybridization assay for detection of rotavirus. *Lancet* **1:** 555.

Greenberg, H.B., A.R. Kalica, A.R. Wyatt, R.W. Jones, A.Z. Kapikian, and R.M. Chanock. 1981. Rescue of non-cultivatable human rotavirus by gene reassortment during mixed infection with ts mutant of a cultivatable bovine rotavirus. *Proc. Natl. Acad. Sci.* **78:** 420.

Kalica, A.R., H.B. Greenberg, R.G. Wyatt, J. Flores, M.M. Sereno, A.Z. Kapikian, and R.M. Chanock. 1981. Genes of human (strain Wa) and bovine (strain UK) rotaviruses that code for neutralization and subgroup antigens. *Virology* **112:** 385.

Kapikian, A.Z., W.L. Cline, H.B. Greenberg, R.G. Wyatt, A.R. Kalica, C.E. Banks, H.D. James, Jr., J. Flores, and R.M. Chanock. 1981. Antigenic characterization of human and animal rotaviruses by an immune adherence hemagglutination assay (IAHA): Evidence for distinctness of IAHA and neutralization antigens. *Infect. Immun.* **3:** 415.

McCrae, M.A. and J.G. McCorquodale. 1982. The molecular biology of rotaviruses. II. Identification of the protein-coding assignments of calf rotavirus genome RNA species. *Virology* **117:** 435.

Characterization of Influenza Virus Glycoproteins Expressed from Cloned cDNAs in Prokaryotic and Eukaryotic Cells

Debi P. Nayak, Alan R. Davis, Masahiro Ueda, Timothy J. Bos, and Natarajan Sivasubramanian
Jonsson Comprehensive Cancer Center
Department of Microbiology and Immunology
UCLA School of Medicine
Los Angeles, California 90024

Influenza is still a major threat to public health because, unlike smallpox, polio, mumps, and measles, it is not yet amenable to effective prophylaxis. Despite the proven value of available inactivated virus vaccines and subunit vaccines, a number of factors, such as short-lived protection and complications including the development of pyrogenic reactions and Guillain-Barre syndrome, have restricted their use to high-risk groups and possibly have limited their effectiveness. One of the modern approaches toward the development of effective vaccines against influenza is to immunize with pure viral surface antigens that can elicit neutralizing antibodies. This approach requires that large quantities of viral surface glycoproteins, namely, hemagglutinin (HA) and neuraminidase (NA), be produced and that antigenic sites that elicit neutralizing antibodies be preserved. To achieve these objectives, recombinant DNA technology offers a unique and novel approach for the development of pure subunit vaccines. As a prelude to this long-range goal, we have expressed both HA and NA from cloned cDNAs in large quantities using both prokaryotic and mammalian cell systems.

Expression of HA in *Escherichia coli*

We have cloned the genes of influenza virus A/WSN/33 by the cDNA cloning method (Davis et al. 1980). Various cDNA clones were screened for different influenza virus genes, and full-length HA cDNA clones were chosen for expression studies. We have expressed HA as a fusion protein using either the *lac UV5* promoter or the *trp* promoter (Davis et al. 1981, 1983b). All our attempts to have the HA protein expressed directly in large quantities using the bacterial promoters have failed (Davis et al. 1981). In fact, many other viral antigens (e.g., hepatitis-B virus surface antigen, vesicular stomatitis virus G protein, and rabies virus glycoprotein), when expressed in *E. coli,* were either unstable or lethal to the cell. Also, since the aminoterminal region of the precursor HA has a hydrophobic signal sequence that interferes with the stable expression of HA in *E. coli,* we decided to express the HA without the aminoterminal signal sequence. For this purpose, the DNA that encodes the signal sequence was deleted, and a new ATG codon was placed in front of the gene (Davis et al. 1981). Subsequently, the modified HA cDNA was fused in phase with the DNA coding for 1005 amino acids of the amino terminus of β-galactosidase or 190 amino acids of the amino terminus of *trp* LE′ protein (Davis et al. 1981, 1983b), using either pβgal13c or pNCV as expression vectors. Appropriate constructions were made (Davis et al. 1983b), and a description of the different constructions used for expression studies is presented in Table 1. Figure 1 shows the partially purified LE′-HA fusion proteins as analyzed by SDS-polyacrylamide gel electrophoresis. These fusion proteins were produced in large quantities by starving the cells for tryptophan, enriched, and purified as described elsewhere (Davis et al. 1983b). The partially purified fusion proteins contained approximately 80% LE′-HA 308 and 60% LE′-HA 396 or LE′-HA 548 as determined by SDS-gel electrophoresis. These partially purified fusion proteins were then tested for both antigenicity and immunogenicity. Table 2 describes the various immunological experiments that were done with the HA fusion proteins. Results show that LE′-HA fusion proteins (LE′-HA 308, 396, and 548) as well as the cyanogen bromide (CNBr) fragment (amino acids 1–226), which is free from the bacterial *trp* LE′ leader peptide, can elicit a relatively high-titer antibody in both mice and rabbits. A number of immunological assays also demonstrate that these antibodies can bind to the HA of detergent-treated virus and intact virions, as well as to the HA present on the surfaces of live cells infected with influenza virus (Davis et al. 1983b). Also, polyclonal antibodies raised against native influenza virus can bind to these bacterial proteins, suggesting that at least some antigenic sites of the native viral HA are present in the fusion protein. In contrast, most of the synthetic peptides of HA cannot react with anti-

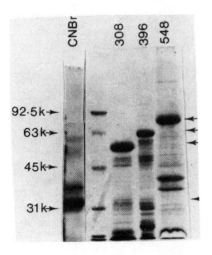

Figure 1
SDS-polyacrylamide gel electrophoresis of partially purified LE′-HA fusion proteins. *E. coli* cells containing pHAT 308, pHAT 396, or pHAT 548 were grown in tryptophan-depleted medium, and *trp* LE′-HA fusion proteins were partially purified and concentrated as described by Davis et al. (1983b). The HA CNBr fragment (leftmost lane) was derived from *trp* LE′-HA-308. M_r values of marker proteins (second lane) are 92,500, 69,000, 45,000, 31,000, 21,500, and 14,400.

Table 1
Primary Structure of HA Proteins Expressed in *E. coli*

Designation	Primary structure[a]			Comment
HA 308	*trp* LE' (190 aa)-Met-Asp .... Ser (1)* (308)			lacks the last 17 amino acids of HA_1 and all of HA_2
HA 396	*trp* LE' (190 aa)-Met-Asp .... Arg-Gly (1) (326)→	..... Phe-8 aa (396)**		lacks the last 151 amino acids of HA_2
HA 548	*trp* LE' (190 aa)-Met-Asp .... Arg-Gly (1) (326)→	.... Ile (548)		complete HA without signal sequence
CNBr 226 of HA 308	Asp .... Met (1) (226)			only a part of HA_1

[a]Asterisk indicates the position (in parentheses) of amino acid residue in HA; arrows indicate the amino terminus of HA_2 after cleavage; and double asterisk indicates the eight amino acids from the pBR322 at the carboxyterminal end.

167

Table 2
Antigenic and Immunogenic Properties of WSN-HA Fusion Proteins in Mice and Rabbits

Antigen	Animal	Relative antibody titer[a]	HI titer[b]	Plaque neutralization[c]	Plaque size (mm)[d]	Immuno-precipitation of WSN viral HA[e]	Antibody binding to infected cells[f]
Mock	mice	0.06	<16	−(23)	n.d.	−	−
	rabbits	n.d.	<16	−(25)	0.3 ± 0.02	−	−
WSN virus	mice	1.0	>128	+(0)	n.d.	+	+
	rabbits	n.d.	>128	+(0)	n.d.	+	+
LE′-HA 308	mice	0.2	<16	−(22)	n.d.	+	+
	rabbits	n.d.	<16	−(27)	0.17 ± 0.02	+	+
LE′-HA 308 CNBr-cleaved	mice	0.38	<16	−(29)	n.d.	+	+
	rabbits	n.d.	<16	n.d.	n.d.	+	+
LE′-HA 396	mice	0.24	<16	−(29)	n.d.	+	n.d.
	rabbits	n.d.	<16	n.d.	n.d.	+	n.d.
LE′-HA 548	mice	0.18	<16	−(32)	n.d.	+	n.d.
	rabbits	n.d.	<16	n.d.	n.d.	+	n.d.

Ten CFW(SW) mice or three New Zealand white rabbits were inoculated with approximately 500 μg or 5 mg of LE′-HA fusion proteins with complete Freund's adjuvant, and a booster was given 4 weeks later. The animals were bled 10 days later, and the antiserum was used for immunological experiments (Davis et al. 1983b). n.d. indicates not done.

[a] Antisera raised against the fusion proteins were tested against WSN virus using the ELISA assay (Davis et al. 1983b).
[b] Reciprocal of hemagglutinin inhibition titer.
[c] + or − indicates whether the serum contains neutralizing antibodies. Numbers in parentheses show the average number of plaques present in culture dishes.
[d] Average diameter of plaques on day 3.
[e] Immunoprecipitation of detergent-treated (1% Triton X-100), labeled WSN virus and analysis by SDS-polyacrylamide gel electrophoresis.
[f] Antibody binding was assayed by immunofluorescence of live infected cells (Davis et al. 1983b).

bodies raised against virus (Green et al. 1982). However, the antibodies raised against fusion proteins are different from those elicited against native viral HA. The level of neutralizing or hemagglutination-inhibiting neutralizing antibodies is low when compared with the levels of neutralizing antibody raised against virus (Table 2). This suggests that the immunogenic properties of the HA fusion proteins are different from those of native viral HA. A number of factors may contribute to the structural difference between bacterial HA and native viral HA. (1) The bacterial HA contains the *trp* LE' peptide (190 amino acids) at its amino terminus. Either the *trp* LE' leader peptide or a different folding of the fusion protein might mask the antigenic epitope(s) involved in eliciting neutralizing antibodies. (2) Bacterial HA is unglycosylated. Carbohydrates are known to modulate the antigenicity by either exposing or masking antigenic sites. Additionally, they may affect the tertiary structure. Since the antibodies to the viral HA can bind to the bacterial HA fusion protein in contrast to synthetic peptides of HA (Green et al. 1982), it is possible that the proper renaturation of these fusion proteins might generate conformation of antigenic epitope(s) similar to that present in native viral HA and thus may elicit neutralizing antibodies.

Expression of HA and NA in Monkey Kidney Cells

Since the bacterial HA fusion protein was unglycosylated and possessed an altered tertiary structure and little biological activity, it was not suitable for studying the structure-function relationship of different domains of the protein. Therefore, the cloned HA cDNA was expressed in a eukaryotic system. For this purpose, we cloned the entire HA cDNA into the late region of SV40 (SV-HA) (Hartman et al. 1982). The SV-HA recombinants lacking the late genes were complemented in lytic infection of monkey kidney cells by the helper function of SV40 early deletion mutants. Influenza HA was expressed as detected by immunofluorescence (Fig. 2) and immunoprecipitation of in-vivo-labeled proteins using either anti-HA polyclonal or monoclonal antibodies. Furthermore, the WSN-HA expressed by the SV-HA recombinants was also glycosylated and had the same molecular weight ($\sim$70,000) as the native viral HA in monkey cells infected with WSN virus (Table 3). Also, the expressed HA molecule migrated to the cell surface as detected by surface immunofluorescence and hemadsorption. Influenza viruses have been shown to bud from the apical surface of the polarized epithelial cells. We also found that in polarized African green monkey kidney (AGMK) cells, HA expressed from cloned cDNA in SV-HA recombinants was accumulated preferentially on the apical surface of the polarized cells (Roth et al. 1983). This suggests that the viral HA possesses all the information necessary for the transport of the molecule to the apical surface of the cell and that the involvement of other influenza virus proteins is not needed for the directional transport of HA.

Neuraminidase, the other influenza virus surface glycoprotein, is also of interest, since structurally it differs from the majority of integral membrane proteins. Whereas HA, like other integral membrane proteins, anchors on the cell membrane via its hydrophobic carboxyl terminus, NA anchors on the membrane by its aminoterminal hydrophobic region. Also, NA does not possess a cleavable signal sequence that is present in HA and other integral membrane proteins. We expressed the WSN-NA from cloned DNA in monkey cells by utilizing the same

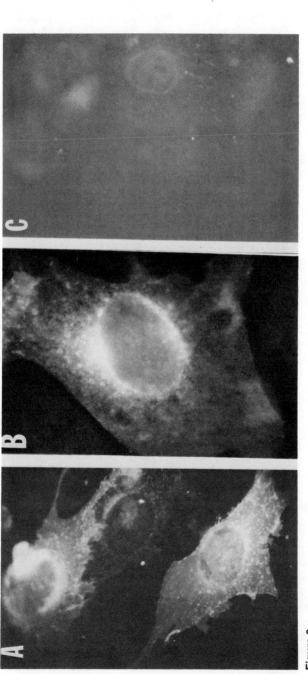

Figure 2
Detection of HA and NA by immunofluorescence. (A) CV-1 cells were infected with SNC(NA) virus, and at 48 hr postinfection, infected cells were used for immunofluorescent staining (Davis et al. 1983a). (B) Secondary AGMK cells were infected with SV-HA₃ (HA), and at 40 hr postinfection, infected cells were used for immunofluorescent staining. (C) Mock-infected cells.

Table 3
Biological Properties of Mammalian Cell Expressed Influenza Surface Proteins

	Viral		Expressed	Expressed NA		
	HA	NA	HA	SNC	SN10	SN26
Synthesis	+	+	+	+	+	−
Glycosylation	+	+	+	+	+	−
Transport to cell surface	+	+	+	+	+	−
Hemadsorption	+	n.a.	+	n.a.	n.a.	n.a.
Enzyme activity	n.a.	+	n.a.	+	+	−
Polarized expression	+	n.d.	+	n.d.	n.d.	n.d.

n.a. indicates not applicable; n.d. indicates not done.

SV40 late replacement vector as above (Davis et al. 1983a). Appropriate SV40-NA recombinant viruses were constructed and complemented in a lytic infection of monkey cells with a helper virus. The NA expressed from cloned cDNA possesses essentially the same properties as the viral NA in WSN-virus-infected cells. NA was detected by immunofluorescence (Fig. 2) as well as by immunoprecipitation of labeled proteins with monoclonal antibodies against NA. In addition, the expressed NA was glycosylated and transported to the cell surface; it possessed enzymatic activity as demonstrated by the cleavage of the sialic acid residue from a-2,3-sialyllactitol. We also replaced the DNA coding for the first 10 aminoterminal acids of NA with SV40 and linker sequences. The NA expressed from this construction (SN10) was similar to the native viral NA, thus suggesting that the first 12 conserved amino acids may not be required for the expression and function of NA. However, when the first 26 amino acids, which includes the hydrophobic anchoring region, were deleted (SN26), no detectable NA was expressed. These results suggest that the aminoterminal hydrophobic region may be necessary for the stable expression of NA. Table 3 describes the biological properties of HA and NA expressed from cDNA in eukaryotic cells. Furthermore, we have also recently shown that the hydrophobic aminoterminal sequence of NA provides, in addition to anchoring function, a signal function in translocation across rough endoplasmic reticulum (Bos et al. 1984).

SUMMARY

We have shown that both glycoproteins (HA and NA) of influenza virus can be expressed from cloned cDNAs. In eukaryotic cells, both HA and NA are synthesized, glycosylated, and transported to the cell surface, and both are biologically active and possess immunological properties similar to those of the native HA and NA in influenza-virus-infected cells. Since cDNA clones can be used for site-specific modification, the eukaryotic expression system will greatly aid in defining the structure-function relationship of different domains of HA and NA.

We have also expressed WSN-HA as a fusion protein in bacteria. Using the *trp* promoter-operator system, we find that HA can be expressed as high as 10–20% of the total bacterial protein when fused to *trp* LE' at the amino terminus. The expressed HA elicits antibodies that are different from those elicited by the native virus or the native HA, suggesting that the structure of bacterial HA may be different from that of the viral HA. Absence of glycosylation in bacteria and the presence of *trp* LE' polypeptides at the amino terminus may affect the tertiary structure and antigenic domains of HA. Therefore, critical experiments are needed to artificially restore the structure of eukaryotic proteins synthesized in bacteria if they are to be used as vaccines. However, bacterially expressed HA may still be useful as a priming antigen to be followed by virus inoculation or a boosting antigen after the initial virus inoculation and thus may reduce the dose of the viral antigen and its toxicity. In addition to humoral antibodies, T cells play a major role in the defense against influenza. The effect of bacterially expressed HA on different subclasses of T cells has yet to be investigated. In summary, influenza HA can be expressed in a rather large amount in bacteria as fusion protein. However, experiments to restore its native structure are critically needed before its potential as a vaccine can be explored.

ACKNOWLEDGMENTS

This work was supported by grants from Wyeth Laboratories, American Home Products, Philadelphia, Pennsylvania, and from National Institutes of Health grant R01-AI-16348. T.J.B. was recipient of U.S. Public Health Service National Research Service Award (GM-07104).

REFERENCES

Bos, T.J., A.R. Davis, and D.P. Nayak. 1984. Aminoterminal hydrophobic region of influenza virus neuraminidase provides the signal function in translocation. *Proc. Natl. Acad. Sci.* (in press).

Davis, A.R., T.J. Bos, and D.P. Nayak. 1983a. Active influenza virus neuraminidase is expressed in monkey cells from cDNA cloned in simian virus 40 vectors. *Proc. Natl. Acad. Sci.* **80:** 3976.

Davis, A.R., A.L. Hiti, and D.P. Nayak. 1980. Construction and characterization of a bacterial clone containing the hemagglutinin gene of the WSN strain (H0N1) of influenza virus. *Gene* **10:** 205.

Davis, A.R., T.J. Bos, M. Ueda, D.P. Nayak, D. Dowbenko, and R.W. Compans. 1983b. Immune response to human influenza virus hemagglutinin expressed in *E. coli. Gene* **21:** 273.

Davis, A.R., D.P. Nayak, M. Ueda, A.L. Hiti, D. Dowbenko, and D.G. Kleid. 1981. Expression of antigenic determinants of the hemagglutinin gene of a human influenza virus in *Escherichia coli. Proc. Natl. Acad. Sci.* **78:** 5376.

Green, N., H. Alexander, A. Olson, S. Alexander, T.M. Shinnick, J.G. Sutcliffe, and R.A. Lerner. 1982. Immunogenic structure of the influenza virus hemagglutinin. *Cell* **28:** 477.

Hartman, J.R., D.P. Nayak, and G.C. Fareed. 1982. Human influenza virus hemagglutinin is expressed in monkey cells using simian virus 40 vectors. *Proc. Natl. Acad. Sci.* **79:** 233.

Roth, M.G., R.W. Compans, L. Guisti, A.R. Davis, D.P. Nayak, M.J. Gething, and J. Sambrook. 1983. Influenza virus hemagglutinin expression is polarized in cells infected with recombinant SV40 viruses carrying cloned hemagglutinin DNA. *Cell* **33:** 435.

Expression in *Escherichia coli* of Capsid Protein VP1 of Poliovirus Type 1

Betty E. Enger-Valk, Jan Jore, and Peter H. Pouwels
Medical Biological Laboratory TNO
2280 AA Rijswijk, The Netherlands

Pieter van der Marel and Toon L. van Wezel
National Institute of Public Health
3720 BA Bilthoven, The Netherlands

Recently, it was shown that the purified capsid polypeptides (VPs) isolated from formalin-inactivated poliovirus induce neutralizing antibodies in animals after two or three injections (van Wezel et al. 1983). These results suggest that several neutralization epitopes are present on the virion. Of the capsid polypeptides isolated from infectious poliovirus type 1 (PV-1), so far only VP1 is able to induce neutralizing antibodies after four to six injections (Blondel et al. 1982; Chow and Baltimore 1982). The identification, using monoclonal antibodies, of a neutralization epitope in this region of PV-3 (Minor et al. 1983) and the finding that a synthetic peptide consisting of amino acids 93–103 of PV-1 VP1 induces neutralizing antibodies (Emini et al. 1983) support the hypothesis that VP1 is important for induction of neutralizing antibodies.

In view of our interest in the possibility of producing a subunit polio vaccine by recombinant DNA techniques, the capsid protein VP1 is a good candidate to clone and express in *Escherichia coli*. PV-1 cDNA has been cloned in *E. coli*, and its nucleotide sequence has been determined (Racaniello and Baltimore 1981; Van der Werf et al. 1981). For cloning of the VP1 gene, we made use of the plasmid pVR104 (Racaniello and Baltimore 1981) kindly provided by Dr. David Baltimore.

DISCUSSION

Cloning of VP1

A *Bam*HI-*Hind*III fragment, comprising the complete VP1 sequence, was subcloned in an expression plasmid, such that expression of VP1 is under the con-

173

trol of the *trp* promoter of *E. coli. trp*-regulated expression in the resulting plasmid pLOP6 is expected to give a fusion protein of 73K, containing 65 amino acids of the *trpE* gene and linker sequences, 117 amino acids of VP3, 302 amino acids of VP1, 149 amino acids of protein 3b, 27 amino acids of protein 5b, and 14 amino acids of *E. coli*. The carboxyterminal 14 amino acids of this polio-coli fusion protein (designated coli-VP1,3) are encoded by vector sequences.

Expression of VP1 in *E. coli*

The expression of VP1 sequences in bacteria containing pLOP6 was analyzed by the immunoblotting technique. Bacterial pellets (2×10^8 to 3×10^8 bacteria) lysed with SDS were electrophoresed on 10% polyacrylamide gels and blotted on nitrocellulose filters. The blots were tested for their reactivity with polyclonal serum against VP1 and with nonimmune serum. Patterns of bacteria containing pLOP6 were compared with those of bacteria containing a control plasmid (e.g., a plasmid not containing polio-specific sequences) or no plasmid. The results (Fig. 1) show that the 73K protein reacts with VP1-specific antibodies, but not with nonimmune serum, and that not only the 73K protein, but also the smaller proteins (e.g., 54K, 43K, and 30K) react specifically with antiserum against VP1. The smaller proteins presumably are degradation products of the 73K protein. The amount of the 73K protein, compared with that of the 54K protein, is different

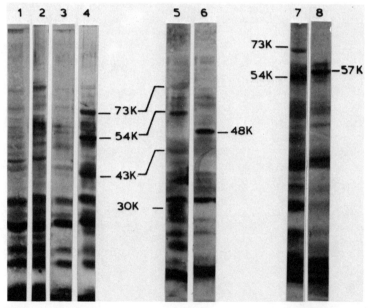

Figure 1
Western immunoblot analysis of bacteria containing plasmids with varying polio-specific sequences. Lanes *1* and *3* were developed with nonimmune serum and lanes *2* and *4–8* with polyclonal serum against VP1. (*1,2*) Bacteria containing a control plasmid; (*3–5, 7*) bacteria containing pLOP6; (*6*) bacteria containing pLOP67; (*8*) bacteria containing pLOP79.

from one bacterial culture to the other. Bacteria cultivated for a shorter period appear to contain more of the 73K protein than bacteria cultivated overnight. Sometimes, the 73K protein is completely degraded, and the largest protein that reacts with antiserum against VP1 is the 54K protein.

From blotting experiments with decreasing amounts of bacterial lysates and from measuring the expression of VP1 sequences by the maxicell system, it also appears (results not shown) that the level of expression is quite low. To obtain more efficient expression of polio-specific proteins and to avoid degradation of fusion proteins, new plasmids were constructed. These plasmids have (1) fewer *trpE* sequences between the promoter and the polio sequence (plasmid pLOP67), (2) fewer polio sequences at the carboxyterminal end of VP1 (pLOP7), (3) fewer polio sequences at the carboxyterminal end of VP1 and a temperature-sensitive origin of replication (pLOP79) such that the gene copy number is increased at 42°C, and (4) a p_l^λ promoter (which can be induced by raising the temperature to 42°C) in place of the *trp* promoter (pLOP671). The expected molecular weights of the VP1 fusion proteins encoded by the different plasmids are 67,000 for pLOP67, 57,000 for pLOP7 and pLOP79, and 67,000 for pLOP671.

The expression of VP1 fusion proteins encoded by the different plasmids is measured in the same way as described for pLOP6. The results obtained with plasmid pLOP67 (see Fig. 1) show that the largest protein reacting with anti-serum against VP1 is a 48K protein. Sometimes a bacterial preparation (not shown) contains a very low amount of a 67K protein, but in all the bacteria containing pLOP67, the 48K protein is present in much higher amounts. This also indicates that the VP1 fusion protein encoded by pLOP67 is rapidly degraded to smaller proteins. Remarkably, the difference in molecular weight between the 48K protein encoded by pLOP67 and the degraded protein of 54K encoded by pLOP6 seems to be approximately the same as the difference in *trpE* amino acids between the two plasmids.

The patterns obtained with the plasmids pLOP7 and pLOP79 are the same, and only the results with pLOP79 are shown (Fig. 1). A protein of 57K specifically reacts with antiserum against VP1, which is a protein of the expected molecular weight. Degradation seems to be less than that for pLOP6. However, the level of expression with pLOP79, measured at 42°C, is comparable to that of pLOP6. The same results are found with plasmid pLOP671, i.e., no increase when expression is under control of the p_l^λ promoter (results not shown).

From the results obtained with the different plasmids, it can be concluded that (1) degradation of a 73K protein to a 54K protein occurs at a site(s) close to the carboxyterminal end of the VP1 gene, (2) degradation of the VP1 fusion protein is less when part of the protein-3b sequence is deleted, and (3) the level of expression is not increased by deletion of *E. coli* (or polio) sequences, by the presence of a temperature-sensitive origin of DNA replication, or by the presence of the p_l^λ promoter.

Isolation of coli-VP1,3

Although the expression of coli-VP1,3 in bacteria containing pLOP6 is low, it was possible to isolate sufficient quantities of the fusion protein to allow immunization experiments. For the isolation and partial purification, advantage was taken of the insolubility of the fusion protein. Bacteria were lysed in such a way that most (>90%) of their protein content became solubilized. After centrifugation of the lysate, the coli-VP1,3 was extracted from the pellet by treatment with 8 M urea, yielding a 10–20-fold purified coli-VP1,3 preparation.

Immunization

Wistar SPF rats were immunized at days 0 and 21 with partially purified coli-VP1,3 (1 mg of protein per injection) with either $AlPO_4$ adjuvant or Freund's adjuvant. Blood samples were taken at days 0, 7, and 28 for serological and immunochemical analyses. Neutralizing antibodies were determined in a neutralization assay using 100 $TCID_{50}$ (tissue-culture-infective doses).

Antibodies raised by the fusion protein reacted in an immunoblotting assay specifically with the virus capsid proteins VP1 and VP3 (results not shown). Apparently, the presence of only part of the VP3 sequence in the fusion protein is sufficient for induction of VP3-specific antibodies.

Table 1 shows that coli-VP1,3 did not induce neutralizing antibodies after two injections (rats 1–4), which is in accordance with the results obtained with VPs isolated from virions (van Wezel et al. 1983). However, injection of coli-VP1,3 at day 0, followed by a second injection at day 21 with a low amount of vaccine (D antigen), which in itself hardly induced neutralizing antibodies (rats 7 and 8), gave rise to a boosterlike production of neutralizing antibodies (rats 5 and 6).

Table 1

Development of Neutralizing Antibodies in Rats after Immunization with Partially Purified coli-VP1,3

Rat no.	Immunization[a]		Neutralization titer		
	day 0	day 21	day 0	day 7	day 28
1	coli-VP1,3 +	coli-VP1,3 +	<2	<2	<2
2	$AlPO_4$	$AlPO_4$	<2	<2	<2
3	coli-VP1,3 +	coli-VP1,3 +	<2	<2	<2
4	CFA	IFA	<2	<2	<2
5	coli-VP1,3 +	5DU +	<2	<2	16
6	$AlPO_4$	$AlPO_4$	<2	<2	16
7	—	5DU +	<2	<2	±2
8	—	$AlPO_4$	<2	<2	±2
9	5DU +	5DU +	<2	2	16
10	$AlPO_4$	$AlPO_4$	<2	2	1024

[a]CFA, complete Freund's adjuvant; IFA, incomplete Freund's adjuvant; 5DU, inactivated polio vaccine, 5 D-antigen units.

This "priming effect" has also been observed for capsid proteins isolated from live or formalin-inactivated virus (van Wezel et al. 1983) and for a synthetic VP1 oligopeptide of 14 amino acids (Emini et al. 1983).

SUMMARY AND CONCLUSIONS

Bacteria containing a plasmid (pLOP6) comprising the VP1 gene and flanking polio sequences are able to synthesize a protein of 73K (coli-VP1,3) that specifically reacts with antibodies against VP1. The efficiency of expression of coli-VP1,3 in *E. coli* is quite low, despite the presence of a strong promoter. Besides, the coli-VP1,3 is rapidly degraded to 54K, 43K, 30K, and smaller proteins. Degradation seems to occur first close to the carboxyterminal end of the VP1 gene and is dependent on the presence of the complete protein-3b sequence. The synthesis of other fusion proteins and/or synthesis in other host organisms will be attempted to improve the production of polio-specific proteins.

The insoluble coli-VP1,3 was partially purified and used for immunization of rats. Like VP1 isolated from infectious virus, coli-VP1,3 does not induce neutralizing antibodies after two injections but is able to prime the immune system for a boosterlike production of neutralizing antibodies upon subsequent injection with a low dose of vaccine. Although the priming effect may be considered as an interesting new trend in vaccinology, further attempts will be undertaken to modulate the conformation of the coli-VP1,3 proteins in such a way that they become able to induce neutralizing antibodies.

REFERENCES

Blondel, B., R. Crainic, and F. Horodniceanu. 1982. Le polypeptide structural VP1 du poliovirus type 1 induit des anticorps neutralisants. *C.R. Acad. Sci.* **294:** 91.

Chow, M. and D. Baltimore. 1982. Isolated poliovirus capsid protein VP1 induces a neutralizing response in rats. *Proc. Natl. Acad. Sci.* **79:** 7518.

Emini, E.A., B.A. Jameson, and E. Wimmer. 1983. Priming for and induction of anti-poliovirus neutralizing antibodies by synthetic peptides. *Nature* **304:** 699.

Minor, P.D., G.C. Schild, S. Bootman, D.M.A. Evans, M. Ferguson, P. Reeve, M. Spitz, G. Stanway, A.J. Cann, R. Hauptmann, L.D. Clarke, R.C. Mountford, and J.W. Almond. 1983. Location and primary structure of a major antigenic site for poliovirus neutralization. *Nature* **301:** 674.

Racaniello, V. and D. Baltimore. 1981. Molecular cloning of poliovirus cDNA and determination of the complete nucleotide sequence of the viral genome. *Proc. Natl. Acad. Sci.* **78:** 4887.

Van der Werf, S., F. Brégérère, H. Kopecka, N. Kitamura, P.G. Rothberg, P. Kourilsky, E. Wimmer, and M. Girard. 1981. Molecular cloning of the genome of poliovirus type 1. *Proc. Natl. Acad. Sci.* **78:** 5983.

van Wezel, A.L., P. van der Marel, A.G. Hazendonk, V. Boer-Bak, and M.A.C. Henneke. 1983. Antigenicity and immunogenicity of poliovirus capsid proteins. *Dev. Biol. Stand.* (in press).

A Direct Cloning-Expression System for Neutralization Antigens of Herpes Simplex Viruses

Wai-Choi Leung, GuoZhong Jing,
Seyed E. Hasnain, ShouChing Tang,
and Maria Leung
Department of Medicine, University of Alberta
Edmonton, Alberta T6G2G3, Canada

Previous experimental approaches to studying the expression of herpes simplex virus (HSV) genes in *Escherichia coli* required a priori the identification of the gene loci in HSV genome. These invariably involved initial genetic mapping, followed by a more refined biochemical analysis that included mapping the location and transcriptional orientation of the mRNA, and, preferably, the analyses of the total nucleotide sequence of the structural gene. This approach was further complicated by the need to remove intervening sequences, should they be present, by site-specific mutagenesis protocol.

We sought to use a direct approach for the cloning and expression of HSV genes to accelerate the studies on the structure and function of HSV-specific proteins. Several considerations were first established for the designing of this experiment: (1) cDNA recombinant clones copied from mRNA, instead of genomic DNA clones, would be used to avoid the presence of intervening sequences that would hinder the expression of cloned genes in *E. coli*. (2) The cloned genes would be ligated downstream to a bacterial promoter to direct the transcription of HSV mRNA in bacteria. (3) The cloned genes would be inserted at the same orientation, preferably in the same reading frame as dictated by the bacterial promoter. (4) The gene products normally repressed in bacteria would be induced to express in high amounts by the presence of inducers. This would increase the possibility of cloning and expressing viral gene products that were toxic to the bacteria. (5) The cloning and simultaneous expression of the HSV genes should be readily identifiable by the expressed gene products. Polypeptide-specific polyclonal antibodies and/or monoclonal antibodies could be used to screen for bacterial colonies expressing the polypeptide. If the suitable anti-

179

bodies were not available, means should be developed to screen for the expressed polypeptide.

Construction of Cloning-Expression Vector

In view of the above considerations, we constructed a new vector, pAH-1, for simultaneous cloning and expression of HSV genes. The key features of pAH-1 was the presence of the pBR322 replicon, an ampicillin resistance gene, and the *lac UV5* promoter. An *Eco*RI restriction endonuclease site was present at the tenth amino acid from the amino terminus of the β-galactosidase gene. Synthetic DNA synthesized chemically by the solid-phase phosphotriester method with a manual DNA synthesizer was inserted into this site to create a stretch of highly hydrophilic peptide sequence, one restriction endonuclease site with a 5' extension (*Sal*I), followed by another site with a 3' extension (*Kpn*I).

When preparing the vector for ligation, the pAH-1 was cut with *Sal*I and *Kpn*I, and the small DNA fragment was removed by chromatography on a Sephacryl S-200 column. A $(dG)_{15}dCdAdGdCdT$ synthetic 20-mer was ligated to the *Sal*I site of the vector, whereas a $dCdAdTdGdG(dA)_{22}$ synthetic 27-mer was joined to the *Kpn*I site. Hence, a protruding single-stranded $(dG)_{15}$ sequence was present at the *Sal*I site and a $(dA)_{22}$ sequence was present at the *Eco*RI site. These two sequences served to align the cDNA at the proper orientation downstream from the *lac* promoter.

Cloning and Expressing cDNA Gene Copies

RNA from HSV-infected cells was extracted by the guanidinium thiocyanate–cesium chloride method, and polyadenylated RNA was selected by oligo(dT)-cellulose chromatography. The first-strand cDNA was synthesized using oligo(dT)$_{12-18}$ as a primer. An oligo(dC) sequence was added to the 3' end of the cDNA by terminal transferase. The dC tailing was performed on the cDNA-mRNA hybrid in order to enrich for the cloning of full-length cDNA. An optional step for further enrichment of full-length cDNA was size selection of the cDNA on alkali sucrose gradient.

The first-strand cDNA was reannealed with the prepared cloning vector pAH-1. The $(dC)_n$ tail of the cDNA hybridized with the $(dG)_{15}$ sequence of pAH-1, whereas the $(dT)_n$ sequence of the cDNA hybridized with the $(dA)_{22}$ sequence of pAH-1. The second-strand cDNA was then synthesized using the $(dG)_{15}$ sequence as a primer and the first-strand cDNA as a template. The recombinant cDNA was used to transform *E. coli* that carried a *lac* repressor and selected for ampicillin-resistant colonies.

Bacterial colonies grown on nitrocellulose filter paper were induced to express the cloned cDNA gene in the presence of isopropylthio-β-D-galactoside (IPTG), lysed with chloroform, and incubated with primary antibody. After extensive washing, they were incubated with ^{125}I-labeled secondary antibody as described by Helfman et al. (1983).

Several HSV-specific cDNA clones were obtained with the antibodies available as screening probe. These include the glycoprotein B (gB) genes HSV-1 and

HSV-2. A polypeptide with a molecular weight of 85,000 was immunoprecipitated from the bacteria expressing the HSV-2 gB gene, which suggests that nearly full-length cDNA clones were obtained for the gB gene.

Screening of HSV cDNA Clones with No Available Antibodies

At present, only a limited number of HSV polypeptides can be screened by the above methods with a limited collection of monoclonal or polypeptide-specific antibodies. However, cDNA clones expressing polypeptides can be detected by the following protocol.

The basic design was to add onto the expressed polypeptide a highly hydrophilic peptide, which would reside on the outer surface of the protein and hence be detected by antibody directed against this peptide. A nine-amino-acid (Glu) polypeptide (least likely to form any structure with any protein of unknown sequence) was inserted near the amino terminus of the *lacZ* gene. We also took advantage of the $(gly)_n$ sequence generated by the cDNA cloning protocol and used it as a spacer arm to extend the hydrophilic sequence out to the surface of the protein. Antipeptide antibodies were raised to this nine-amino-acid peptide by immunizing rabbits. The antibodies were then used to immunoprecipitate HSV polypeptides expressed in the cDNA library.

We are currently using this antibody as an immunoabsorbent to purify the HSV polypeptide. The HSV polypeptide can then be used as antigen for the production of monoclonal or polypeptide-specific antibodies. The cDNA clones can be used to map the gene loci for these polypeptides. We believe that it will provide a simple and efficient way to assess the genes and gene products of herpesviruses.

CONCLUSION

The above findings suggest a cDNA cloning-expression system for the efficient screening of recombinant cDNA using antibody probes. It has the advantages over other published methods (Helfman et al. 1983; Young and Davis 1983) in the directional insertion of cDNA downstream from the bacterial promoter and the avoidance of the use of restriction endonuclease during the cloning protocol. An additional hydrophilic peptide was inserted in front of the expressed polypeptide in order to fish out an unknown protein, should no polypeptide-specific antibody be available. We envision that such cloning-expression systems can be constructed for yeast and mammalian cell promoters.

ACKNOWLEDGMENT

This study was supported by the Alberta Heritage Foundation of Medical Research, National Cancer Institute of Canada, and Medical Research Council of Canada.

REFERENCES

Helfman, D.M., J.R. Feramisco, J.C. Fiddes, G.P. Thomas, and S.H. Hughes. 1983. Identification of clones that encode chicken tropomyosin by direct immunological screening of a cDNA expression library. *Proc. Natl. Acad. Sci.* **80:** 31.

Young, R.A. and R.W. Davis. 1983. Efficient isolation of genes by using antibody probes. *Proc. Natl. Acad. Sci.* **80:** 1194.

High-level Production in *Escherichia coli* of Hybrid Proteins Expressing Parts of Coding Sequences of HSV Glycoproteins

Egon Amann, Michael Bröker, and Florian Wurm
Research Laboratories, Behringwerke AG
D-3550 Marburg 1, Federal Republic of Germany

Herpes simplex viruses (HSV) are among the most common infectious agents of man. There are at least two distinct serotypes (HSV-1 and HSV-2), and both cause persistent and latent infections, including recurrent cutaneous disease, lethal neonatal disease, and viral encephalitis (Nahmias et al. 1981). To date, inactivated viral particle vaccines and subunit vaccines have shown therapeutic effects in the treatment of HSV-1 and HSV-2 infections, although clinical double-blind studies have not yet been completed.

It has been established that HSV-1 and HSV-2 infectivity can be neutralized in vitro with antisera directed against each of the major glycoproteins of the virus (gA/B, gC, gD, and gE). Antisera directed against gD prepared from either virus are capable of neutralizing both HSV-1 and HSV-2 infectivity in vitro and in vivo. Since the DNA sequence of gC and gD and their location on the HSV-1 genome have been determined (Frink et al. 1983; Watson et al. 1982), we chose to express these two proteins in *Escherichia coli* in order to test the utility of genetically engineered HSV antigens for active immunization.

Attempts to Express Directly gC and gD

We have constructed *E. coli* expression vectors that allow the regulated high-level expression of cloned genes using the efficient hybrid *trp-lac* ("*tac*") promoter (Amann et al. 1983). The *tac* promoter carries the *lac* operator sequence and therefore can be repressed in *lacI*q strains and can be induced by isopropylthio-β-ᴅ-galactoside (IPTG). Some of our expression vectors carry, in addition to the *tac* promoter, the efficient *lacZ* ribosome binding site followed by unique cloning sites. These vectors can be used to express cloned genes directly, i.e., in an unfused, naturally occurring state.

The genes for gC (HSV-1 strain F) and gD (HSV-1 strain McIntyre) were sub-cloned from larger clones and identified by restriction enzyme mapping, and the DNA was partially sequenced. We observed several strain differences (comparing strain F and strain KOS for gC and strain Patton and strain McIntyre for gD) at the DNA level, which, in most cases, are single base changes at third codon positions ("silent mutations").

Upon introduction of gC- and gD-coding sequences into the unique cloning sites behind the *tac* promoter and subsequent induction with IPTG of cultures harboring such plasmids, no gC- or gD-specific expression was observed either on Coomassie-blue-stained polyacrylamide gels or in more sensitive radioimmunoassays. With several of our constructs, however, we observed growth inhibition of bacterial cultures upon induction with IPTG. This might be attributed to a low-level expression of gC- and gD-specific sequences and "toxic" effects of the highly hydrophobic sequences at the aminoterminal and carboxyterminal ends of the proteins.

Low-level Expression of gC and gD Sequences after Removal of Aminoterminal Hydrophobic Sequences

We removed with restriction enzymes the DNA sequences coding for the hydrophobic aminoterminal regions of gC and gD. *Hind*III linkers were introduced to serve as adaptors for fusing the remaining coding sequences to an aminoterminal portion of the bacteriophage λcI repressor gene (see Fig. 1 for the amount of deleted DNA in the case of gD). The cI gene carries a unique *Hind*III site, and its gene product (m.w. 26,000) is stable in *E. coli*. It can be expressed by the *tac* promoter at a rate of up to 30% of the total cellular *E. coli* protein and therefore should be well suited to serve as an aminoterminal "acceptor" to which HSV coding sequences can be fused.

Fusion of gC and gD sequences, now missing 150–250 bp at their 5' ends but retaining all of their carboxyterminal sequences, to the *Hind*III site of the cI gene in the correct translational reading frame results in the immunologically detectable production of chimeric proteins. These proteins are rapidly degraded in *E. coli* and show marked toxic effects to the *E. coli* cell, i.e., upon induction with IPTG, growth inhibition occurs and, with some of our constructs, lysis of bacterial cultures is observed. From these findings, we conclude that not only the aminoterminal, but also the carboxyterminal hydrophobic sequences are detrimental to the cell and cannot be expressed at high levels in *E. coli*.

High-level Production of Stable, Tripartite gC and gD Fusion Proteins

Next, we wanted to replace the carboxyterminal hydrophobic sequences of gC and gD with a large carboxyterminal moiety of the *E. coli* β-galactosidase (βgal) protein. To enable such manipulations, we first constructed cI/βgal fusion vectors under *tac* promoter control. Figure 2 shows the result of an induction experiment with bacteria carrying a cI/βgal fusion plasmid (pMF2). A protein with a molecular

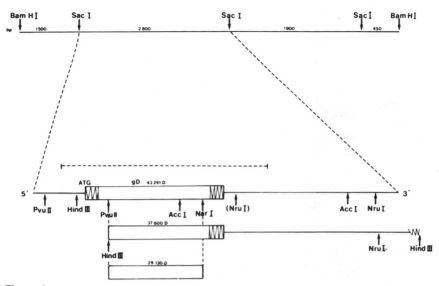

Figure 1
Restriction map of HSV-1 gD gene. A 6600-bp *Bam*HI fragment cloned in pACYC184 served as the source of gD-specific sequences. A 2800-bp *Sac*I fragment was subcloned and mapped with restriction enzymes. Top boxed area corresponds to the coding sequence of gD. Middle boxed area corresponds to the region fused to *cI* (see text). The *Pvu*II site in the gD-coding sequence has been changed to a *Hind*III site by insertion of a *Hind*III linker to match the *Hind*III site in the *cI* gene (see text). Bottom boxed area corresponds to the expressed region in the *cI/gD/βgal* fusion plasmid pMF100 (see text). Zigzag lines at the amino and carboxyl termini of gD depict the hydrophobic areas. Dashed line corresponds to the sequenced region (Watson et al. 1982). The *Nru*I site in parentheses is present in the HSV-1 Patton strain but absent in the McIntyre strain, all other sites are present in both strains.

weight of 125,000, of which 17,000 are *cI*-specific sequences and which has *β*gal activity, can be observed. The vectors can be opened at the junction between *cI* and *β*gal sequences and additional DNA can be inserted (Fig. 3). Since the translational reading frame at the cloning sites is known, the reading frame of the incoming DNA can be aligned by choosing the correct restriction sites or by introducing appropriate DNA linkers.

We constructed in this manner several *cI/gC/β*gal and several *cI/gD/β*gal fusion plasmids. An example of the structure of a plasmid encoding a *cI/gD/β*gal fusion protein is presented in Figure 3, and the corresponding IPTG-induced protein is shown in Figure 2. The fusion protein has a molecular weight of 155,000, of which approximately 30,000 correspond to gD-specific sequences. Figure 1 shows the location and extent of gD-specific sequences expressed in pMF100 (*Hind*III/*Nar*I fragment). Upon induction with IPTG, massive amounts of the fusion proteins are synthesized which form extractable precipitating particles.

The *cI/gC/β*gal and *cI/gD/β*gal fusion proteins appear to be stable and no longer toxic to *E. coli*. We interpret these findings such that removal of the hydrophobic

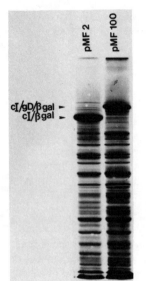

Figure 2
SDS-polyacrylamide gel electrophoresis of total protein extracts of IPTG-induced *E. coli* cultures harboring plasmids coding for a cI/βgal fusion protein (pMF2) and for a cI/gD/βgal fusion protein (pMF100). Arrows indicate the positions of the fusion proteins.

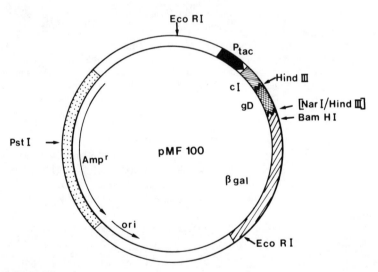

Figure 3
Structure of the cI/gD/βgal expression plasmid pMF100. The *tac* promoter and its direction of transcription are shown as a thick black arrow. Crosshatched area corresponds to an 800-bp, gD-specific HindIII/NarI fragment fused at its 5′ end to the aminoterminal sequence of the bacteriophage λcI repressor gene and at its 3′ end to a large carboxyterminal sequence of the *E. coli* βgal gene. Both fusions occur in the correct translational reading frame with gD sequences. Hatched areas correspond to cI and βgal sequences, respectively. Dotted area corresponds to the ampicillin resistance gene. (ori) Origin of replication.

sequences avoids strong toxic effects of gC and gD sequences to *E. coli* and that fusion to βgal protects these sequences from proteolytic degradation.

Initial Characterization of Antigenic Properties of gC and gD Fusion Proteins

For immunization experiments, we partially purified *cI/gC/βgal* and *cI/gD/βgal* fusion proteins and for control, a *cI/βgal* fusion protein. Proteins of approximately 60–80% homogeneity were used to immunize rabbits and mice (three injections). Blood samples were tested in an ELISA specific for HSV envelope antigen. In the case of the *cI/gD/βgal* protein, anti-gD antibody titers of 1/160 were observed, whereas the *cI/βgal* control protein and preimmune samples were negative (titer < 1/10). Experiments with *cI/gC/βgal* proteins are still in progress, and results have not yet been obtained.

DISCUSSION

We failed to produce authentic, unfused HSV-1 gC and gD proteins in *E. coli*. After removal of aminoterminal and carboxyterminal hydrophobic sequences of gC and gD, large parts of the coding sequences could be expressed at a high level as tripartite fusion proteins. Partial purification of *cI/gD/βgal* fusion protein and immunization of mice and rabbits resulted in anti-gD antibody production. Currently, we are performing protection experiments in mice, which, after immunization with *cI/gC/βgal* and *cI/gD/βgal* fusion proteins, will be challenged with HSV-1. These experiments should answer the question, if the approach followed here will result in the production of specific viral antigens in a prokaryotic host. One might envision the direct vaccination with highly purified fusion proteins or, as an alternative, the in vitro proteolytic degradation of the fusion proteins to obtain smaller peptides that possibly resemble authentic viral antigens more closely. In parallel to this approach we are planning to produce HSV antigens in eukaryotic systems.

ACKNOWLEDGMENTS

We thank J. Hilfenhaus for help with the immunization experiments, G. Polastri for critical reading of the manuscript, and M. Fach for excellent technical assistance.

REFERENCES

Amann, E., J. Brosius, and M. Ptashne. 1983. Vectors bearing a hybrid *trp-lac* promoter useful for regulated expression of cloned genes in *E. coli. Gene* **25:** 167.

Frink, R.J., R. Eisenberg, G. Cohen, and E.K. Wagner. 1983. Detailed analysis of the portion of the herpes simplex virus type 1 genome encoding glycoprotein C. *J. Virol.* **45(2):** 634.

Nahmias, A.J., J. Dannenbarger, C. Wickliffe, and J. Muther. 1981. In *The human herpesviruses: An interdisciplinary perspective* (ed. A.J. Nahmias et al.), p. 3. Elsevier, New York.

Watson, R.J., J.H. Weis, J.S. Salstrom, and L.W. Enquist. 1982. Herpes simplex virus type-1 glycoprotein D gene: Nucleotide sequence and expression in *E. coli. Science* **218:** 381.

Production of an HSV Subunit Vaccine by Genetically Engineered Mammalian Cell Lines

Laurence A. Lasky, Donald Dowbenko, Christian Simonsen,* and Phillip W. Berman
Departments of Vaccine Development and Molecular Biology, Genentech, Inc. South San Francisco, California 94080*

The problem of herpes simplex virus (HSV) infection has grown to epidemic proportions in the United States (Corey et al. 1983). Although the biology of these viruses has been extensively studied for some time, little progress has been made in terms of a treatment or cure for this malady. Although no immunotherapies are currently available, it is likely that a vaccine against HSV infection would provide a needed prophylactic measure. In this paper, we describe a new method by which a subunit vaccine against HSV infection has been produced using genetically engineered mammalian cells.

Glycoprotein D

Although the HSV-1 genome is large and codes for a variety of proteins, it has been shown that most of the host immune response against HSV infection is directed against the glycoproteins found on the surface of the virus. At least four glycoproteins are encoded by the virus: gA/B, gC, gD, and gE. Although neutralizing antibodies can be produced against any of these antigens, considerable evidence suggests that glycoprotein D (gD) is probably the most important neutralizing determinant (Norrild 1980). Observations that support this view are (1) gD from HSV-1 and HSV-2 share a number of antigenic determinants so that antibodies induced by one type of glycoprotein will cross-neutralize both viruses, (2) passively transferred anti-gD polyclonal and monoclonal antibodies have been shown to protect mice against HSV-1 and HSV-2 challenges, and (3) immunization of mice with purified HSV-1 gD protects them from a lethal HSV-1 or HSV-2 challenge. Taken together, these results indicate that a subunit vaccine made

189

from gD should serve to protect the immunized host from infection by both HSV-1 and HSV-2.

Cloning and Expression of the HSV-1 gD Gene in Mammalian Cells

The information available suggests that if sufficient quantities of gD were produced by recombinant DNA techniques, then a subunit vaccine against HSV infection would be feasible. To express the protein in a suitable host-vector system, the gene was cloned and the DNA sequence was determined. Analysis of the hydrophilic and hydrophobic regions of the protein sequence derived from the DNA sequence revealed that gD contained features typical of other membrane-bound glycoprotein sequences. Thus, an aminoterminal hydrophobic signal sequence was followed by a long stretch of sequence that contained three potential N-linked glycosylation sites. The carboxyl terminus of the protein encoded a hydrophobic membrane-binding domain followed by a hydrophilic cytoplasmic anchor sequence.

Previous work on the influenza hemagglutinin protein revealed that deletion of the carboxyterminal membrane-binding domain from the protein resulted in the secretion of this protein from cells when tested in short-term DNA-transfection assays (Gething and Sambrook 1982). Although significant quantities of hemagglutinin were produced in this short-term assay, the construction of continuous cell lines for the production of a secreted viral antigen would, undoubtedly, result in a more economic process for the production of a subunit vaccine. Cell lines producing such a secreted antigen would provide a novel approach to studying subunit vaccines because the product could be isolated directly from the culture medium, a procedure that would considerably simplify the isolation of the vaccine and would obviate the need to destroy the cells producing the vaccine.

Figure 1 illustrates the scheme for the construction of a vector system that establishes permanent mammalian cell lines that produce a secreted form of gD. Cleavage at the *Hin*fI site at amino acid 300 resulted in the removal of the carboxyterminal membrane-binding domain from gD. The *Hin*dIII-*Hin*fI fragment containing the bulk of the gD gene was isolated and then incorporated into a mammalian-cell expression vector as described in Figure 1. This plasmid, pgDtrunc•DHFR, contained the following features: (1) the truncated gD gene under the transcriptional control of the SV40 early promoter and utilizing the 3' termination and polyadenylation signals of the hepatitis-B surface antigen gene (Simonsen and Levinson 1983a), (2) a cDNA encoding the murine dihydrofolate reductase (DHFR) sequence under the transcriptional control of a second SV40 early promoter that allows for the selection of DHFR-deficient cell lines (Simonsen and Levinson 1983b), and (3) a bacterial vector containing the ampicillin resistance gene and bacterial origin of replication derived from the plasmid pBR322.

The plasmid described in Figure 1 was transfected onto DHFR-deficient Chinese hamster ovary (CHO) cells, and cell lines capable of growth in media lacking hypoxanthine, glycine, and thymidine were selected. Several cell lines were cloned, and the cells from two of the cloned lines were metabolically labeled with [^{35}S]methionine. Figure 2 illustrates the results of immunoprecipitation

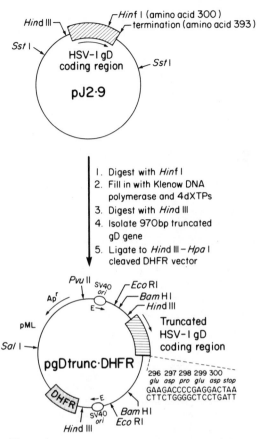

Figure 1
Diagram of the plasmid pgDtrunc•DHFR, constructed for the expression of a secreted form of gD. The expression plasmid consisted of the pBR322 bacterial origin of replication and ampicillin resistance gene, a cDNA clone encoding DHFR under the transcriptional control of the SV40 early promoter, and a *Hind*III-*Hin*fI fragment that encodes the first 300 amino acids of gD under the transcriptional control of a second SV40 early promoter. The *Hind*III site of this fragment lies 74 bp to the 5′ side of the gD initiator methionine. This *Hind*III site is also 250 bp to the 3′ side of the Goldberg-Hogness box of the SV40 early promoter. The *Hin*fI site, blunted with the DNA polymerase I Klenow fragment and the four deoxyribonucleotide triphosphates, was ligated to the *Hpa*I site in the 3′ nontranslated region of the hepatitis-B virus surface antigen gene (Simonsen and Levinson 1983a). The resultant plasmid was transfected into DHFR-deficient CHO cells using the calcium phosphate precipitation method.

experiments with intra- and extracellular extracts from these cell lines. Immunoprecipitations of intracellular extracts revealed that a discrete band at approximately 37,000 daltons could be immunoprecipitated with rabbit anti-HSV-1 antiserum. When the cell media were similarly analyzed, a diffuse band migrating at

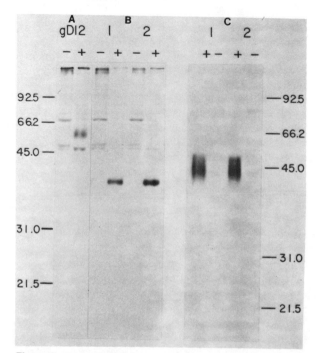

Figure 2

Radioimmunoprecipitation of cell-associated and secreted forms of gD. Cells were grown in Ham's F12 medium (GIBCO) lacking hypoxanthine, glycine, and thymidine and supplemented with 7% commercially dialyzed bovine fetal serum (GIBCO), penicillin (100 units/ml), and streptomycin (100 units/ml). When the cultures were approximately 80% confluent, the medium was removed, the cells were washed twice with phosphate-buffered saline (PBS), and labeling medium (Dulbecco's modified Eagle's medium containing one-tenth the normal concentration of methionine) was added to a final volume of 0.05 ml/cm^2. [^{35}S]Methionine (SJ.204; Amersham) was added to a final concentration of 50–75 μCi/ml, and the cells were grown for an additional 18–20 hr. After labeling, the medium was harvested, and the cells were washed twice in PBS and removed from the culture dish by treatment with PBS containing 0.02% EDTA. The cells were then solubilized in the lysis buffer containing PBS, 3% NP-40, 0.1% bovine serum albumin, 5×10^{-5} M phenylmethylsulfonyl fluoride, and 0.017 TIU/ml of aprotinin, and the resultant lysate was clarified by centrifugation at 12,000g. For immunoprecipitation reactions, cell lysates were diluted threefold with PBS, and aliquots (typically 180 μl) were mixed with 2–5 μl of serum and incubated at 4°C for 30 min. Immune complexes were then absorbed to fixed *Staphylococcus aureus* cells according to the method of Kessler (1975) and were precipitated by centrifugation at 12,000g for 30 sec. The *S. aureus* cells were then washed three times with wash buffer (PBS, 1% NP-40, 0.3% SDS), and the immune complexes were eluted with 20 μl of polyacrylamide sample buffer (62.5 mM Tris-HCl buffer, pH 6.8, containing bromphenol blue) at 90°C for 3 min. After centrifugation at 12,000g for 30 sec, the supernatants were applied to 10% polyacrylamide slab gels according to the method of Laemmli (1970). (*A*) Immunoprecipitation of membrane-bound gD. (*B*) Immunoprecipitation of the intracellular form of the truncated gD from lysates of two independently derived cell lines (1 and 2). (*C*) Immunoprecipitation of the truncated gD from the culture supernatants of the middle two cell lines. – indicates control rabbit antiserum; + indicates rabbit anti-HSV-1 antiserum (Dako Corp.).

192

about 45,000 daltons was detected. The difference in molecular weights found for the intra- and extracellular forms of the antigen appeared to represent a pre-cursor-product relationship between unglycosylated and glycosylated forms of gD. The secreted antigen was immunoprecipitated with a number of different rabbit and human polyclonal anti-HSV antibodies as well as several anti-gD monoclonal antibodies. It thus appears that the cell lines described here produce a gD that is synthesized, glycosylated, and transported to the extracellular medium and is antigenically similar to the native, membrane-bound form of gD.

Immunogenicity of Secreted gD

Although the secreted gD was found to be antigenically similar to native gD, in vivo experiments were performed to determine whether the secreted antigen would function as a subunit vaccine in the mouse. Vaccination and boosting of BALB/c mice were done as described in Table 1. At the end of the vaccination period, the mouse sera were tested for the ability to neutralize HSV-1 and HSV-2 in vitro. As shown in Table 1, sera from mice vaccinated with secreted gD were able to neutralize both HSV-1 and HSV-2, although the titers to HSV-2 were somewhat lower. To determine whether mice vaccinated with secreted gD would be protected from an HSV challenge, gD-vaccinated and control mice were inoculated with 1×10^7 plaque-forming units of HSV-1. Table 1 shows that although 80% of the control mice were either paralyzed or died from HSV-1 infection, 100% of the gD-vaccinated mice were protected from HSV-1-induced illness. These animal studies demonstrate that the secreted gD provides complete immunity to HSV-1 infection in the mouse.

Table 1
Immunogenicity of Secreted gD in Mice

Antigen[a]	Number	In vitro neutralization[b] titers ($\log_2$)		HSV-1 challenge[c,d]		
		HSV-1	HSV-2	paralyzed	dead	normal
HSA	13	<3	<3	3	7	3
Secreted gD	11	7	3.4	0	0	11

[a]Eight-week-old female BALB/c mice were injected at multiple intradermal and subcutaneous sites with approximately 3 µg of secreted gD emulsified in complete Freund's adjuvant. Four weeks after the primary immunization, the mice were boosted with the same amount of antigen incorporated in Freund's incomplete adjuvant. Control mice were matched to the experimentals with regard to age, sex, and strain and were immunized according to the same procedure, with the exception that 3 µg of human serum albumin (HSA) replaced the secreted gD. Serum samples were taken 19 days after boosting and were used for in vitro neutralization studies. Both groups of mice were challenged with virus 42 days after boosting.

[b]For in vitro neutralization studies, mouse sera serially diluted ($\log_2$ dilution range of 3–14) with Dulbecco's modified Eagle's medium containing 10% fetal calf serum were incubated with 40 pfu of HSV-1 or HSV-2 for 1 hr at 37°C in a volume of 200 µl. Aliquots (175 µl) of antibody-treated virus were applied to 4×10^4 VERO cells in each well of 96-well microtiter tissue-culture plates. After 4 days, the culture medium was removed, and the plates were stained with 0.5% crystal violet. Neutralization titers were calculated by determining the highest serum dilution that prevented virus growth.

[c]Mice were challenged by intraperitoneal injection of 1×10^7 pfu of HSV-1 (MacIntyre strain). Challenged mice were observed for a period of three weeks and were scored for HSV-1-induced paralysis and mortality.

[d]Significant at $p = 0.002$ level.

DISCUSSION

The results reported here provide the first demonstration of the usefulness of genetically engineered mammalian cell lines for the production of subunit vaccines. The encouraging animal results we have obtained suggest that an efficacious subunit vaccine for HSV infection may now be a reality.

REFERENCES

Corey, L., H. Adams, Z. Brown, and K. Holmes. 1983. Genital herpes simplex virus infections: Clinical manifestations, course, and complications. *Ann. Intern. Med.* **98:** 958.

Gething, M. and J. Sambrook. 1982. Construction of influenza hemagglutinin genes that code for intracellular and secreted forms of the protein. *Nature* **300:** 598.

Kessler, S. 1975. Rapid isolation of antigens from cells with a staphylococcal protein A-antibody adsorbent: Parameters of the interaction of antibody-antigen complexes with protein A. *J. Immunol.* **115:** 1617.

Laemmli, U. 1970. Cleavage of structural proteins during the assembly of the head of bacteriophage T4. *Nature* **227:** 680.

Norrild, B. 1980. Immunocytochemistry of herpes simplex virus glycoproteins. *Curr. Top. Microbiol. Immunol.* **90:** 67.

Simonsen, C.C. and A.D. Levinson. 1983a. Isolation and expression of an altered mouse dihydrofolate reductase cDNA. *Proc. Natl. Acad. Sci.* **80:** 2495.

———. 1983b. Analysis of processing and polyadenylation signals of the hepatitis B virus surface antigen gene using SV40-HBV chimeric plasmids. *Mol. Cell. Biol.* **3:** 2250.

Expression of Feline Panleukopenia Virus Antigens in *Escherichia coli*

Jonathan Carlson, Ian Maxwell,
Francoise Maxwell, Alistair Mcnab,
Keith Rushlow, Mike Mildbrand,
Yosh Teramoto, and Scott Winston
Syngene Products and Research
Fort Collins, Colorado 80524

Feline panleukopenia virus (FPV) is an autonomous parvovirus that infects the lymphoid and blood-forming tissues and the gastrointestinal mucosa of the cat, causing a drop in the white blood cell count and severe enteritis. The virus has given rise to at least two known variants that cause a similar disease in other host animals. In the late 1940s, an outbreak of severe enteritis in mink was shown to be due to a parvovirus (mink enteritis virus, MEV) that is very closely related to FPV. In the late 1970s, another variant, canine parvovirus (CPV), caused widespread outbreaks of enteritis in dogs and myocarditis in puppies. CPV is closely related to FPV on both the antigenic and nucleic acid levels as shown by comparative serological and restriction endonuclease mapping studies (Tratschin et al. 1982). CPV is thought to be of recent origin, since antibodies to the virus have not been detected in dog sera collected before 1976. Vaccines based on either inactivated or modified live FPV or CPV have been shown to confer protection in dogs against CPV. Conventional vaccines, however, suffer from the possibility of outbreaks of disease caused by incompletely inactivated or attenuated virus. FPV and CPV are known to be immunosuppressive under some situations and can therefore increase susceptibility to other infectious agents. This suggests that caution must be used in administration of vaccines based on whole virus preparations. An alternate approach to immunization is to use parvoviral antigens produced in bacteria by the use of recombinant DNA methods as the immunogen. Vaccines produced in this way should eliminate any problems associated with whole virus preparations, since complete virus would never be involved in the preparation.

195

Autonomous parvoviruses contain a single-stranded DNA genome of about 5 kb in length. The virions contain three proteins with approximate molecular weights of 83,000, 64,000, and 61,000. The largest species comprises about 10% of the virion protein. The other two proteins make up the remainder, although the relative proportions can vary considerably. The 61-kD protein is derived from the 64-kD protein by proteolytic cleavage. Most, if not all, of the amino acid sequences of the two smaller proteins are also contained in the large 83-kD protein. Since these structural proteins must contain the epitopes required for neutralization, our efforts were directed at cloning and expressing the gene coding for these proteins.

DISCUSSION

Cloning of FPV Sequences

The 3' end of DNA isolated from parvovirus contains inverted repeat sequences that form a hairpinlike structure at the end of the DNA. This terminal hairpin was used as a primer template by *Escherichia coli* DNA polymerase to convert the single-stranded viral DNA to double-stranded DNA. This product was used as a source for the portion of the genome between the *Eco*RI site at map position 20 and the *Pst*I site at position 58 (Fig. 1). This fragment was ligated to pBR322, which had been digested with *Eco*RI and *Pst*I to form the plasmid pEP19. The

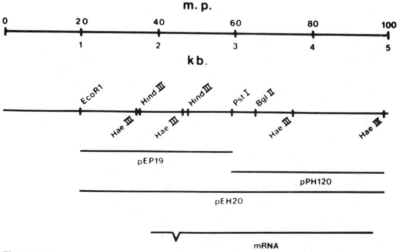

Figure 1

Portions of the FPV genome contained in the recombinant plasmids constructed from FPV DNA. The 5-kb linear genome runs from map position (m.p.) 0 at the 3' end to m.p. 100 at the 5' end. A simplified restriction map is shown along with the portions of the genome contained in plasmids pEP19, pPH120, and pEH20, which were constructed as described in the text. The bottom line indicates the position of the major FPV-specific mRNA on the genome.

portion of the genome between the *Pst*I site at position 58 and the *Hae*III site at position 96 (see Fig. 1) was cloned from replicative form DNA by digestion of the DNA with *Pst*I and then partial digestion with *Hae*III. This mixture of fragments was ligated with pBR322 that had been cut with *Eco*RI, treated with DNA polymerase to fill in the ends, and then cut with *Pst*I. One plasmid, pPH120, contained the desired insert.

A plasmid (pEH20) containing the entire FPV sequence from the *Eco*RI site at position 20 to the *Hae*III site at position 96 was constructed by ligating the *Pst*I-*Eco*RI insert from pEP19 and the *Pst*I-*Hind*III insert from pPH120 with pBR322 digested with *Eco*RI and *Hind*III. Restriction digests of the cloned FPV DNA have with minor exceptions confirmed the map published for MEV (Tratschin et al. 1982).

Single-strand-specific Nuclease Mapping of FPV Transcripts

The sequences coding for FPV-specific mRNA were mapped as follows. Cytoplasmic RNA from FPV-infected CFK cells was hybridized with single-stranded FPV DNA. The nonhybridized nucleic acids were digested with mung bean nuclease, and the protected fragments were run on alkaline agarose gels, blotted onto DBM paper, and annealed with ^{32}P-labeled nick-translated probes. This procedure allows sizing of the fragments of DNA complementary to the RNA. When this procedure was carried out using the pEP19 insert, fragments of about 270 bp and 660 bp were protected from digestion by mung bean nuclease. When FPV DNA between the *Hind*III sites at positions 34 and 48 was used in this procedure, fragments of about 270 bp and 100 bp were protected. When the pEH20 insert was used, fragments of about 270 bp and 2500 bp were protected by the RNA (data not shown). These results, together with results from similar experiments using restriction fragments labeled with ^{32}P at the 5′ ends, indicate that the major FPV-specific RNA consists of a 270-bp 5′ portion mapping between the *Hind*III sites spliced to a 2500-bp 3′ portion extending from about position 46 to about position 95. The major mRNA of FPV is therefore complementary to the 5′ half of the FPV genome as shown in Figure 1. This transcriptional map is similar to that for parvovirus MVM (minute virus of mice), as shown by single-strand-specific, nuclease-mapping experiments (Pintel et al. 1983). In parvovirus H1, this region of the genome codes for the three virion proteins as shown by hybrid-arrested translation experiments (Rhode and Paradiso 1983). Presumably, the virion proteins are coded by the 5′ half of the genome in FPV as well.

Synthesis of FPV Protein Sequences in *E. coli*

Expression of the cloned FPV DNA in *E. coli* was carried out using the methods and plasmids developed by Guarente et al. (1980). DNA sequences to be expressed were fused to the portion of the *E. coli* β-galactosidase gene that codes for the enzymically active carboxyterminal region of the protein. A portable transcriptional and translational control region consisting of the *E. coli lac* operator, promoter, ribosome binding site, and first eight codons of β-galactosidase was inserted into the FPV DNA after cleavage by an appropriate restriction enzyme and resection with BAL-31 nuclease. Bacteria were transformed with these plasmids, and expression of the hybrid gene was detected using agar plates containing an indicator for β-galactosidase activity. Restriction digests of plasmid DNA isolated from several transformants positive for β-galactosidase synthesis indicated that FPV DNA ranging from about 800 to 2000 bp in length was inserted between the *lac* promoter and the β-galactosidase gene. Four clones containing FPV inserts of about 800 bp (11Z24), 1100 bp (11Z13), 1400 bp (34.9), and 1800 bp (34.1) were selected for further characterization. A map of plasmid 11Z24 is shown in Figure 2A, and the portion of the FPV genome in the four β-galactosidase fusion plasmids is shown in Figure 2B.

We have also constructed an expression plasmid in which the FPV sequence extending from the *Hpa*II site at position 56 to the *Hae*III site at position 96 is fused to an *Hpa*II site in the *E. coli trp* LE' gene as shown in Figure 2 A and B. This plasmid places expression of the FPV protein sequences under control of the efficient *trp* promoter and leader peptide ribosome binding site. Furthermore, the LE' amino terminus renders fusion proteins insoluble and therefore less susceptible to proteolytic degradation (Kleid et al. 1981).

Lysates of bacteria transformed with these expression plasmids were subjected to electrophoresis in SDS-polyacrylamide gels. Two of the β-galactosidase fusion plasmids gave new Coomassie-blue-staining bands (Fig. 3A). In 11Z24, a prominent band at about 145 kD was present. This is about the size of the fusion protein, which would be expected from the size of the FPV DNA insert in 11Z24. In bacteria containing plasmid 34.1, a faint band at 165 kD is evident. This is somewhat smaller than the protein expected from this construction. Cells transformed with ptrpLEFPV in which the *trp* promoter had been induced by growth in the absence of tryptophan contain a new Coomassie-blue-staining protein based at about 69 kD (Fig. 3B). This is the expected molecular weight for the LEFPV fusion protein.

Gels identical to the stained gels shown in Figure 3, A and B, were blotted onto nitrocellulose. The blots were reacted first with rabbit antiserum raised against SDS-disrupted FPV and then with peroxidase-conjugated goat anti-rabbit IgG. Bands were visualized using diaminobenzidine as a substrate. As shown in Figure 3A, the new fusion protein bands in 11Z24 and 34.1 react strongly with the antiserum. In addition, a faint band is evident in the 34.1 lysate at about 175 kD to 180 kD. This is about the size of the fusion protein expected for 34.1. Some lower-molecular-weight bands also react with the serum. These are probably proteolytic degradation products of the fusion proteins, since they are not present in the control lysate. Similarly, the 69-kD band in the ptrpLEFPV lysate reacts with the serum as do a number of lower-molecular-weight degradation products (Fig. 3B). The FPV antigen synthesized by the ptrpLEFPV plasmid makes up approximately 5% of the protein in the lysates as quantitated by ELISA. The 11Z24 and 34.1 fusion proteins account for about 0.5% and 0.2%, respectively, of the total cellular protein. All three of the fusion proteins are insoluble and sediment to the pellet upon centrifugation at 10,000g. The proteins can be dissolved in either 0.5% SDS or 6 M urea.

A partially purified preparation of the 11Z24 protein was tested for its ability to raise antibodies against FPV in dogs. Two dogs that were immunized with five injections of protein developed serum neutralization titers of 1:128 and 1:256, whereas the titer of a contact control dog remained less than 1:2. However, reliable immunization of animals with this protein has proven difficult, and immunogenicity studies with the 34.1 and LEFPV proteins are in progress.

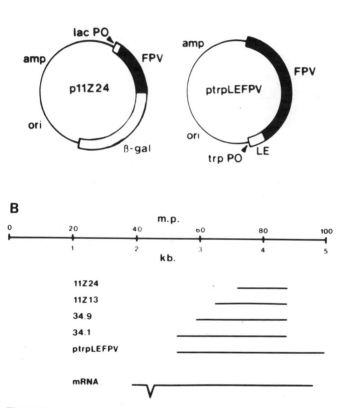

Figure 2
Plasmids that express FPV antigens. (*A*) Plasmids 11Z24 and ptrpLEFPV. The genes coding for the fusion proteins are represented as thicker regions. (■) FPV DNA; (□) bacterial sequences. (*B*) Regions of the FPV genome contained in the various expression plasmids. (*Top*) Linear map of the FPV genome; (*middle*) portions of the genome contained in the various plasmids. 11Z24, 11Z13, 34.9, and 34.1 are all fused to β-galactosidase at about position 84, 17 codons before the termination codon of the FPV protein. The *lac* promoter and ribosome binding site were fused to the FPV DNA at the left end of the lines drawn in the figure for these plasmids. The *trp* promoter and the amino terminus of the LE' gene were fused to the FPV DNA at the left end of the line labeled ptrpLEFPV. (*Bottom*) Position of the major FPV-specific mRNA shown for reference.

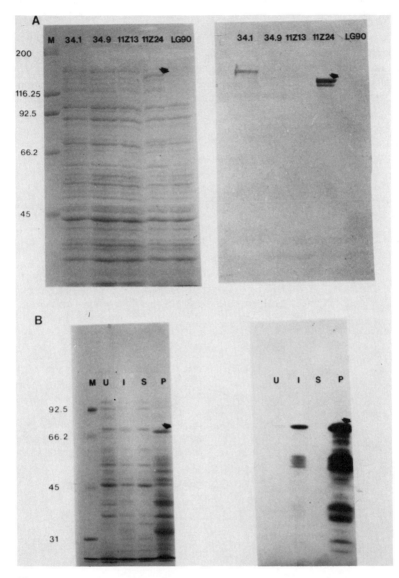

Figure 3
FPV fusion proteins produced in bacteria. (*A, left*) Coomassie-blue-stained SDS-polyacry-lamide gel of total lysates of bacteria transformed with the various β-galactosidase fusion plasmids. (M) Markers with the molecular weights indicated at the left; (LG90) a lysate of bacteria that contains no plasmid. (*A, right*) Nitrocellulose blot of an identical gel reacted with rabbit antiserum raised against SDS-disrupted FPV and developed as described in the text. Arrows indicate the 11Z24 fusion protein in both the gel and the blot. (*B, left*) Coomassie-blue-stained SDS-polyacrylamide gel of preparations from bacteria trans-formed with ptrpLEFPV. (U,I) Total lysates from uninduced and induced cells, respectively. (S,P) Supernatant and pellet fractions of a 10,000*g* centrifugation of an induced lysate. (*B, right*) Blot of an identical gel developed as described in the text. Arrows indicate the 69K LEFPV fusion protein.

SUMMARY

We have constructed recombinant DNA plasmids that contain about 80% of the FPV genome. These plasmids include the gene coding for the major virion protein. Plasmids that express portions of this gene as fusion proteins with either β-galactosidase or the *trp* LE' protein have been constructed. Studies are under way to determine whether or not these fusion proteins can raise a neutralizing antibody response against FPV and CPV in animals. These studies should help us to determine the position and the nature of the neutralizing epitopes of FPV and CPV and hopefully allow us to develop a safer, more effective vaccine against these viruses.

REFERENCES

Guarente, L., G. Lauer, T.M. Roberts, and M. Ptashne. 1980. Improved methods for maximizing expression of a cloned gene: A bacterium that synthesizes rabbit β-globin. *Cell* **20:** 543.

Kleid, D.S., D. Yansura, B. Small, D. Dowbenko, D.M. Moore, M.J. Grubman, P.D. McKercher, D.O. Morgan, B.H. Robertson, and H.L. Bachrach. 1981. Cloned viral protein vaccine for foot-and-mouth disease: Responses in cattle and swine. *Science* **214:** 1125.

Pintel, D., D. Dadachanji, C.R. Astell, and D.C. Ward. 1983. The genome of minute virus of mice, and autonomous parvovirus, encodes two overlapping transcription units. *Nucleic Acids Res.* **11:** 1019.

Rhode, S.L. III and P.R. Paradiso. 1983. Parvovirus genome: Nucleotide sequence of H-1 and mapping of its genes by hybrid-arrested translation. *J. Virol.* **45:** 173.

Tratschin, J.D., G.K. McMaster, G. Kranauer, and G. Siegl. 1982. Canine parvovirus: Relationship to wild-type and vaccine strains of feline panleukopenia virus and mink enteritis virus. *J. Gen. Virol.* **61:** 33.

The Rabies Glycoprotein Gene Is Expressed in *Escherichia coli* as a Denatured Polypeptide

Lawrence T. Malek, Gisela Soostmeyer,
Robert T. Garvin, and Eric James
Genetic Engineering Group
Connaught Research Institute
Willowdale, Ontario, Canada

Antibodies raised against purified rabies virus glycoprotein have been shown to neutralize infectious rabies virus, and the purified glycoprotein was about 70-fold more immunoprotective when used *alone* than when virally bound (Dietzschold et al. 1978). Rabies would therefore appear ideal for the application of genetic engineering methods in order to develop a superior subunit vaccine (for a recent review of rabies subunit vaccines, see Wunner et al. 1983). Accordingly, we have cloned the coding sequence of the rabies glycoprotein and have expressed this gene in *Escherichia coli* using a powerful prokaryotic promoter.

RESULTS

Synthesis and Sequence of the Rabies Glycoprotein Gene

A full-length DNA copy of the glycoprotein gene for the rabies virus ERA strain was obtained by oligonucleotide-primed synthesis from the genomic RNA template. After cloning the gene into pBR322, the complete DNA sequence was determined. The sequence is nearly identical to the one reported by Anilionis et al. (1981), having but three single-base substitutions and only one amino acid change. The amino acid change, a proline for a leucine at position 8 from the amino terminus of the mature glycoprotein, has been confirmed both by the DNA sequence of an independent gene subclone and by the amino acid sequence of the glycoprotein itself (Dietzschold et al. 1982).

Construction of an Expression Plasmid for the Rabies Glycoprotein Gene

To ensure the expression of biosynthetic rabies glycoprotein (BRG), the terminal *Eco*RI-*Hind*III DNA fragment of the cloned glycoprotein gene was replaced with

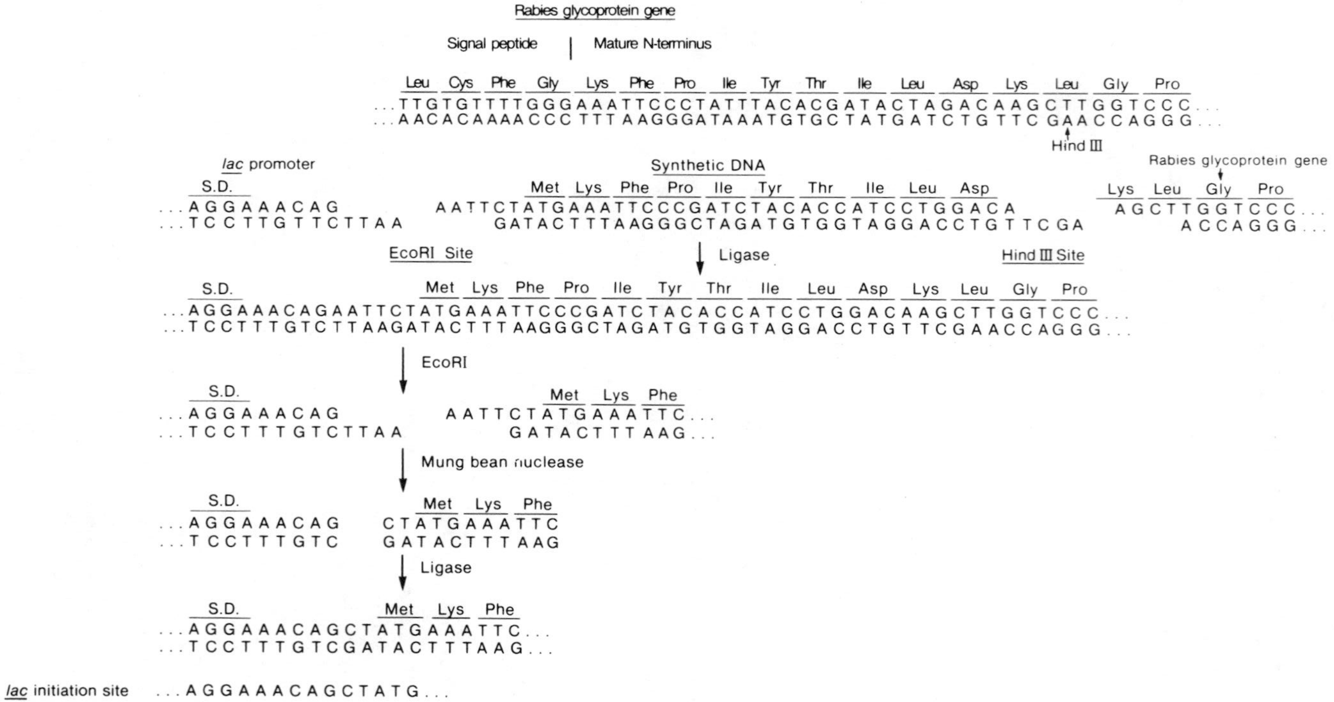

Rabies glycoprotein gene

Signal peptide | Mature N-terminus

Leu Cys Phe Gly Lys Phe Pro Ile Tyr Thr Ile Leu Asp Lys Leu Gly Pro
...TTGTGTTTGGGGAATTCCCTATTTACACGATACTAGACAAGCTTGGTCCC...
...AACACAAAACCCTTTAAGGGATAAATGTGCTATGATCTGTTCGAACCAGGG...
                                                    Hind III

Rabies glycoprotein gene

                                                    Lys Leu Gly Pro
                                                    AGCTTGGTCCC...
                                                    ACCAGGG...

Synthetic DNA

              Met Lys Phe Pro Ile Tyr Thr Ile Leu Asp
              AATTCTATGAAATTCCCGATCTACACCATCCTGGACA
              GATACTTTAAGGGCTAGATGTGGTAGGACCTGTTCGA
EcoRI Site   Hind III Site

              │ Ligase
              ▼
         Met Lys Phe Pro Ile Tyr Thr Ile Leu Asp Lys Leu Gly Pro
...AGGAAACAGAATTCTATGAAATTCCCGATCTACACCATCCTGGACCTGTTCGAACCAGGG...
...TCCTTTGTCTTAAGATACTTTAAGGGCTAGATGTGGTAGGACCTGGACCTGTTCGAACCAGGG...

S.D.
lac promoter

...AGGAAACAG
...TCCTTTGTCTTAA

S.D.

       │ EcoRI
       ▼
                Met Lys Phe
              AATTCTATGAAATTC...
              GATACTTTAAG...

S.D.
...AGGAAACAG
...TCCTTTGTCTTAA

       │ Mung bean nuclease
       ▼
                Met Lys Phe
              CTATGAAATTC
              GATACTTTAAG

S.D.
...AGGAAACAG
...TCCTTTGTC

       │ Ligase
       ▼
                Met Lys Phe
...AGGAAACAGCTATGAAATTC...
...TCCTTTGTCGATACTTTAAG...

S.D.

lac initiation site   ...AGGAAACAGCTATG...

Figure 1

Construction of an expression plasmid for the rabies glycoprotein gene. A segment of the glycoprotein gene, coding for the eukaryotic signal peptide and the first amino acids of the mature glycoprotein, was replaced with a 37-bp synthetic DNA fragment lacking the signal sequence. The modified glycoprotein gene was then joined to a lac UV5 promoter without altering the sequence of the lac initiation site. The glycoprotein amino acid sequence is indicated above the corresponding coding region sequence. The Shine-Dalgarno (S.D.) sequence is overlined.

204

a 37-bp synthetic oligonucleotide (Fig. 1). This not only removed the coding region for the signal peptide—a region known to be deleterious to vesicular stomatitis virus (VSV) glycoprotein expression in *E. coli* (Rose and Shafferman 1981)—but also positioned the initiator ATG next to the first codon of the mature rabies glycoprotein. The modified glycoprotein gene was inserted into a plasmid containing the *lac UV5* promoter, via the *Eco*RI site and a *Bam*HI site, which was positioned immediately after the natural stop codon. The natural *lac* initiation site was then restored by successive digestions with *Eco*RI and mung bean nuclease, followed by ligation of the resulting blunt ends (Fig. 1). Thus, both the natural spacing between the Shine-Dalgarno sequence and the initiator ATG and the natural sequence of the *lac* initiation site were preserved. This construction was intended to provide the inducible expression of a 58K, full-length (505 amino acid) BRG with no intervening leader at the amino terminus.

Expression and Identification of BRG in *E. coli*

Cultures of *E. coli* strain JM103 containing the rabies expression plasmid were grown in the presence or absence of the isopropylthio-β-D-galactoside (IPTG) inducer, and whole-cell protein extracts were analyzed by SDS-polyacrylamide gel electrophoresis (SDS-PAGE). A unique protein was present in the induced culture (Fig. 2, lane 3) but was absent in either the uninduced culture (lane 4) or an induced culture of JM103 harboring an analogous expression plasmid containing the human proinsulin structural gene (lane 2). The size of this protein, approximately 58K, agrees closely with that predicted for an unglycosylated product of the glycoprotein gene. The 58K BRG was more readily observed by analyzing the insoluble proteins of *E. coli* following disruption of the cells by sonication. The BRG was quantitatively recovered in the disrupted cell pellet of the induced culture (Fig. 2, lane 5) but was undetected in that of the uninduced culture (lane 6). The level of BRG expression from the *lac UV5* promoter was estimated to be 2–5% of the total *E. coli* protein.

The BRG was further characterized by Western blot analysis, using rabbit antisera prepared against authentic rabies virus glycoprotein, which had been purified by SDS-PAGE. The antisera reacted uniquely with the BRG, which was present in a culture expressing the glycoprotein gene (Fig. 2, lane 9) but was absent in a control culture expressing the human proinsulin gene (lane 8). The antisera also reacted with authentic 64K glycoprotein from the virus (lane 7). Western blot analysis was performed using total cellular *E. coli* or rabies virus proteins, which were separated by SDS-PAGE, as represented in Figure 2, lanes 1–3. Thus, preliminary biochemical and immunological data suggest that the product of the cloned rabies glycoprotein gene is an unglycosylated form of the rabies glycoprotein.

The BRG Produced in *E. coli* Is Not Immunocompetent

The BRG as produced by our gene construction in *E. coli* is *not* immunocompetent in mice. Since this material, with the possible exception of an aminoterminal *N*-formyl methionine, has an amino acid sequence identical to that of mature rabies glycoprotein, the failure of BRG to elicit a protective response could be

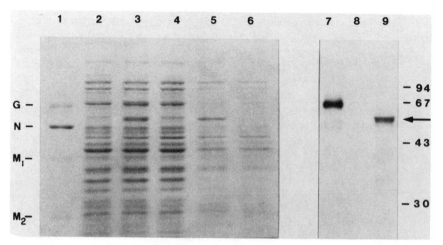

Figure 2
Expression and identification of BRG in *E. coli*. Cellular proteins from induced or uninduced cultures of *E. coli* JM103 were analyzed by 10% SDS-PAGE. (*1*) Rabies virus; (*2*) induced JM103 containing human proinsulin expression plasmid; (*3,4*) induced and uninduced JM103 containing BRG expression plasmid; (*5,6*) insoluble protein fraction of cells shown in lanes *3* and *4*, respectively. Western blot analysis (lanes *7–9*) of an SDS-gel (represented by lanes *1–3*) was performed using rabbit antisera prepared against authentic rabies glycoprotein. The four major rabies virus proteins shown in lane *1* are labeled at the left. Migration of marker proteins is indicated at the right by their molecular weights (in kilodaltons). Arrow indicates the position of BRG.

due either to the lack of glycosylation or to the inability of BRG to achieve the native glycoprotein conformation. Of these two possibilities, we believe the latter to be the more likely explanation for the following reasons. (1) Glycosylation has so far not been shown to be determinative of immunocompetence in any genetically engineered system known to us. (2) After mild reduction, rabies glycoprotein loses 95% of its immunological activity (Dietzschold et al. 1982). (3) Cytoplasmic proteins in *E. coli* are made reduced, i.e., proteins with stable disulfide bonds have not been detected in *E. coli* cytoplasmic extracts; however, β-lactamase is folded with the formation of one disulfide bond as it is transported into the periplasmic space (Pollitt and Zalkin 1983).

Oxidative Renaturation of BRG

The BRG expressed in *E. coli* does not elicit a protecting response and is presumably denatured. Therefore, the BRG needs to be renatured under conditions favoring disulfide bond formation. Accordingly, the partially purified glycoprotein obtained from the disrupted cell pellet (Fig. 2, lane 5) was dissolved in 7 M guanidine-HCl, dialyzed against 4 M urea and 2 mM dithiothreitol (DTT), and finally against buffer containing no urea and 0.1 mM DTT. A parallel dialysis was also performed in the presence of detergent. The solubility of BRG was monitored throughout the dialysis by SDS-PAGE and Western blot analyses. In the presence of detergent, BRG was completely soluble, whereas in the absence of detergent, only about half was soluble. In contrast, BRG, as produced in *E. coli,* is only soluble in denaturing solvents. Although solubility is rather inconclusive evidence for proper renaturation, only the water-soluble BRG gave positive results in the single radial diffusion (SRD) test for vaccine potency.

DISCUSSION

We have described the cloning, expression, and characterization of a biosynthetic rabies glycoprotein and have reported preliminary results of oxidative renaturation of the BRG directed toward the production of a genetically engineered subunit vaccine for rabies. In addition, we have drawn attention to the often overlooked question of oxidative folding of eukaryotic proteins and especially to the fact that disulfide bond formation does not occur when the protein is cytoplasmically expressed in *E. coli.* It is therefore apparent that *E. coli* will prove suitable as a host-vector system for the cytoplasmic expression of eukaryotic proteins only when the biologically active conformation is not dependent on the formation of disulfide bonds; in all cases of eukaryotic proteins needing disulfide bond formation for the attainment of native conformation, biological activity will only be observed if oxidative refolding is effected in vitro or if the address of the expressed protein is periplasmic.

The problem of renaturing the BRG and other eukaryotic proteins may be circumvented by the use of yeast or other eukaryotic cells as host systems. The cytoplasmic environment of these cells allows disulfide bond formation, and in the proper host cell, the protein may also be secreted, processed, and glycosylated. Host choice should therefore be of major consideration when contemplating the expression of eukaryotic proteins for use as vaccines, especially in those situations where the immunodominant epitopes are a consequence of secondary structure.

Note Added in Proof

The aminoterminal amino acid sequence determined for BRG was NH_2-Met-Lys-Phe-Pro-. This amino acid sequence, identical to that predicted from the DNA sequence, proves that the initiator methionine was not removed from BRG when expressed in *E. coli.* The presence of an aminoterminal methionine could be a cause for the apparent nonimmunogenicity of BRG.

ACKNOWLEDGMENTS

We thank Drs. Joel Haynes, Shi-Hsiang Shen, and Richard Elliott for obtaining the DNA sequence of the cloned rabies glycoprotein gene, Ms. Susan Meakin for technical assistance, Mr. Richard Hertler for providing rabies-virus-infected BHK cell media, and Miss Lynne-Marie McKay for secretarial assistance. This work was supported by a PILP grant from the National Research Council of Canada.

REFERENCES

Anilionis, A., W.H. Wunner, and P.J. Curtis. 1981. Structure of the glycoprotein gene in rabies virus. *Nature* **284:** 275.

Dietzschold, B., J.H. Cox, and G. Schneider. 1978. Structure and function of rabies glycoprotein. *Dev. Biol. Stand.* **40:** 45.

Dietzschold, B., T.J. Wiktor, R. Macfarlan, and A. Varrichio. 1982. Antigenic structure of rabies virus glycoprotein: Ordering and immunological characterization of the large CNBr cleavage fragments. *J. Virol.* **44:** 595.

Pollitt, S. and H. Zalkin. 1983. Role of primary structure and disulfide bond formation in β-lactamase secretion. *J. Bacteriol.* **153:** 27.

Rose, J.K. and A. Schafferman. 1981. Conditional expression of the vesicular stomatitis virus glycoprotein gene in *Escherichia coli. Proc. Natl. Acad. Sci.* **78:** 6670.

Wunner, W.H., B. Dietzschold, P.J. Curtis, and T.J. Wiktor. 1983. Rabies subunit vaccines. *J. Gen. Virol.* **64:** 1649.

Hepatitis-B Vaccine: Characterization of Hepatitis-B Antigen Particles Produced in Yeast

Pablo Valenzuela, Patricia Tekamp-Olson,
Doris Coit, Ulrike Heberlein, George Kuo,
Frank R. Masiarz, Maria A. Medina-Selby,
and Steve Rosenberg
*Chiron Research Laboratories, Chiron
Corporation, Emeryville, California 94608*

Joanne Whitney, Al Burlingame,
and William J. Rutter
*Department of Biochemistry and
Biophysics, University of California
San Francisco, California 94143*

Hepatitis-B virus (HBV) causes both acute disease (hepatitis) and late disease (chronic hepatitis, cirrhosis, and hepatocellular carcinoma). The worldwide impact of these diseases is tremendous. Most morbidity, as well as mortality amounting to several hundred thousand deaths per year, is associated with the late manifestations (Francis 1983). The control of HBV-related diseases by a safe and efficient vaccine would significantly improve world health.

A formalin-inactivated HBV vaccine has been produced in several laboratories (Francis 1983). The source of material for these vaccines has been the 22-nm lipoprotein particles (hepatitis-B surface antigen, HBsAg) derived from plasma of chronic HBV carriers. Such a source presents potential hazards in view of unknown factors that may be present in the plasma. In addition, as high-risk populations are immunized, sources of plasma containing large quantities of HBsAg will become scarce. These problems could be eliminated by alternative ways of producing HBsAg particles. This possibility became a reality when molecular cloning and nucleotide sequencing of the HBV DNA revealed the organization of the viral genome and the amino acid sequence of the two structural proteins of the virus (Valenzuela et al. 1979, 1980). Using this information, we were able to design and construct recombinant plasmids that induce yeast cells to produce hepatitis-B surface protein. These molecules then assembled with other species inside the yeast cell to produce highly immunogenic HBsAg particles (Valenzuela et al. 1982). Similar results have been confirmed by others (Hitzeman et al. 1983;

Miyanohara et al. 1983). The similarity in structure of the yeast particle to bona fide 22-nm particles isolated from sera of carriers and the high immunogenicity in animals emphasized the value of the yeast HBsAg particle as a vaccine.

Synthesis of HBsAg Particles in Yeast

At Chiron we have developed a technology that allows the efficient synthesis of this antigen in yeast, and we have genetically engineered yeast strains presently employed by scientists at Merck, Sharp, and Dohme in the development of a second-generation hepatitis-B vaccine that has been successfully tested in animals (McAleer et al. 1984). Briefly, these in vitro genetic manipulations are as follows (Fig. 1A): (1) We have modified the HBsAg coding region, deleting 5'-untranslated sequences that have proved deleterious for expression. (2) We have isolated and used several new yeast promoters to drive efficiently the transcription apparatus in yeast, especially those from the glycolytic enzymes glyceraldehyde 3P dehydrogenase and pyruvic kinase, which have proved to be very active at high cell densities. Using promoters that can be regulated, such as those from copper-chelatin and pho-5 genes, we have been able to regulate the

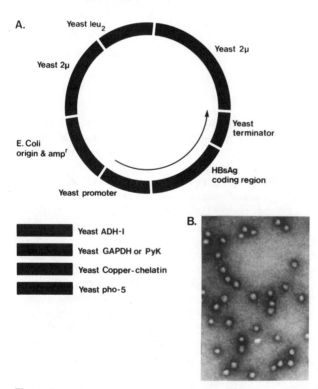

Figure 1
(*A*) Structure of plasmid vectors for the expression of HBsAg in yeast. (*B*) Electron micrographs of yeast HBsAg purified by immunoabsorption.

expression of HBsAg by changing the concentration of Cu^{++} or phosphate, respectively. (3) We have introduced 3'-flanking regions from homologous yeast genes to terminate efficiently transcription at the proper sites. (4) Finally, we have utilized new vectors that allow the stable maintenance of the plasmid in high copy number in the absence of selective medium. Using this system, it is possible to produce particles such as those shown in Figure 1B at very high yields.

Structure of the Yeast HBsAg Particle

Several experiments indicate that the particles produced in yeast represent a lipoproteic structure assembled by the specific interactions of the surface protein and membrane phospholipids from the yeast cell: (1) Particles can be obtained by mechanic disruption of the yeast cells with glass beads or by gentle osmotic shock of yeast spheroplasts, suggesting that the particle formation is not related to the extraction procedure used. Yields from osmotically shocked cells increase considerably in the presence of low (0.1–0.01%) concentrations of the nonionic detergent Triton X-100. These concentrations of Triton X-100 do not solubilize membranes and are probably necessary to disaggregate the particles from other cell components. (2) Velocity and equilibrium sedimentation studies in sucrose and CsCl gradients, respectively, indicate relatively homogeneous particles with

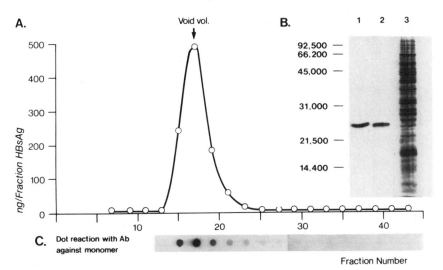

Figure 2
Gel filtration and SDS gel electrophoresis of yeast extracts containing HBsAg. (*A,C*) Gel filtration in Sephacryl S-200; fractions were assayed for particle using the Abbott AUSRIA test and for monomer by a dot assay using a specific monoclonal antibody. (*B*) SDS gel electrophoresis of purified yeast HBsAg particles and of crude yeast extracts. (*1*) HBsAg-containing yeast extracts were subjected to SDS gel electrophoresis, transferred to nitrocellulose, and developed with monoclonal antibody against surface protein; (*2*) SDS gel electrophoresis of immunoaffinity-purified yeast HBsAg particles; (*3*) SDS gel electrophoresis of yeast extracts containing HBsAg.

a sedimentation coefficient of about 40S and a density of 1.19 g/ml, values that are practically identical to those of particles isolated from serum. (3) Direct observation by electron microscopy (Fig. 1B) shows that the sizes of the particles synthesized in yeast and isolated either by velocity sedimentation or by immunoaffinity chromatography are quite homogeneous (16–26 nm) and are not randomly broken membrane pieces. No particles are detected by electron microscopy after centrifugation of extracts from control yeast cells lacking the expression plasmid. This indicates that the synthesis of the surface protein monomer is a requisite to the formation of the particles. (4) Only one protein species with a molecular weight of about 25,000 is obtained by SDS gel electrophoresis of highly purified particles (Fig. 2B).

The fraction of surface protein present as the HBsAg particle in the cell extracts has been determined using a monoclonal antibody able to react efficiently not only with the HBsAg particle, but also with the surface protein monomer. Using this antibody, it is possible to detect the 25K surface protein after blotting SDS gels into nitrocellulose filters (Fig. 2B). Analysis by gel filtration of cell extracts solubilized in mild detergent indicates that all of the surface protein material (assayed either by the Abbott AUSRIA [Fig. 2A] test or by a dot assay using the monoclonal antibody [Fig. 2B]) is present in the high-molecular-weight form. This high-molecular-weight fraction is quantitatively retained by immunoaffinity columns and determined by electron microscopy to be formed of 18–24-nm particles (not shown). These results indicate that in contrast to a recent report (Hitze-

Table 1
Partial Lipid Composition of Biosynthetic HBsAg Particle

	Yeast (%)		Mammalian (%)	
Lipids	particle	cells	particle	cells
Sterols				
and sterol esters				
ergosterol	97	100	—	—
cholesterol	3	—	100	100
16:0	42	55	60	
16:1	23	35	40	
18:0	21	10	—	
18:1	14	—	—	
Triglycerides				
16:0	30	21	48	44
16:1	45	42	17	23
18:0	9	6	16	14
18:1	16	32	19	20
Phosphoryl choline				
16:0; 16:0	18	22		
16:1; 16:0	36	43		
16:1; 16:1	—	—		
16:0; 18:0	36	26		
18:0; 18:0	9	9		

Comparison of the values obtained by mass spectrometry of lipid fractions from particles isolated from recombinant yeast and mammalian cells (Laub et al. 1983), as well as membranes from both host cells.

man et al. 1983), most, if not all, of the surface protein in the cell extract is assembled into the HBsAg particles.

We have initiated the characterization of the lipidic components of the HBsAg particles synthesized in yeast and in mammalian cells by mass spectrometry. Preliminary results (see Table 1) indicate a significant similarity between the lipidic molecules of the yeast particle and those from the mammalian particle; there are differences such as the prevalence of unsaturated fatty acids and the presence of ergosterol instead of cholesterol in yeast. These experiments indicate that both particles have grossly similar structures but with distinct differences due to the specific host cell where they are synthesized.

CONCLUSION

Our studies indicate that genetically engineered yeast cells efficiently synthesize and assemble bona fide HBsAg particles. These particles constitute an excellent material for the preparation of a second-generation hepatitis-B vaccine that is safer than that obtained from previous sources and is available in unlimited quantities. The vaccine produced in yeast using this technology has proven to be highly efficacious in animals (McAleer et al. 1984). Clinical trials in humans are in progress.

REFERENCES

Francis, D.P. 1983. Selective primary health care: Strategies for control of disease in the developing world. III. Hepatitis B virus and its related diseases. *Infect. Dis. Rev.* **5:** 322.

Hitzeman, R.A., C.Y. Chen, F.E. Hagie, E.J. Patzer, C.C. Liu, D.A. Estell, J.V. Miller, A. Yaffe, D. Kleid, A.D. Levinson, and H. Oppermann. 1983. Expression of hepatitis B virus surface antigen in yeast. *Nucleic Acids Res.* **11:** 2745.

Laub, O., L.B. Rall, M. Truett, Y. Shaul, D.N. Standring, P. Valenzuela, and W.J. Rutter. 1983. Synthesis of hepatitis B surface antigen in mammalian cells. Expression of the entire gene and the coding region. *J. Virol.* **48:** 271.

McAleer, W.J., E.B. Buynak, R.Z. Maigetter, E. Wampler, and W.J. Miller. 1984. Human hepatitis B vaccines from recombinant yeast. *Nature* **307:** 178.

Miyanohara, A., A. Toh-e, C. Nozaki, F. Hamada, N. Ohtomo, and K. Matsubara. 1983. Expression of hepatitis B surface antigen in yeast. *Proc. Natl. Acad. Sci.* **80:** 1.

Valenzuela, P., A. Medina, W.J. Rutter, G. Ammerer, and B.D. Rutter. 1982. Synthesis and assembly of hepatitis B virus surface antigen particles in yeast. *Nature* **298:** 347.

Valenzuela, P., M. Quiroga, J. Zaldivar, P. Gray, and W.J. Rutter. 1980. The nucleotide sequence of the hepatitis B viral genome and the identification of the major viral genes. In *Animal virus genetics* (ed. B.N. Fields et al.), p. 55. Academic Press, New York.

Valenzuela, P., P. Gray, M. Quiroga, J. Zaldivar, H.M. Goodman, and W.J. Rutter. 1979. Nucleotide sequence of the gene coding for the major protein of the hepatitis B virus surface antigen. *Nature* **280:** 815.

Genetically Engineered Vaccine against Avian Infectious Bronchitis Virus with the Advantages of Current Live and Killed Vaccines

**David Cavanagh, Matthew M. Binns,
Michael E.G. Boursnell, and T. David K. Brown**
*Department of Microbiology
Houghton Poultry Research Station
Houghton, Huntingdon, Cambs.
PE17 2DA, England*

Avian infectious bronchitis virus (IBV) is a disease of chickens and is of considerable economic importance. It results in the loss of egg production in layers and in reduced weight gain and death due to secondary infection with *Escherichia coli* and other bacteria in broilers. Nonrespiratory tissues, e.g., oviduct and kidney, can also be damaged. The disease is generally controlled by live-virus vaccines. These are relatively inexpensive to produce, are conveniently and cheaply administered, and have been generally successful. However, stability is low, they can have adverse effects on the kidneys and reproductive tract, and they predispose young chickens to secondary infection by bacteria. Most reports have indicated that killed IBV vaccines are poor inducers of respiratory tract protection, although they have been used successfully to boost a primary response induced by a live vaccine. Although costly to produce and administer, they lack the disadvantage of the live vaccine.

The greater efficacy of live vaccines compared with that of killed vaccines has not been explained. One factor may be that live vaccines efficiently induce protection because the virus replicates at the tracheal mucosa and stimulates local immunity. Ideally, what is required is a vaccine that not only stimulates good immunity, but also is cheap, stable, convenient to use, and safe.

Design of a Novel Vaccine

We propose to develop a vaccine in which there is a live component (*E. coli*) replicating at a mucosal surface (the gut) and producing the viral protection-inducing peptides (PIPs; equivalent to a killed vaccine). The bacterium would be applied in food or drinking water. A nonpathogenic bacterium replicating in a

215

region of the respiratory tract might be the best vector, since IBV replicates principally in the respiratory tract. However, little is known about their use for genetic manipulation.

The gut and respiratory mucosae of some mammals are known to form part of a common mucosal immune system (Bienenstock et al. 1981). If this exists in the chicken, then it would be expected that some IBV-specific immune cells that are stimulated in the gut would populate the respiratory tract and protect it against IBV infection. This aspect of the chicken's immune system is being studied. Also, nonpathogenic strains of *E. coli* capable of colonizing the gut of chickens are being evaluated for their suitability as hosts for plasmid vectors that will express the PIPs.

Role of IBV Proteins in Immunity

IBV is a coronavirus comprising a lipid membrane, a single-stranded RNA genome, and three protein structural elements: the nucleocapsid (N) protein, associated with the RNA; a transmembrane glycosylated membrane (M) protein; and teardrop-shaped surface projections or spikes (S). The S protein comprises equal amounts of two glycopolypeptides S1 (m.w. 90,000) and S2 (m.w. 84,000) (Cavanagh 1983b). The polypeptide moiety of S1 and S2 is approximately 60K (Cavanagh 1983a). Each spike contains two, possibly three, copies of S1 and S2, and a model for S has recently been proposed (Fig. 1) (Cavanagh 1983c).

The S, M, and N proteins of IBV have been separated using nonionic detergent (Cavanagh 1983b); lyophilized and resolubilized S was in the shape of rosettes formed by aggregation of the molecules at their hydrophobic ends (Cavanagh 1983c). Intramuscular inoculation of chickens with 20-μg quantities of S, M, or N with Freund's adjuvant on three occasions resulted in the induction of serum-virus-neutralizing (SN) and hemagglutination-inhibiting (HI) antibodies in chickens vaccinated with S, but not with M or N (D. Cavanagh and J.H. Darbyshire, in prep.). The maximum SN and HI titers were similar to those obtained by infection of chickens. However, the chickens were not resistant to live-virus challenge.

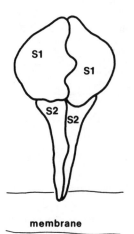

membrane

Figure 1
A speculative model for the S protein of IBV. (Reprinted, with permission, from Cavanagh 1983c.)

Low titers of anti-M protein-complement-dependent neutralizing antibody have been reported for some coronaviruses; the importance of these in vivo has yet to be determined. Studies with several coronaviruses have indicated that S is largely responsible for the induction of neutralizing antibody and, in one study (Hasony and Macnaughton 1981), for protection. Whether the PIPs are contained within S1, S2, or both is unknown. An anti-S neutralizing monoclonal antibody has recently been shown to bind S1 and not S2 (A.P.A. Mockett et al., in prep.).

Cloning of IBV Genes

The IBV mRNA that contains the S-precursor gene forms a very small proportion of the total IBV-specific mRNA in chick kidney cells (Stern and Kennedy 1980; T.D.K. Brown and D. Cavanagh, unpubl.). IBV genomic RNA—a single-stranded molecule of approximately 20 kb with a 3' poly(A) tail—can be obtained in much greater quantity from purified IBV grown in embryonated eggs. Therefore, genomic RNA was used to produce double-stranded cDNA corresponding to the first 3.3 kb from the 3' end, using oligo(dT) priming and reverse transcriptase; this sequence, some of which has been determined, includes the N and M genes (Boursnell and Brown 1983). An oligonucleotide primer was made that corresponded to a sequence of 13 nucleotides approximately 150 bases in from the 5' terminus of the cDNA. This is currently being used to produce more cDNA that will encompass the S-precursor gene.

Protection-inducing Antigenic Determinants of IBV

Identification of the protection-inducing determinants of IBV is being undertaken using some of the approaches referred to elsewhere in this volume. Consideration of serological protection studies of IBV raises an interesting point. IBV shows extensive antigenic variation and has been divided into serotypes on the basis of in vitro neutralization tests; strains of one serotype show little or no cross-neutralization of strains of other serotypes (see Darbyshire et al. 1979). However, vaccination of chickens with one serotype can result in protection of the respiratory tract against other serotypes. Although this does not apply to all IBV isolates, it does indicate that some of the protection-inducing determinants of IBV are common to isolates of several serotypes. This implies that the identification of those antigenic determinants that induce neutralizing antibody (determined in vitro) will not concurrently identify those antigenic determinants responsible for the induction of protection in vivo. The identification and further study of conserved regions of IBV polypeptides may therefore be very important. We are currently devising a protocol for the in vivo testing of the protection-inducing capacity of IBV peptides.

SUMMARY

Our approach, in which a live bacterium would be used to produce PIPs within the alimentary tract of chickens, has been adopted because of the necessity of combining the efficacy and cheapness of conventional live vaccines with the greater stability and safety of killed vaccines. If detrimental and unavoidable processing of the PIPs occurs in bacteria, then the use of viral vectors can be examined.

ACKNOWLEDGMENT

This research was carried out under research contract GBI-2-011-UK of the Biomolecular Engineering Programme of the Commission of the European Communities.

REFERENCES

Bienenstock, J., A.D. Befus, and M. McDermott. 1981. Mucosal immunity. In *The mucosal immune system* (ed. F.J. Bourne), p. 5. The Hague, Martinus Nijhoff Publishers.

Boursnell, M.E.G. and T.D.K. Brown. 1983. DNA sequencing studies of genomic cDNA clones of avian infectious bronchitis virus. In *Coronaviruses: Molecular biology and pathogenesis* (ed. P.J.M. Rottier et al.). Plenum Press, London. (In press.)

Cavanagh, D. 1983a. Coronavirus IBV glycopolypeptides: Size of their polypeptide moieties and nature of their oligosaccharides. *J. Gen. Virol.* **64:** 1187.

———. 1983b. Coronavirus IBV: Further evidence that the surface projections are associated with two glycopolypeptides. *J. Gen. Virol.* **64:** 1787.

———. 1983c. Coronavirus IBV: Structural characteristics of the spike protein. *J. Gen. Virol.* **64:** 2577.

Darbyshire, J.H., J.G. Rowell, J.K.A. Cook, and R.W. Peters. 1979. Taxonomic studies on strains of avian infectious bronchitis virus using neutralization tests in tracheal organ cultures. *Arch. Virol.* **61:** 227.

Hasony, J.H. and M.R. Macnaughton. 1981. Antigenicity of mouse hepatitis virus strain 3 subcomponents in C57 strain mice. *Arch. Virol.* **69:** 33.

Stern, D.F. and S.I.T. Kennedy. 1980. Coronavirus multiplication strategy. I. Identification and characterization of virus-specified RNA. *J. Virol.* **24:** 665.

Cloning and Expression of the Surface Glycoprotein gp195 of Porcine Transmissible Gastroenteritis Virus

Sylvia Hu, Joan Bruszewski,
Thomas Boone, and Larry Souza
Amgen, Thousand Oaks, California 91320

Transmissible gastroenteritis virus (TGEV) causes acute and highly contagious enteric disease in pigs. Although pigs of all ages are susceptible to TGEV infection, the effects on newborn piglets and lactating sows are most severe. Clinical signs include vomiting, diarrhea, and dehydration, and most pigs that die of TGEV do so in 3–5 days. The mortality rate in newborn pigs frequently approaches 100%. Although accurate statistics are not available, extensive epidemics of TGEV occur every winter in the swine belt. There is no safe and effective vaccine or practical method of treatment (Bohl 1975).

TGEV is an enveloped RNA-containing virus that belongs to the group called coronaviruses. The genome of TGEV is an 18.5-kb single-stranded RNA of positive polarity. This RNA is associated with the 55-kD nucleocapsid protein. There are two major glycoproteins present in the virion of TGEV: gp31 is found mostly embedded within the membrane, whereas gp195 forms the surface projections that protrude from the membrane. Only one serotype of TGEV is known so far, and this is determined by gp195. Virions lacking gp195 are not infectious. A semipurified preparation of gp195, when injected into pigs, elicited a neutralizing immune response that was protective against the challenge of TGEV (Garwes et al. 1978/1979). These properties of gp195 imply that it might be used as an effective subunit vaccine. When in vivo glycosylation of gp195 is inhibited by tunicamycin, or when most of the sugar moiety on gp195 is cleaved off by endoglycosidase H, a 145-kD protein is generated (Fig. 1). These results showed that the protein component of gp195 is 145 kD, and a gene coding for protein of this size is estimated to be about 3.9 kb.

By inhibiting host-cell RNA synthesis with actinomycin D, we have identified

219

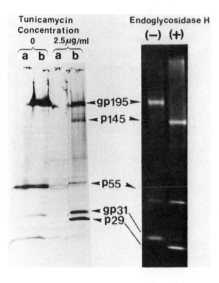

Figure 1
(*Left*) SDS-polyacrylamide gel electrophoresis of TGEV proteins immunoprecipitated from infected cells with or without tunicamycin treatment using normal pig serum (*a*) and neutralizing pig serum (*b*). (*Right*) Shift of migration in gel of the two immunoprecipitated TGEV glycoproteins when they were digested with endoglycosidase H.

six discrete virus-specific poly(A)-containing RNAs in TGEV-infected cells. The sizes of these mRNAs are 18.5 (genomic), 9.4, 5.3, 4.3, 2.9, and 2.0 kb. It is known that for coronaviruses, all of these RNAs are messengers, but that expression occurs by translation of only the 5'-terminal part of the RNA not present in the next smaller RNA (Fig. 2). It is obvious that only the 18.5 and 9.4 kb mRNAs of TGEV are large enough to encode a 3.9-kb (gp195) gene.

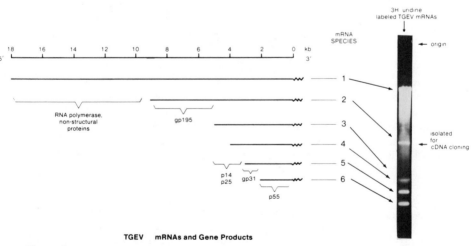

Figure 2
Transcriptional scheme of TGEV and the six discrete-size TGEV mRNAs identified by gel electrophoresis.

After isolating each TGEV mRNA species, we performed in vitro translation with the rabbit reticulocyte lysate system, followed by immunoprecipitation of the translation product with TGEV-specific antiserum. Only the 9.4-kb mRNA served as a template to synthesize a 145-kD protein that is in turn immunoprecipitable (data not shown). We therefore concluded that the gp195 gene was located near the 5' end of the 9.4-kb mRNA. Our later cloning and expression of this region directly confirmed this map location for gp195.

We purified the 9.4-kb and the 18.5-kb (genomic) TGEV mRNAs by sucrose gradient and subjected them to the cDNA cloning protocol originated by Okayama and Berg (1982). One cDNA clone obtained from the genomic RNA contained 9.4 kb of TGEV sequences starting at the 3' end. A restriction endonuclease cleavage map of this clone was constructed (Fig. 3). Partial nucleic acid sequence analysis revealed one unique, translational open reading frame that probably extended continuously for 3.9 kb in the predicted gp195 coding region, starting 8 bases downstream from the second 5' *Hpa*I site and ending 80 bases upstream of the unique *Xba*I site. Later experiments showed that translation of the entire 3.9-kb region gave rise to a single polypeptide chain, confirming that this region contained one common open reading frame. Several interesting features were noted from the sequences. First, the amino acid sequences are generally very hydrophobic, with many potential carbohydrate attachment sites (Asn-X-Ser or Asn-X-Thr). Second, the aminoterminal 20 amino acids resemble typical "signal-peptide" sequences for secretory proteins (Inouye and Halegoua 1980). Third, sequences around the amino terminus are ACC<u>AUG</u>A, and sequences around the carboxyl terminus are GCC<u>AUG</u>A; in both cases, the AUG codons fulfill the characteristics of a translation initiation codon (Kozak 1981). Further-

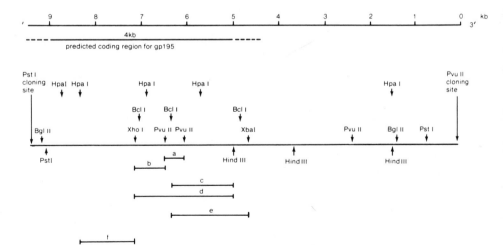

Figure 3
Restriction endonuclease cleavage map of the 9.4-kb TGEV sequences starting from the 3' end of the genome. (*a–f*) Fragments that have been subcloned for expression in *E. coli.*

more, analysis of the translational reading frame indicated that the UGA codons in frame one serve as the termination for translating the genes upstream, whereas the AUG codons in a different frame could initiate the translation of the downstream proteins.

To express the entire region coding for gp195 in *Escherichia coli*, the fragments (Fig. 3; *Hpa*I-*Xho*I, *Xho*I-*Pvu*II, *Pvu*II-*Pvu*II, *Bcl*I-*Hind*III, *Bcl*I-*Xba*I, and *Xho*I-*Hind*III) were first cloned into M13 to determine the sequences and therefore the open reading frame. Utilizing additional restriction endonuclease cleavage sites found in the adjacent M13 sequences, the various fragments were then cloned into a plasmid, pFM414, that carries a temperature-sensitive mutation in plasmid copy number control, so that 50- to 100-fold excess of plasmid-coded gene products can be induced by temperature shift. The *E. coli trp* promoter and the aminoterminal coding region of another gene having a restriction site in the same reading frame as the TGEV-M13 fragment were cloned simultaneously (utilizing three-way ligation) with pFM414, allowing TGEV fusion proteins to be formed. With all constructions, fusion proteins of full predicted size were synthesized with no smaller by-products. The levels of expression varied and were inversely related to the size of the products, generally between 2% and 10% of the total cellular protein. These TGEV-related proteins were isolated (Fig. 4) and tested for their antigenicity and immunogenicity in rabbits and rats. They were all antigenic and raised humoral antibodies in immunized animals that not only bind to the original immunogen, to the intact TGEV, but also specifically immunoprecipitated gp195. The neutralizing titers of these immune sera against TGEV are now being tested.

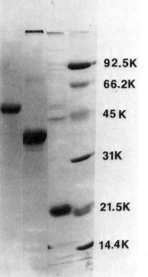

Figure 4
SDS-polyacrylamide gel electrophoresis of three of the purified TGEV proteins expressed in *E. coli*. (a–c) Products coded by fragments a–c in Fig. 3.

REFERENCES

Bohl, E.H. 1975. Transmissible gastroenteritis. In *Diseases of swine* (ed. H.W. Dunne and A.D. Leman), p. 168. Iowa State University Press, Ames, Iowa.

Garwes, D.J., M.H. Lucas, D.A. Higgins, B.V. Pike, and S.F. Cartwright. 1978/1979. Antigenicity of structural components from porcine transmissible gastroenteritis virus. *Vet. Microbiol.* **3**: 179.

Inouye, M. and S. Halegoua. 1980. Secretion and membrane localization of proteins in *Escherichia coli. CRC Crit. Rev. Biochem.* **7**: 339.

Kozak, M. 1981. Possible role of flanking nucleotides in recognition of the AUG initiator codon by eukaryotic ribosomes. *Nucleic Acids Res.* **9**: 5233.

Okayama, H. and P. Berg. 1982. High-efficiency cloning of full-length cDNA. *Mol. Cell Biol.* **2**: 161.

In Vitro Genetic Constructions Devised to Express Given Antigenic Determinants at the Surface of Gram-negative Bacteria

**Bernadette Bouges-Bocquet, Jean-Luc Guesdon,
Christian Marchal, and Maurice Hofnung**
Unité de Programmation Moléculaire et
Toxicologie Génétique CNRS LA.271, INSERM U.163
Institut Pasteur, 75015 Paris, France

It has been shown that it is possible to change the cellular location of a bacterial cytoplasmic protein, β-galactosidase, by constructing hybrid proteins with the aminoterminal part of an outer membrane protein (for review, see Hall and Silhavy 1981). One consequence of this work could be to expose an immunological polypeptide at the surface of a gram-negative bacterium. This could, for example, result in a new type of vaccine, but it would also be a good test of our knowledge of the rules governing protein localization. Therefore, we have started the construction of hybrid molecules between an outer membrane protein, which could act as a carrier to the outer membrane, and immunogenic polypeptides. We chose maltoporin (LamB protein) as the outer membrane protein.

In this paper, we describe our attempts to construct hybrid proteins through the intermediate of fusions with β-galactosidase, and we present an analysis of the sites affecting location, stability, and toxicity of modified LamB proteins. We also describe the early results of hybrid construction with a fragment of the surface antigen, HBs, of hepatitis-B virus, as immunogenic polypeptide.

Cloning through the Intermediate of Fusions with β-Galactosidase

Proximal fragments of the *lamB* gene of different lengths have been fused with the *lacZ* gene coding for β-galactosidase (for review, see Hall and Silhavy 1981; Benson and Silhavy 1983). The fused genes produce hybrid proteins that— whenever the *lamB*-proximal gene fragment corresponds to more than 70 aminoterminal amino acids—are localized, in part, on the outer membrane (Benson

225

and Silhavy 1983). Conversely, hybrid proteins carrying a peptide X at the carboxyterminal end of β-galactosidase have also been constructed; X represents
proinsulin, as described by Ullrich et al. (1977), and somatostatin, as described
by Itakura et al. (1977). These hybrid proteins are not transferred to membranes
but remain cytoplasmic.

We attempted to use these constructions to produce trihybrid proteins LamB-
LacZ-X in order to bring X to the outer membrane (Fig. 1). The gene fusions were
made in vitro, and their structures were identified by restriction analysis (Marchal
1983). However, when the constructions were introduced into E. coli, they became highly unstable. After growth, even under noninduced conditions, the only
clones that survived had deleted the DNA in the fusion region, preventing production of the trihybrid protein. We suspected that the trihybrid proteins LamB-
LacZ-X, which were shown to be synthesized in a Zubay-type system, were highly
toxic to the bacteria. Synthesis of the largest LamB-LacZ fusions used (42–12
and 42–18, see Fig. 1) or the LacZ-X fusion proteins did not affect bacterial growth
to a great extent. We thus assumed that the cellular location of the trihybrid
proteins was the cause of their toxicity. At least two hypotheses could be proposed: (1) The protein LamB-LacZ-X, either for conformational or for energetic
reasons, remains stuck at some stage of the secretory process and jams the
system (for review, see Michaelis and Beckwith 1982). This explanation would
contradict a model proposed to account for the outer membrane location of the
largest LamB-LacZ hybrid proteins (Hall and Silhavy 1981). This model assumes
that the LacZ part of the hybrid protein does not cross the membrane during
export. Insertion of X should not then affect the process. (2) The insertion of the
protein on the outer membrane induces lysis of the bacterium (abnormal folding
in the membrane).

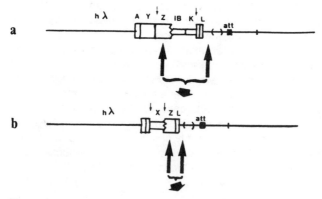

Figure 1
In vitro construction of bacteriophage λ recombinants with *lamB-lacZ-X* gene fusions. (a)
lamB-lacZ gene fusion under the control of *L8 UV5* promoter. Three different fusions (see
Hall and Silhavy 1981) were used: 42–1 carries about the proximal half of LamB and 42–12
and 42–18, about two thirds of LamB. (b) *lacZ-X* gene fusion (Marchal 1983). X is somatostatin or proinsulin (see text). *Sac*I fragments of the vectors (b) were replaced by *Sac*I
fragments of donors (a), yielding six different trihybrid proteins (Marchal 1983). Up arrows
indicate the *Sac*I site; down arrows indicate the *Eco*RI site. (A) *lacA;* (Y) *lacY;* (Z) *lacZ;* (IB)
lamB; (K) *malK;* (L) *lac* promoter *L8 UV5;* (att) λ attachment site.

Further studies involving small modifications of the *lamB* gene were undertaken in order to identify which structures are toxic to the cell and to propose a strategy for constructing hybrid proteins that are efficiently localized on the outer membrane.

Properties of Modified LamB Proteins

To allow construction of genes coding for proteins that might be lethal, the *lamB* gene was cloned on a plasmid with a *tac* promoter (a gift from Egon Amann [this volume]). This plasmid was introduced into a strain with a *lacI*^{Q1} mutation that overproduces the repressor of the *lac* (and *tac*) promoters. This allows a low level of basal expression and a high level of induction (Bouges-Bocquet et al. 1983).

The *lamB* gene was modified by linker insertions, resulting either in the insertion of a few amino acids or in a phase shift in the reading frame and premature termination of the protein shortly after the linker insertion. Some deletions were obtained either spontaneously or by ligation between two restriction sites. One large insertion (47 amino acids of exogenous peptide) was also constructed as a cloning intermediate (pBG4; see below).

The properties of these modified proteins are shown in Tables 1 and 2. Isopropylthio-β-D-galactoside (IPTG) induces modified proteins on the plasmid; thus, sensitivity to IPTG characterizes sensitivity to overproduction of modified proteins. The wild-type protein encoded by plasmid pBB0 is slightly toxic to the bacteria when overproduced. A likely explanation would be that when wild-type LamB protein is overproduced, lysis occurs because the outer membrane is overloaded with this protein (overproduction of periplasmic proteins does not induce lysis; P. Duplay, pers. comm.).

None of the modified proteins thus far studied were found in the inner membrane (Tables 1 and 2, last line), using the constructions presented in this paper. It was thus proposed that increased sensitivity to IPTG results from incorrect folding of the modified proteins in the membrane (Bouges-Bocquet et al. 1983). The lethality of proteins where only the last ten amino acids at the carboxyl terminus have been changed (pBBa3, pBBa8) suggests that the last ten amino acids play a key role in the folding of the protein in the membrane (possibly, since these residues are hydrophobic in the wild type, by a direct interaction with the membrane). For proteins of premature termination (Table 1), sensitivity to IPTG decreases with the length measured on gel. This is probably due to a decrease in protein stability (Table 1).

The six deletion proteins studied (Table 2) are rather stable, but all are very toxic to the bacterium. In contrast, insertions into at least three different positions hardly modify the properties of the protein. Plasmid pBG4 is of particular interest. It codes for a hybrid protein (47 exogenous amino acids inserted at amino acid 183 of the LamB protein) that is stable and nontoxic to the bacterium.

The efficient localization on the outer membrane of proteins encoded by plasmids pBBm1 (deletion of amino acids 183–240), pBBs1 (192–294), and pBBe2 (above 294) shows that the first 183 amino acids of LamB code for all the information required for proper and efficient routing of the protein. This is consistent with the results of Benson and Silhavy (1983). Insertion of other exogenous polypeptides was thus attempted at amino acid 183, which corresponds to a proline-glycine turn of LamB protein.

Table 1
Properties of Modified LamB Proteins (Modified Carboxyl Terminus)

				Modified carboxyl terminus					
	pBB0	pBBa8	pBBh1	pBBa4	pBBe2	pBBn6	pBBm5	pBBc1	pBBh7
Mutagenesis site (in amino acids)	421	411	321	306	294	279	183	132	28
Predicted length	421	432	326	323	302	299	189	140	32
Apparent m.w. on gel in kD	47.8	48.9	38	38	36.3	34.3	25.1	n.t.	n.t.
in amino acids	421	431	335	335	320	302	221	n.t.	n.t.
Sensitivity to IPTG	S	SSS	SS	SS	S	S	S	R	R
Approximate half-time (min) before degradation	>60	>60	~40	~40	~20	n.t.	2	<1	<1
Location according to Osborn gradient	OM	OM	OM	OM	OM	n.t.	n.t.	n.t.	n.t.

n.t. indicates not tested; S, sensitive; R, resistant; OM, outer membrane.

Table 2
Properties of Modified LamB Proteins (Deletions and Insertions)

	Deletions							Insertions		
	pBBa3	pBBa6	pBBs1	pBBm1	pBBc5	pBBc2	pBBe3	pBBm2	pBG4	pBBc7
Mutagenesis site (in amino acids)	411	306	192	183	132	132	294	183	183	132
Predicted length	~420	316	309	~340	~425	350	425	429	468	425
Apparent m.w. on gel in kD	47.8	35.5	38	37.1	47.8	n.t.	47.8	n.t.	51.5	47.8
in amino acids	421	313	335	327	421	n.t.	421	n.t.	462	421
Sensitivity to IPTG	SSS	SSS	SSS	SSS	SSS	SSS	SS	S	S	SS
Approximate half-life (min)	>60	~40	>60	~40	>60	n.t.	>60	n.t.	>60	>60
Location according to Osborn gradient	OM	OM	OM	OM	OM	n.t.	OM	n.t.	n.t.	OM

n.t. indicates not tested; S, sensitive; OM, outer membrane.

Hybrid Protein with a Fragment of the Surface Antigen of Hepatitis

The gene fragment coding for amino acids 111 to 155 of the surface antigen of hepatitis was fused to the gene fragment coding for the first 183 amino acids of LamB. The construction, verified by DNA sequencing, proved to code for the fused protein. The carboxyterminal part of LamB is out of phase. The resulting hybrid protein LamB-HBs could be detected on SDS gels after immunoprecipitation with anti-LamB serum (Fig. 2). It is not toxic to the bacterium. However, consistent with the above results on modified proteins, the half-life of the protein is short (a few minutes).

CONCLUSIONS

To export a given polypeptide efficiently to the outer membrane of the bacterium, several conditions are likely to be important:

1. The fragment of carrier protein, LamB in our study, should code for all the determinants involved in localization to the outer membrane. According to our results, the 183 aminoterminal amino acids of the LamB protein seem to be sufficient.

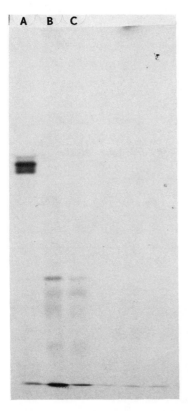

Figure 2
Immunoprecipitation with anti-LamB serum of whole cellular extracts. Cells at $DO_{600} = 0.8$ were induced for 10 min with 10^{-3} M IPTG and then labeled for 2 min with [^{35}S]methionine. (A) Plasmid pBB0 carrying wild-type *lamB* gene; (B,C) plasmids carrying gene fusions with a fragment of HBs.

2. The hybrid protein should be stable in order to give immunological responses. The longer the fragment of LamB protein, the better the stability. The carboxy-terminal part of the LamB protein also seems to increase stability.
3. To allow DNA stability, the hybrid protein encoded by the fused genes should not be too toxic to the bacterium. The folding of the protein seems to play a key role in this toxicity.

We described here two hybrid proteins. One contains a 47-amino-acid insert at amino acid 183 of LamB protein. This protein, which contains the carboxyter-minal part of LamB, is stable and not toxic to the bacteria. The second hybrid protein contains the 183 aminoterminal amino acids of LamB followed by 44 immunogenic amino acids of HBs. The carboxyterminal part of LamB is not in phase in this construction. The resulting protein is not toxic, but it is stable for only a few minutes.

Other hybrids, including the aminoterminal and carboxyterminal sequences of LamB, are under construction. In addition, immunological tests should be developed to screen for hybrid proteins that, meeting the preceding criteria, expose the immunogenic polypeptide at the surface of the bacteria with the correct conformation.

ACKNOWLEDGMENTS

This work was supported by grants from the Délégation Général á la Recherche Scientifique et Technique and the Centre National de la Recherche Scientifique (CP-960002), NATO (grant 1297), the Fondation pour la Recherche Médicale, the Ligue National Française contre le Cancer, and the Association pour le Développement de la Recherche sur le Cancer.

REFERENCES

Benson, S.A. and T.J. Silhavy. 1983. Information within the mature LamB protein necessary for localization to the outer membrane of *E. coli* K12. *Cell* **32:** 1325.

Bouges-Bocquet, B., H. Villarroya, and M. Hofnung. 1983. Linker mutagenesis in the gene of an outer membrane protein of *E. coli*, LamB. *J. Cell. Biochem.* (in press).

Hall, M.N. and T.J. Silhavy. 1981. Genetic analysis of the major outer membrane proteins of *E. coli*. *Annu. Rev. Genet.* **15:** 91.

Itakura, K., T. Hirose, R. Grea, A.D. Riggs, H. Heyneker, F. Bolivar, and H. Boyer. 1977. Expression in *E. coli* of a chemically synthesized gene for the hormone somatostatin. *Science* **198:** 1056.

Marchal, C. 1983. "Etude d'une protéine de membrane externe chez *E. coli* K12." Thése de doctorat d'Etat, Paris.

Michaelis, S. and J. Beckwith. 1982. Mechanism of incorporation of cell envelope proteins in *E. coli*. *Annu. Rev. Microbiol.* **36:** 435.

Ullrich, A., J. Shire, J. Chirgwin, R. Pictet, E. Tischer, W.J. Rutter, and H.M. Goodman. 1977. Rat insulin genes: Construction of plasmids containing the coding sequences. *Science* **196:** 1313.

Synthesis and Secretion of Hepatitis-B Surface Antigen Particles in Transfected Animal Cells

Marie-Louise Michel,[*][†] **Eliane Sobzack,**[*]
Didier Lamy,[†][‡] **and Pierre Tiollais**[†]
*Groupement de Génie Génétique and
†Unité de Recombinaison et Expression Génétique
INSERM U.163, CNRS LA.271, Institut Pasteur
75724 Paris Cedex 15, France*

The development of a vaccine against hepatitis B is important because of the high prevalence of chronic hepatitis-B virus (HBV) infection, the severity of the related liver diseases, and the relationship between HBV and liver cancer. The restricted host range of the virus and the lack of a cell-culture system for HBV propagation have greatly impeded the understanding of the molecular genetics of the virus, as well as the production of a vaccine that is actually prepared from defective viral particles present in the sera of chronic carriers.

Hepatitis-B Virus

Infected plasma contains varying amounts of viral particles of different sizes and forms (Tiollais et al. 1981). The complete infectious virion (or Dane particles) is 42 nm in diameter. It consists of an envelope that carries the hepatitis-B surface antigen (HBsAg) and a 27-nm nucleocapsid that carries the hepatitis-B core antigen (HBcAg) and contains a circular molecule of DNA. The 22-nm spherical and filamentous particles represent free envelopes of the virus. Some sera contain only free viral envelopes and are therefore noninfectious; even when a serum contains infectious virions, free envelopes remain present in a large excess. In this case, a soluble antigen related to the capsid, the hepatitis-e antigen (HBeAg), is also present. The HBsAg in the viral envelope has one group-specific determinant *a* and two sets of mutually exclusive subtype determinants *d/y* and *w/r*. Thus, the four major subtypes of HBsAg are denoted *adw, ayw, adr,* and *ayr.*

‡Present address: Institut Mérieux, 69260 Marcy l'Etoile, France.

The HBV genome has an unusual structure in that there is a single-stranded region of variable length ranging from 50% to 100% the length of the L strand. The maintenance of the circular structure is assured by base pairing of the 5' ends of the two strands over a length of about 260 bp. A DNA polymerase associated with the capsid is capable of repairing the single-stranded region by elongating the 3' end of the S strand.

A general presentation of the genetic organization of HBV can be deduced from the comparative analysis of the nucleotide sequences of cloned genomes (Fig. 1). The L strand carries all or virtually all of the protein-coding capacity of the genome and can be considered as the minus strand.

Translation of gene S, the coding sequence of the major protein of the envelope, gives rise to a polypeptide 226 amino acids in length. Theoretical analysis of its primary structure shows that the polypeptide can be divided into three hydrophobic segments separated by two hydrophilic ones. Most of the amino acid variations observed for genomes of different serological subtypes occur mostly in the hydrophilic segments. In addition, the presence of some amino acid is correlated with the HBsAg subtype determinant. The two hydrophilic regions therefore contain most or all HBsAg determinants.

HBsAg is a dimer of the polypeptide encoded by gene S and is stabilized by disulfide bonds. One of the two polypeptides of the dimer is glycosylated, the site being Asn-146 within the sequence Asn-Cys-Thr. The number of dimers present in a 22-nm particle is about 50–100. This dimer structure in a particular form is essential for full antigenicity and immunogenicity of HBsAg.

Future Alternatives for a Vaccine

The HBV vaccine that is actually available consists of 22-nm free viral envelopes purified from the sera of chronic carriers. Its efficacy and safety have been well documented. Nevertheless, the technical procedure presently used for the vaccine is restricted by the unavailability of large quantities of infected human plasma. Moreover, stringent and laborious control processes are necessary to avoid contamination by infectious HBV particles or propagation of possible viral agents that could be present in the serum.

Recombinant DNA technology offers different new possibilities. Viral 22-nm particles can be produced in eukaryotic cells (animal cells [Dubois et al. 1980; Moriarity et al. 1981] or yeast [Valenzuela et al. 1982; Hitzeman et al. 1983; Miyanohara et al. 1983]) transfected with cloned HBV DNA. A polypeptide (the major polypeptide of the envelope or a hybrid polypeptide with HBsAg activity) can be synthesized in transformed bacteria (Burrell et al. 1979; Charnay et al. 1980). A short oligopeptide carrying an HBsAg determinant can also be chemically synthesized (Lerner et al. 1981; Bhatnager et al. 1982; Dreesman et al. 1982; Prince et al. 1982). Finally, a live vaccine using another virus (e.g., vaccinia) as vector (Smith et al. 1983) and propagation of HBsAg are also conceivable.

The choice of procedure depends on several factors, including efficacy, cost of production, and safety. The animal cell system is attractive because in this system, HBsAg is assembled as 22-nm particles that are glycosylated and secreted. These particles seem to be identical to the 22-nm particles present in human serum.

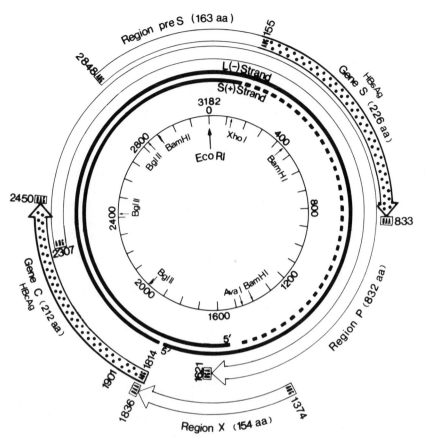

Figure 1
Genetic organization of the HBV genome. The cloned HBV genome shown is that of the
ayw subtype. Some restriction sites present in this clone are indicated. The broad arrows
surrounding the genome correspond to the four large open regions of the L minus-strand
transcript. These four potential coding sequences are termed region S (divided into pre-S
region and gene *S*), gene *C*, region P, and region X. The number of amino acids in parentheses corresponds to the length of the hypothetical polypeptides encoded by this HBV
clone. Dotted areas indicate the two sequences coding for HBsAg and HBcAg.

Gene-*S* Expression in Animal Cells

To study gene-*S* expression in animal cells, we used a model consisting of cell
lines in which cloned HBV DNA fragments have been integrated. This can be
obtained by cotransfection of cells with HBV DNA and the gene of a recessive or
a dominant marker. After selection of the transfected cells, cellular clones are
screened for gene-*S* expression by radioimmunoassay for HBsAg. Using this
technique, the HBsAg transcription unit, including the promoter, was localized.
By studying the capacity of HBV DNA recombinants to elicit HBsAg synthesis in
transfected mouse cells, an HBsAg promoter was localized. The HBsAg poly(A) +
mRNA was characterized by Northern blot and mapped on the HBV genome.

This RNA is about 2.3 kb long. Studies on the control mechanism of gene-*S* expression have shown that expression of this gene is constitutive. Optimization of HBsAg production was studied using gene-*S* amplification. The bovine papilloma virus (BPV) is a suitable nonlytic vector for that purpose, since the viral DNA establishes itself in many copies as an extrachromosomal element. The HBsAg transcription unit was inserted in the late genes of BPV.

Antigenicity and Immunogenicity of HBsAg 22-nm Particles

One of the many advantages of the animal cell system is that it enables us to obtain a continuous secretion of HBsAg particles without lysis of the cell. Particles present in the cell supernatant can be easily purified by ultracentrifugation in CsCl and sucrose gradients (Fig. 2).

Purification of large quantities of HBsAg particles permits us to study the chemical structure, antigenicity, and immunogenicity of the particles. They have the same morphology, diameter, and density as those of the 22-nm particles of human origin. They contain the major polypeptide of the envelope in the two glycosylated and nonglycosylated forms and are agglutinated by specific anti-HBs antibodies. Both the group and subtype determinants were present on the particles. When injected into mice, the particles induced formation of anti-HBs. Antibody titers of several hundred IU/ml were obtained. The constant affinity of these antibodies to human HBsAg particles was about 1×10^{-8} moles/liter. The anti-HBs antibodies react specifically with both the group and the subtype HBsAg determinants.

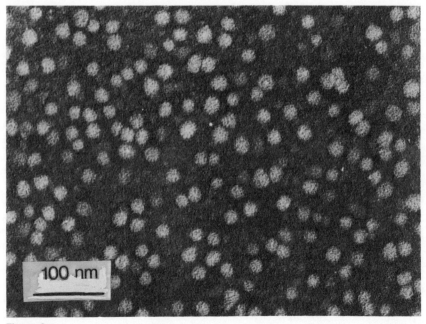

Figure 2
HBsAg 22-nm particles secreted from animal cells transfected with cloned HBV DNA.

CONCLUSION

The animal cell system enables us to obtain synthesis, glycosylation, and assembly of HBsAg in a particular form. These HBsAg particles are secreted in the cell supernatant without lysis of the cells. It is therefore possible to collect large quantities of HBsAg particles. These particles have the same structure and antigenic and immunogenic properties as those of human origin. They therefore constitute a suitable material for a future vaccine.

ACKNOWLEDGMENT

This work was supported by Institut Mérieux (Lyon, France) and Institut Pasteur Production (Marnes la Coquette, France).

REFERENCES

Bhatnagar, P.K., E. Papas, H.E. Blum, D.R. Milich, D. Nitecki, M.J. Karels, and G.N. Vyas. 1982. Immune response to synthetic peptide analogues of hepatitis B surface antigen specific for the a determinant. *Proc. Natl. Acad. Sci.* **79:** 4400.

Burrell, C.J., P. Mackay, P.J. Greenaway, P.H. Hofschneider, and K. Murray. 1979. Expression in *Escherichia coli* of hepatitis B virus DNA sequences cloned in plasmid pBR322. *Nature* **279:** 43.

Charnay, P., M. Gervais, A. Louise, F. Galibert, and P. Tiollais. 1980. Biosynthesis of hepatitis B surface antigen in *Escherichia coli. Nature* **286:** 893.

Dreesman, G.R., Y. Sanchez, I. Ionescu-Matiu, J.T. Sparrow, H.R. Six, D.L. Peterson, F.B. Hollinger, and J.L. Melnick. 1982. Antibody to hepatitis B surface antigen after a single inoculation of uncoupled synthetic HBsAg peptides. *Nature* **295:** 158.

Dubois, M.F., C. Pourcel, S. Rousset, C. Chany, and P. Tiollais. 1980. Extraction of hepatitis B surface antigen particles from mouse cells transformed with cloned viral DNA. *Proc. Natl. Acad. Sci.* **77:** 4549.

Hitzeman, R.A., C.Y. Chen, F.E. Hagie, E.J. Patzer, C.C. Liu, D.A. Estell, J.V. Miller, A. Yaffe, D.G. Kleid, A.D. Levinson, and H. Oppermann. 1983. Expression of hepatitis B surface antigen in yeast. *Nucleic Acids Res.* **9:** 2745.

Lerner, R.A., N. Green, H. Alexander, F.T. Liu, G. Sutcliffe, and T.M. Shinnick. 1981. Chemically synthesized peptides predicted from the nucleotide sequence of the hepatitis B virus genome elicit antibodies reactive with the native envelope protein of Dane particles. *Proc. Natl. Acad. Sci.* **78:** 3403.

Miyanohara, A., A. Toh-E, C. Nozaki, F. Hamada, N. Ohtomo, and K. Matsubara. 1983. Expression of hepatitis B surface antigen in yeast. *Proc. Natl. Acad. Sci.* **80:** 1.

Moriarty, A.M., B.H. Hoyer, J.W.K. Shih, J.L. Gerin, and D.H. Hamer. 1981. Expression of the hepatitis B surface antigen gene in cell culture by using a simian virus 40 vector. *Proc. Natl. Acad. Sci.* **78:** 2606.

Prince, A.M., H. Ikram, and T.P. Hopp. 1982. Hepatitis B virus vaccine: Identification of HBsAg/a and HBsAg/d but not HBsAg/y subtype antigenic determinants on a synthetic immunogenic peptide. *Proc. Natl. Acad. Sci.* **79:** 579.

Smith, G.L., M. Mackett, and B. Moss. 1983. Infectious vaccinia virus recombinants that express hepatitis B virus surface antigen. *Nature* **302:** 490.

Tiollais, P., P. Charnay, and G.N. Vyas. 1981. Biology of hepatitis B virus. *Science* **213:** 406.

Valenzuela, P., A. Medina, W.J. Rutter, G. Ammerer, and B.D. Hall. 1982. Synthesis and assembly of hepatitis B surface antigen in yeast. *Nature* **298:** 347.

Expression of Hepatitis-B Surface Antigen in Eukaryotic Cells Using Viral Vectors

Christian Stratowa, Johannes Doehmer, Yuan Wang,* and Peter H. Hofschneider
Max-Planck-Institut für Biochemie
Am Klopferspitz, D-8033 Martinsried
Federal Republic of Germany

The only available source of antigenic material to prepare a vaccine against hepatitis-B virus (HBV) is the sera of human chronic carriers of hepatitis-B surface antigen (HBsAg). For obvious reasons, it is desirable to avoid the use of human serum as a source for HBsAg and to employ methods in gene technology.

Several host systems have been tested for expression of the viral genome, in particular that part encoding the HBsAg. When *Escherichia coli* was used as the host organism, at best only low-level production of unglycosylated HBsAg was achieved. Given that the bacterial environment does not seem suitable for proper expression and modification of many eukaryotic genes and gene products, it will be important to develop and utilize eukaryotic gene expression systems based on higher organisms.

Here, we report the use of the transforming fragment of extrachromosomally replicating bovine papilloma virus (BPV) DNA and of the integrated proviral form of Moloney murine sarcoma virus (Mo-MSV) as eukaryotic vectors for introducing the HBsAg into NIH-3T3 mouse fibroblasts. We also describe the establishment of mouse cell lines that continuously express high levels of HBsAg.

DISCUSSION

Construction of the Recombinant Plasmids

Cloned HBV DNA, subtype *adw*, was isolated from the plasmid pAO1-HBV (Cummings et al. 1980) and recircularized to restore its genomic organization. By

---

*Present address: Shanghai Institute of Biochemistry, Chinese Academy of Sciences, Shanghai, China.

cleavage of the circular HBV genome with *Bg*/II, the complete HBsAg gene, including the promoter and polyadenylation site necessary for transcription, was obtained. This fragment was ligated to the *Bam*HI site of the plasmid vector pBPV$_{T69}$, which contains the 69% *Bam*HI-*Hind*III transforming region of BPV (Sarver et al. 1981). The recombinant plasmid is named pBPVHBsR/8 (Wang et al. 1983).

Bg/II-cleaved HBV DNA was inserted into the unique *Bg*/II site of Mo-MSV DNA. Two recombinant plasmids were characterized by restriction enzyme analysis. One plasmid, pMSVHBs4, contains a single *Bg*/II fragment, encoding the HBsAg gene; the other plasmid, pMSVHBs9, contains two copies of the large *Bg*/II fragment in a head-to-tail orientation, separated by the small *Bg*/II fragment (Stratowa et al. 1982).

The recombinant plasmids were transfected onto NIH-3T3 mouse fibroblasts using the calcium phosphate technique. From foci, which appeared 3 weeks after transfection, cell lines could be established that produce HBsAg.

Cell Lines Producing HBsAg

Three cell lines were studied in detail: Y1, transformed with pBPVHBsR/8; J1, transformed with pMSVHBs4; and J2, transformed with pMSVHBs9. HBsAg production from these cell lines was measured and compared with an established human hepatoma cell line (PLC/PRF/5; Alexander et al. 1976) under conditions where cells were kept in maintenance medium (Fig. 1A) or where medium was changed every day (Fig. 1B). Surface antigen secreted into the culture medium was assayed by radioimmunoassay (AUSRIA II; Abbott), and the quantity of HBsAg was determined by comparison with a known standard (HBsAg/*adw* from human serum, 17 μg/ml; Max von Pettenkofer-Institut, Munich). The results are shown in Table 1.

The relatively high production rate for HBsAg is mainly due to amplification of the HBsAg gene in the case of the BPV-HBV recombinant because of episomal replication. For the Mo-MSV-HBV recombinants, the high production rate might be explained by the presence of the retroviral large terminal repeats that contain a so-called enhancer sequence.

Characterization of the Gene Product

The biophysical properties of the HBsAg secreted into culture medium were the same as those reported for HBsAg of human serum. After equilibrium sedimentation through a discontinuous CsCl gradient, HBsAg was present in a fraction corresponding to a buoyant density of 1.2 g/ml. Examination of the surface antigen by electron microscopy revealed spherical particles with a mean diameter of 22 nm.

To determine the polypeptide composition, biosynthetically labeled HBsAg was immunoprecipitated and analyzed by electrophoresis on a polyacrylamide gel. In agreement with recently published data for purified HBsAg from human serum

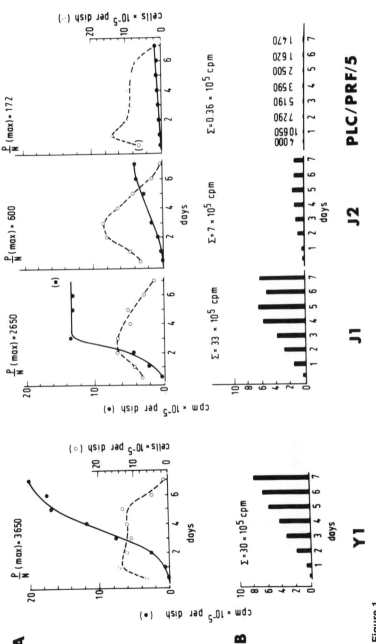

Figure 1

Production kinetics for cell lines Y1, J1, J2, and PLC/PRF/5. (A) Cells were seeded at 5×10^5 per 35-mm petri dish in DME medium/10% newborn calf serum. Cells were fed with 2 ml of medium after overnight cultivation (time 0). At the indicated times, medium was removed, volume was measured, and medium was assayed for HBsAg. Cells were removed from the same dish by trypsinization and counted with a hematocytometer. Values shown are the average of two determinations. (B) Cells were seeded as described above. Medium was changed every day and assayed for HBsAg. (Reprinted, with permission, from Stratowa et al. 1983.)

241

Table 1
Production Rates for Cell Lines Y1, J1, J2, and
PLC/PRF/5

Cell line	Production rate	
	ng/ml/day	ng/10⁷ cells/day
Y1	420	6000
J1	400	4500
J2	60	800
PLC/PRF/5	10	200

(Stibbe and Gerlich 1982), Figure 2 shows four polypeptides with molecular weights of 24,000, 28,000, 34,000, and 37,000. As already known, the 28K molecule is the glycosylated form of the single 24K HBsAg molecule.

For immunogenicity studies, four guinea pigs were inoculated subcutaneously with 20 μg of purified HBsAg in the presence of $Al(OH)_3$. After 2 weeks, the inoculation was repeated. As shown in Table 2, increasing antibody titers in guinea pigs could be detected by radioimmunoassay (AUSAB; Abbott).

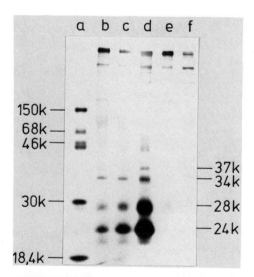

Figure 2
Electrophoretic analysis of immunoprecipitated HBsAg polypeptides. ³⁵S-labeled proteins from cell line Y1 and from untransfected NIH-3T3 cells were incubated with preimmune guinea pig serum or with high-titered anti-HBsAg serum from guinea pigs and precipitated with protein A–Sepharose CL-4B. Proteins were analyzed by polyacrylamide gel electrophoresis and autoradiography. (*a*) ¹⁴C-labeled protein standards: globulins (150K); bovine serum albumin (68K); ovalbumin (46K); carbonic anhydrase (30K); lactoglobulin A (18.4K). (*b–d*) Proteins from cell line Y1 incubated with 0.1 μl (*b*), 1 μl (*c*), and 10 μl (*d*) anti-HBsAg serum. (*e*) Proteins from cell line Y1 incubated with 10 μl preimmune serum. (*f*) Proteins from untransfected NIH-3T3 cells incubated with 10 μl anti-HBsAg serum. (Reprinted, with permission, from Wang et al. 1983.)

Table 2
Anti-HBsAg Titer Obtained in Serum of Guinea Pigs Immunized with HBsAg Particles from Y1 Cells

Weeks[a]	Titer in guinea pig[b]			
	1	2	3	4
0	0	0	0	0
2	96	100	62	76
4	352	20,800	6,120	6,480
6	88	35,200	5,760	7,200
8	100	56,000	5,400	12,100
12	800	70,000	–	11,200
18	1,000	200,000	–	34,600

[a]The first injection of HBsAg was done at time 0 and the second one, 2 weeks later.
[b]Titers are in radioimmunoassay units calculated according to the specifications of the manufacturer.

CONCLUSION

The results presented here indicate that the HBsAg produced by mouse fibroblasts is indistinguishable from HBsAg found in human serum: It is found in the culture medium as 22-nm spherical particles, it is glycosylated, and it is immunogenic in guinea pigs. Therefore, it might serve as a safe and essentially unlimited source for HBsAg. It still needs to be demonstrated in a challenge experiment that chimpanzees can be successfully immunized with HBsAg produced by mouse fibroblasts.

REFERENCES

Alexander, J.J., E.M. Bey, E.W. Geddes, and G. Lecatsas. 1976. Establishment of a continuously growing cell line from primary carcinoma of the liver. *S. Afr. Med. J.* **50:** 2124.

Cummings, I.W., J.K. Browne, W.A. Salser, G.V. Tyler, R.L. Snyder, J.M. Smolec, and J. Summers. 1980. Isolation, characterization, and comparison of recombinant DNAs derived from genomes of human hepatitis B virus and woodchuck hepatitis virus. *Proc. Natl. Acad. Sci.* **77:** 1842.

Sarver, N., P. Gruss, M.-F. Law, G. Khoury, and P.M. Howley. 1981. Bovine papilloma virus deoxyribonucleic acid: A novel eukaryotic cloning vector. *Mol. Cell. Biol.* **1:** 486.

Stibbe, W. and W.H. Gerlich. 1982. Variable protein composition of hepatitis B surface antigen from different donors. *Virology* **123:** 436.

Stratowa, C., J. Doehmer, Y. Wang, and P.H. Hofschneider. 1982. Recombinant retroviral DNA yielding high expression of hepatitis B surface antigen. *EMBO J.* **1:** 1573.

Stratowa, C., J. Doehmer, Y. Wang, M. Schaefer-Ridder, and P.H. Hofschneider. 1983. Construction of cell lines producing hepatitis B surface antigen using eukaryotic viral vectors. In *Second International Symposium on Viral Hepatitis: Extended Abstracts* (ed. F. Deinhardt). Marcel Dekker, New York.

Wang, Y., C. Stratowa, M. Schaefer-Ridder, J. Doehmer, and P.H. Hofschneider. 1983. Enhanced production of hepatitis B surface antigen in NIH 3T3 mouse fibroblasts by using extrachromosomally replicating bovine papillomavirus vector. *Mol. Cell. Biol.* **3:** 1032.

Production of Hepatitis-B Recombinant Vaccines

W. Neal Burnette, Babru Samal,
Jeffrey K. Browne, Dennis Fenton,
and Grant A. Bitter
Amgen, Thousand Oaks, California 91320

Hepatitis B is a disease of global significance—more than 200 million people are believed to be persistently viremic. Primary infection is a major cause of acute liver disease; the carrier state is responsible for chronic disease, such as cirrhosis, and is strongly associated with hepatocellular carcinoma. The hepatitis-B virus (HBV), or Dane particle, is a 42-nm enveloped structure containing a partially double-stranded circular DNA genome. The genome is known to encode a DNA polymerase, a viral core protein, and a surface antigen (HBsAg). The most prevalent structure in the sera of chronic carriers of the disease is a 22-nm particle that contains only HBsAg embedded in a spherical (sometimes filamentous) membrane. These particles have been shown to elicit a protective immune response and have become the basis for current vaccines (Krugman 1982).

Although these vaccines are highly efficacious (Szmuness et al. 1980), their production is very sensitive to the availability of suitable chronic carriers for plasmapheresis and subsequent recovery of sufficient HBsAg material for vaccine formulation. The nature of the source of the starting material necessitates that each vaccine lot be highly purified, stringently inactivated, and subjected to an extensive safety-testing program in chimpanzees (Hilleman et al. 1982). The subsequent cost of these vaccines effectively places them out of reach of people in the highly endemic regions of the Third World. We therefore sought to produce an equally efficacious yet accessible vaccine by recombinant DNA technology.

HBsAg Expression in Yeast

A general yeast expression vector was constructed using the promoter for the highly expressed yeast glyceraldehyde-3-phosphate dehydrogenase (GPD) gene

(G. Bitter and K. Egan, in prep.). The plasmids also contain selective markers and origins of replication for both *Escherichia coli* and yeast. For the expression of HBsAg in yeast, the gene for the *adw* serotype of HBsAg was cloned downstream from the GPD promoter (Fig. 1A). The 5' portion of this gene was replaced with a chemically synthesized DNA segment that restored the native GPD untranslated leader and utilized optimal yeast codons for the first 32 amino acids of the surface antigen.

This plasmid was then used to transform *Saccharomyces cerevisiae*. Analysis of whole-cell lysates by SDS-polyacrylamide gel electrophoresis (SDS-PAGE) revealed that HBsAg comprises about 1–2% of the total cell protein. The effect of resynthesizing the GPD untranslated leader and the 5' coding region of the HBsAg gene appeared to be an increase of at least tenfold in antigen expression (G. Bitter and K. Egan, in prep.). Gradient analyses indicated that surface antigen released on cell lysis is found embedded in lipid particles similar in biophysical properties to those isolated from human carriers. Electron microscopy revealed a striking resemblance between yeast particles and the 22-nm human HBsAg particles.

HBsAg Expression in Mammalian Cells

For expression in mammalian cells, we constructed an SV40 vector in which the HBsAg gene replaced the early-region T-antigen functions of the viral genome (Fig. 1B). This chimeric genome was then used to transfect monkey kidney (COS) cells that constitutively express the SV40 T-antigen functions to complement the replication of the defective virus. Stock virus from the transfection was used for subsequent infection of COS cells and the production of HBsAg. The antigen was found secreted into the extracellular culture medium as 22-nm particles. The level of expression totals about 2×10^8 HBsAg molecules per cell, or 9 μg per 10^6 cells, during the 7–10-day course of the infection.

Purification, Micelle Formation, and Formulation with Adjuvant

For the mass production of vaccines, it was important to develop rapid and scalable methods for purifying HBsAg materials. HBsAg particles were recovered from clarified yeast cell lysates or mammalian cell cultures by a variety of adsorption and precipitation methods. The resuspended precipitates were subjected to isopycnic gradient centrifugation in potassium bromide gradients, where the lipoprotein HBsAg particles were separated from cellular or medium components by flotation. Residual contaminants were removed by rate-zonal sedimentation in sucrose gradients. When purified in this manner and subjected to SDS-PAGE (Fig. 2), the COS-cell-derived HBsAg appears as a doublet at about 25,000 and 22,000 daltons (Fig. 2, left), similar to that seen in human material where there are both glycosylated and nonglycosylated forms of the antigen (Peterson 1981). The yeast-derived HBsAg (Fig. 2, right) migrates as a single band of about 22,000 daltons, consistent with it being nonglycosylated in yeast.

It has been demonstrated that protein micelles can be prepared from the integral membrane proteins of a number of enveloped viruses (Helenius and von Bonsdorff 1976); it was subsequently shown that these micelles can be highly

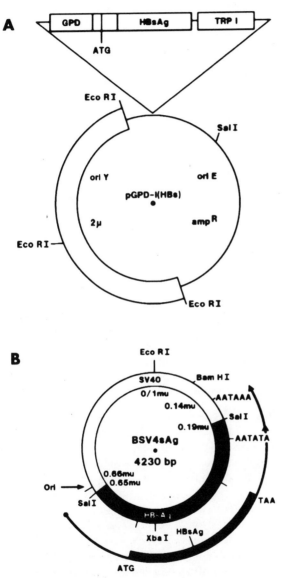

Figure 1

HBsAg expression vectors. (A) Yeast expression vector is a derivative of pBR322 carrying the yeast 2μ plasmid and gene. The surface antigen gene was inserted downstream from the yeast GPD promoter, and a chemically synthesized DNA segment was substituted for the untranslated leader and first 32 codons of the surface antigen gene as described in the text. (B) Mammalian (COS) cell expression vector was constructed from the SV40 genome by replacing the early region with the surface antigen gene. Arrow indicates the transcript and the two possible polyadenylation signals.

COS-DERIVED   YEAST-DERIVED
   HBsAg   HBsAg

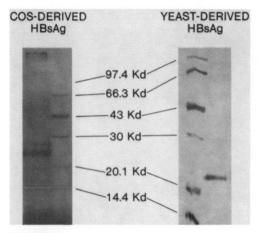

Figure 2
SDS-PAGE analysis of HBsAg. COS-cell-derived and yeast-cell-derived surface-antigen-containing particles were purified as described in the text and subjected to electrophoresis in 10% polyacrylamide–SDS gels. The gels were subsequently stained with silver.

effective immunogens (Morein et al. 1978). In fact, protein micelles derived from human HBsAg-containing particles proved to be significantly more immunogenic on a weight basis than the particles themselves (Skelly et al. 1981). We adapted the original protocol of Helenius and von Bonsdorff (1976) to produce protein micelles from both the yeast- and mammalian-cell-derived HBsAg particles. Briefly, the particles were delipidated with a nonionic detergent and the detergent removed by centrifugation of the material into a detergent-free sucrose gradient. This allows the free polypeptides to self-associate by hydrophobic interactions into protein micellar forms.

Antigens are generally much more immunogenic when administered with an adjuvant. We adsorbed each of our particle and protein micellar preparations to alum, one of the most widely used adjuvants for human vaccines. For the purposes of storage and immunogenicity testing, each adjuvanted vaccine was suspended in phosphate-buffered saline and thimerosal.

Immunogenicity of HBsAg

The immunogenicity of hepatitis-B vaccine materials in mice is generally predictive of the protective immune response in man. A standard mouse potency study (Office of Biologics, FDA) was conducted to determine the relative immunogenicity of our preparations. Briefly, 27-day-old Swiss white female mice were inoculated intraperitoneally with varying dosage levels of the adjuvanted materials. Twenty-eight days postinoculation, sera were collected and assayed for anti-HBsAg titer with a commercial radioimmunoassay kit.

Table 1 summarizes the data obtained from the mouse study. All groups of mice were more than 90% seroconverted by HBsAg doses of 625 ng or greater. Even at the lowest dose of 39 ng, each material was able to elicit an immune

Table 1
Immunogenicity of rDNA-derived Hepatitis-B Vaccines in Mice

		Seroconversion			
Vaccine material	dose $(\mu g)^a$	no. of mice[b]	%	GMT[c]	ED_{50}^d (ng)
Yeast HBs particles	10	14/14	100	1804	112
	2.5	15/15	100	2214	
	0.625	15/15	100	359	
	0.156	6/15	40	4.5	
	0.039	10/15	67	7.5	
Yeast HBs micelles	10	9/9	100	1706	22[e]
	2.5	10/10	100	1599	
	0.625	9/9	100	646	
	0.156	8/10	80	28	
	0.039	6/10	60	13	
Mammalian HBs particles	10	14/14	100	2001	98
	2.5	14/15	93	501	
	0.625	14/15	93	90	
	0.156	6/15	40	4.4	
	0.039	3/15	20	1.7	
Mammalian HBs micelles[f]	0.625	9/9	100	696	25[e]
	0.156	9/10	90	192	
	0.039	6/10	60	15	

[a]Determined by immunoassay.
[b]Number of mice seroconverted per number of mice in group.
[c]GMT = geometric mean titer in RIA units.
[d]ED_{50} = effective dose required to seroconvert 50% of mice.
[e]Extrapolated value.
[f]No doses of 10 μg and 2.5 μg given.

response in a significant number of mice. Estimates of the effective dose necessary to seroconvert 50% of the animals (ED_{50}) were made from linear regression analyses of the lower doses in each experimental set. The ED_{50} values of the particulate vaccine materials were 98 ng and 112 ng for the mammalian-cell-derived and yeast-derived materials, respectively. The micellar vaccines, on the other hand, appeared to be about four times as effective with ED_{50} values of 25 ng and 22 ng, respectively.

DISCUSSION

Our results indicate that it is possible to produce, by recombinant DNA methodology, defined and highly immunogenic vaccine materials for immunization against hepatitis B. The purified protein micellar preparations appear to offer an advantage over particulate materials because of their enhanced immunogenicity. The ability to generate large quantities of HBsAg material, particularly by fermentation of yeast, holds great promise for the worldwide control of hepatitis-B-related acute and chronic liver disease and associated hepatocellular carcinoma.

ACKNOWLEDGMENT

We thank K. Egan, R. Smalling, and C. Wong for technical assistance.

REFERENCES

Helenius, A. and C.H. von Bonsdorff. 1976. Semliki Forest virus membrane proteins: Preparation and characterization of spike protein octamers soluble in detergent-free medium. *Biochim. Biophys. Acta* **436:** 895.

Hilleman, M.R., E.B. Buynak, W.J. McAleer, A.A. McLean, P.J. Provost, and A.A. Tytell. 1982. Hepatitis A and hepatitis B vaccines. In *Viral hepatitis: 1981 International Symposium* (ed. W. Szmuness et al.), p. 385. The Franklin Institute Press, Philadelphia, Pennsylvania.

Krugman, S. 1982. The newly licensed hepatitis B vaccine: Characteristics and indications for use. *J. Am. Med. Assoc.* **247:** 2012.

Morein, B., A. Helenius, K. Simons, R. Pettersson, L. Kaariainen, and V. Schirrmacher. 1978. Effective subunit vaccines against an enveloped animal virus. *Nature* **276:** 715.

Peterson, D.L. 1981. Isolation and characterization of the major protein and glycoprotein of hepatitis B surface antigen. *J. Biol. Chem.* **256:** 6975.

Skelly, J., C.R. Howard, and A.J. Zuckerman. 1981. Hepatitis B polypeptide vaccine preparation in micelle form. *Nature* **290:** 51.

Szmuness, W., C.E. Stevens, E.J. Harley, E.A. Zang, W.R. Oleszko, D.C. William, R. Sadovsky, J.M. Morrison, and A. Kellner. 1980. Hepatitis B vaccine: Demonstration of efficacy in a controlled clinical trial in a high-risk population in the United States. *N. Engl. J. Med.* **303:** 833.

Hepatitis-B Vaccine Purification by Immunoaffinity Chromatography

D. Eugene Wampler, Eugene B. Buynak,
B. Jeffrey Harder, Alan C. Herman,
Maurice R. Hilleman, William J. McAleer,
and Edward M. Scolnick
Merck, Sharp and Dohme Research Laboratories
West Point, Pennsylvania 19486

There are an estimated 170,000,000 hepatitis-B carriers in the world, and approximately 1,000,000 of them are in the United States. Individuals who remain chronically infected run a high risk of developing chronic liver disease and hepatocellular carcinoma. Because of the prevalence and severity of this disease, there was an intensive effort over the past 10 years to develop a commercial vaccine. This was accomplished in 1982 with the introduction of vaccines made in the United States and in Europe.

These "first-generation" vaccines are made from the blood plasma of humans who are chronic carriers of the hepatitis-B surface antigen (HBsAg). In the early 1970s, Dr. Saul Krugman (New York University Medical Center) demonstrated that boiled serum could be used to protect institutionalized children against hepatitis-B infection. Since that time, a variety of procedures have been used to isolate the HBsAg from plasma and to prepare experimental vaccines.

Dr. John Gerin (Georgetown University) exploited the unusual hydrodynamic properties of the HBsAg in a purification scheme based primarily on isopycnic and rate-zonal centrifugation. Dr. Edda DeRizzo and collaborators (Baylor College of Medicine) used fractional precipitation with polyethylene glycol 6000 and polyelectrolyte 60. Dr. A.R. Neurath and collaborators (New York Blood Center) have used affinity chromatography with concanavalin A and ω-aminononane as the immobile ligands. The French vaccine is prepared using a procedure that relies almost entirely on large-scale centrifugation (Maupas et al. 1978).

The group at Merck, headed by Dr. Hilleman, developed a manufacturing procedure that includes conversion of plasma to serum, ammonium sulfate fractionation, two centrifugation steps, treatment with pepsin and urea, and finally gel chromatography (Hilleman et al. 1982). The Merck vaccine comes as close to a pure antigen as anything available.

Because only about 2 out of 10,000 individuals have plasma with a high enough titer to be suitable for vaccine manufacture, alternate antigen sources have recently been considered. Two such sources of "second-generation" vaccines are human transformed cells grown in cell culture and recombinant yeast cells. Both of these sources provide an unlimited supply of raw material but impose new requirements on the purification process.

Human plasma used in vaccine manufacture has an antigen concentration of about 400 μg/ml. Since the total serum protein concentration is about 60 mg/ml, only a 150-fold purification is required. Both the hepatoma cell line and yeast culture express relatively low concentrations of antigen at relatively low purity. An additional disadvantage of yeast as a source of antigen is that a crude yeast extract is a very complex mixture of impurities. In the plasma case, a single component, albumin, makes up 65% of the contaminating protein. Because of the lower titers and lower purity of these alternate sources, we have reexamined the purification procedure. The hepatoma cell line used in this work was originally isolated by Dr. J.J. Alexander (Alexander et al. 1976) and was given to us by Dr. R.J. Daemer (National Institutes of Health). The recombinant yeast strain was developed in a joint effort by Dr. Rutter's laboratory in San Francisco, Dr. Hall's laboratory in Seattle, and the Merck laboratories. The genetic construction of this yeast strain has been described previously (Valenzuela et al. 1982).

At Merck, we have used polyclonal antibodies purified from the sera of goats that had been hyperimmunized with the human plasma antigen. The specific anti-HBsAg antibodies are separated from other goat antibodies by immunoaffinity chromatography using purified plasma antigen as the immobile phase. The purified anti-HBsAg is then attached to cyanogen bromide (CNBr)-activated Sepharose and poured into a column. A clarified yeast cell extract or hepatoma cell culture fluid containing antigen is passed over the column at a flow rate of 2 column volumes/hr. Adsorption and elution of HBsAg from the goat antibody column can be followed by the absorbance of 280 nm, and a typical pattern is shown in Figure 1.

Most of the protein is not bound to the column and can be seen in the off-scale optical density tracing. Unadsorbed debris is washed away with hypertonic buffer as the optical density returns to baseline. HBsAg is then eluted with NH_4SCN. As the antigen comes off, it gives a typical optical spike that settles down to the plateau absorbance of thiocyanate. Thiocyanate is then washed away and the column is ready for reuse. The fractions containing antigen are pooled, and thiocyanate is removed either by dialysis or by ultrafiltration.

The product of a single pass over such an immunoaffinity column is essentially pure hepatitis antigen. SDS gel electrophoresis of the cell culture antigen is shown in Figure 2A, which compares plasma antigen purified by the conventional procedure and the cell culture antigen. Antigens from both of these mammalian sources show two major bands at 25,000 and 28,000 daltons, typical of the plasma antigen. Both of these major bands are expressions of the same polypeptide chain, the slower migrating one being the glycosylated form. Although other bands are present, all of the bands react with antibody to HBsAg as shown by Western blot analysis. Our interpretation is that the higher-molecular-weight

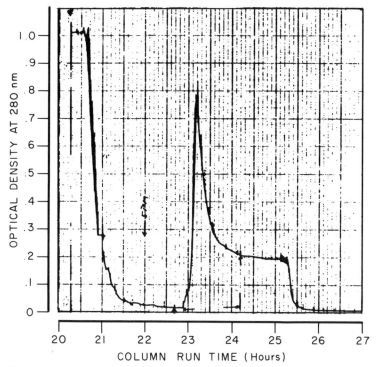

Figure 1
A typical optical density pattern for the adsorption and elution of HBsAg using a goat anti-body column. The fluid containing the antigen passed through the column from hr 0 to hr 20. The column was washed with hypertonic buffer from hr 20 to hr 22.75; 3 M NH₄SCN was applied from hr 22.75 to hr 25.25.

bands are dimers and higher-order aggregates of the basic monomer that have been incompletely disaggregated. The yeast antigen, shown in Figure 2B, displays only the nonglycosylated band. The sample in lane 3 is the yeast extract that was charged to the column and gives an indication of the strength of this one-step purification procedure. Despite this absence of the glycosylated subunit, the purified yeast antigen has the typical 20-nm particle appearance when viewed by electron microscopy (Fig. 3).

Both the yeast and cell culture products have been formulated into vaccines. In both cases, vaccine formulation was the same as for the plasma antigen, i.e., treatment with formaldehyde and adsorption to alum with thimerosal added as a preservative. The vaccines pass the standard safety tests and are antigenic in mice as shown in Table 1. Groups of ten mice were vaccinated with 1 ml of vaccine, in a fourfold dilution series. The number of mice that responded by developing anti-HBsAg antibodies is given in the numerator. The ED_{50} is a statistical estimate of the amount of antigen protein required to seroconvert 50% of the mice. Smaller numbers indicate greater potency, but the apparent greater potency of the yeast vaccine is not statistically significant at the 95% level.

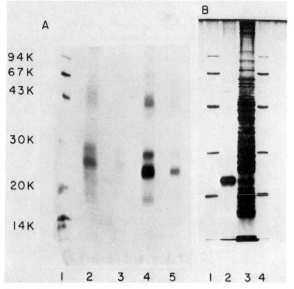

Figure 2
SDS-PAGE analysis of cell culture (A) and yeast (B) antigens (silver stain). (A, Lane 1) Molecular-weight markers; (lane 2) HBsAg purified from plasma by the method of Hilleman et al. (1982); (lane 4) HBsAg purified from cell-culture fluid by immunoaffinity chromatography. (B, Lanes 1,4) Molecular-weight markers; (lane 2) purified antigen from yeast extract; (lane 3) crude yeast extract.

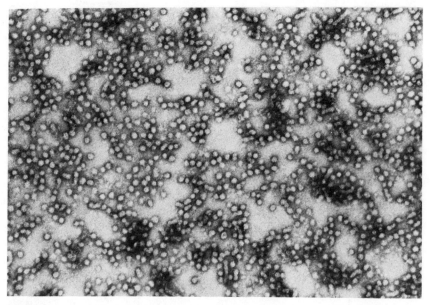

Figure 3
Electron micrograph of HBsAg purified from yeast by immunoaffinity chromatography. Magnification, 76,000×.

Table 1
Antigenic Activity in Mice of HBsAg Purified from Human Plasma, from
Cell Culture, and from Yeast Cells

Dose	Number of positive mice/total		
(μg/mouse)	human plasma	human cell culture	yeast
10	8/10	8/10	8/10
2.5	9/10	8/10	8/10
0.625	4/10	7/10	6/10
0.156	0/10	0/9	1/10
0.0375	—	—	0/10
ED_{50}	0.81 μg	0.79 μg	0.40 μg

The yeast product is not only a potent antigen, it also gives long-lasting antibody titers. The results of an experiment in grivet monkeys, shown in Table 2,
show that antibody titers remain high 52 weeks after vaccination with the yeast
antigen.

In conclusion, immunoaffinity chromatography is a practical method of purifying HBsAg to make a vaccine. The antigen produced is of high purity, has the
typical physicochemical properties of HBsAg, and is fully immunogenic in animals. The columns are expensive because high-purity antibody must be used,
but if used repeatedly, immunoaffinity columns can be economical.

ACKNOWLEDGMENTS

We thank Dr. E.D. Lehman and M. Mudri for the SDS-PAGE analysis; W. Miller
and R. Machlowitz for analytical support; Dr. B. Wolanski and R. Ziegler for electron microscopy; and H.E. Darmofal, J.T. Deviney, K.I. Guckert, R.R. Roehm, and
L.W. Stanton for assistance in the animal tests.

REFERENCES

Alexander, J.J., E.M. Bay, E.W. Geddes, and G. Lecatsos. 1976. Establishment of a continuously growing cell line from primary carcinoma of the liver. *S. Afr. Med. J.* **50:** 2124.

Table 2
Duration of Antibody Response in Grivet Monkeys Vaccinated with
HBsAg Purified from Yeast

Dose	Anti-HBsAg response (geometric mean titer)		
(μg/injection)	week 4	week 8	week 52
40	88	1,078	11,554
10	184	877	4,984
2.5	225	1,168	10,868
.625	109	925	313

Hilleman, M.R., E.B. Buynak, W.J. McAleer, A.A. McLean, P.J. Provost, and A.A. Tytell. 1982. Hepatitis A and hepatitis B vaccines. In *Viral hepatitis* (ed. W. Szmuness et al.), p. 385. The Franklin Institute Press, Philadelphia, Pennsylvania.

Maupas, P., A. Coudeau, P. Coursaget, J. Drucker, F. Barin, and M. Andre. 1978. Immunization against hepatitis B in man: A pilot study of two years' duration. In *Viral hepatitis* (ed. G.N. Vyas et al.), p. 539. The Franklin Institute Press, Philadelphia, Pennsylvania.

Valenzuela, P., A. Medina, W.J. Rutter, G. Ammerer, and B.D. Hall. 1982. Synthesis and assembly of hepatitis B virus surface antigen particles in yeast. *Nature* **298:** 347.

Antigenic Determinants in the Poliovirus Capsid Protein VP1

Marie Chow, James L. Bittle,
James Hogle, and David Baltimore
Center for Cancer Research and
The Whitehead Institute for Biomedical Research
Massachusetts Institute of Technology
Cambridge, Massachusetts 02139;
Department of Molecular Biology, Scripps Clinic and
Research Foundation, La Jolla, California 92037

The human population is protected from poliovirus infection by vaccination with one of two types of trivalent polio vaccines developed in the 1950s: a killed vaccine (the Salk vaccine) or a live attenuated virus vaccine (the Sabin vaccine). Both vaccines, which contain all three poliovirus serotypes, present problems. The Salk vaccine uses wild-type virus that is inactivated by treatment with formalin. Improperly or incompletely killed batches of virus could result in infecting the vaccinees with active wild-type virus. Thus, elaborate safety testing is a crucial and costly part of the production process. Also, the vaccine must be given by syringe inoculation and must be given in multiple doses. The live Sabin vaccine, made from attenuated strains obtained by serial passage of a wild-type virus through monkey kidney tissue culture, carries the risk that virus may revert to neurovirulence. In addition, the vaccine presents special dangers to immune-compromised individuals. These safety risks can be minimized through the development of a subunit vaccine, e.g., a vaccine that does not contain intact viral particles or possess the polioviral genome. Before a subunit vaccine can be developed, however, the neutralizing antigens must first be defined and characterized.

Neutralizing Antigen VP1

There are four proteins, VP1, VP2, VP3, and VP4, in the polio capsid. These proteins are encoded at the 5' end of the genome, and they are synthesized as a large precursor, 1a, that is subsequently cleaved to yield the four proteins associated as a complex within the infected cell. Recently, it has been shown that

257

VP1, in a denatured form, will elicit neutralizing antibodies in rats (Chow and Baltimore 1982) and in rabbits (Blondel et al. 1982). Under identical immunization conditions, the capsid proteins VP2 and VP3 failed to elicit neutralizing antibodies, although antisera that recognized the cognate proteins were obtained. The anti-VP1 neutralizing response is extremely weak compared with that observed with virions. This difference in response may be due to the antigenic differences in denatured versus native VP1 or they may reflect other antigenic determinants on the virion due to the presence of the other capsid proteins. Nevertheless, the anti-VP1 serum is serotype-specific and thus reflects the serotypic response seen in the antivirion sera. By characterizing poliovirus variants that escape neutralization by neutralizing antivirion monoclonal antibodies, Minor et al. (1983) showed also that VP1 contained a major neutralizing determinant.

Antigenic Regions in VP1

To define the antigenic regions in VP1 that can induce neutralizing antibodies, a number of peptides were synthesized that cover in the aggregate most of the type-1 VP1 protein sequence. This was possible since the nucleic acid sequences for the capsid regions have recently been determined for the genomes of the wild-type poliovirus type-1 Mahoney (Racaniello and Baltimore 1981; Kitamura et al. 1981), type-3 Leon (Minor et al. 1983), and all three of the Sabin

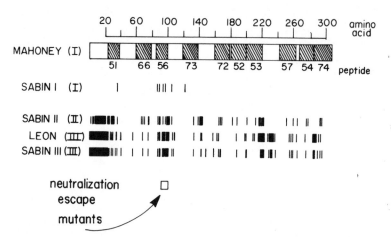

Figure 1
Location of the synthetic peptides within the VP1 sequence. The locations of the synthetic peptides are denoted by the shaded regions along the linear VP1 amino acid sequence for the type 1, Mahoney strain; the amino acid sequence was determined from the nucleotide sequence (Racaniello and Baltimore 1981). The amino acid residues are numbered with the amino terminus of VP1 being 1, and residue 302 is at the carboxyl terminus of VP1. The regions where the VP1 sequences for the type 3, Leon, and Sabin 1, 2, and 3 strains differ from the type 1, Mahoney strain, are shaded below the peptide map. The VP1 region neutralizing determinant for poliovirus type 3 that was localized by mapping viral mutants resistant to neutralizing monoclonal antibodies is delineated by the box (Minor et al. 1983).

vaccine serotypes (A. Nomoto, pers. comm.). The placement of the peptides within the VP1 sequence is shown in Figure 1. The peptides coupled to keyhole limpet hemocyanin (KLH) in complete Freund's adjuvant were injected into rabbits or Lewis rats and subsequently boosted with the coupled peptide in incomplete Freund's adjuvant. After three booster injections, the animals were bled and assayed for neutralizing antibodies (Table 1). Three antipeptide sera possessed neutralizing activity. Although the neutralizing titers were low (barely detectable for peptide 57) and varied from animal to animal, the three rats injected with a particular peptide gave qualitatively similar results. In addition, similar neutralizing titers were observed with antipeptide sera obtained from rabbits. Thus, no neutralizing titers were observed for antisera against peptides 51, 53, 54, 56, 72, 73, and 74. Although no neutralizing titers have been observed with peptide 56, other data presented below indicate that there is a neutralizing determinant located in the region of the VP1 protein, which partially overlaps with the carboxyl terminus of this peptide. This is consistent with the observations of Minor et al. (1983) that a major neutralizing determinant is located between amino acids 96 and 104. We are presently retesting peptide 56 and a number of new peptides that encompass this region to clarify this apparent discrepancy.

Several observations are noteworthy. The three peptides that induce neutralizing antibodies are located in quite separate segments of the VP1 sequence; thus, they may represent distinct neutralization sites within the virion. Alternatively, the peptides may be located adjacent to each other in the VP1 tertiary structure, forming one neutralization determinant. Further studies will be needed to distinguish between these alternatives. Similar neutralization titers were observed whether the immunizations were carried out in rabbits or rats. Thus, the antigenic responses observed are qualitatively independent of the animal species immunized and are a characteristic of the peptide antigen. The antipeptide sera show serotype specificity. This indicates that it will be possible to obtain serotype-specific responses using VP1 protein fragments.

VP1 Antigenic Determinants Found in Antivirion Sera

To characterize the VP1 antigenic determinants found in antisera made against mature poliovirus virions, peptides were used to compete the neutralizing activity found in antivirion sera. The antisera were incubated with a large molar excess of peptides and then incubated with a constant amount of infectious polioviral particles. The amount of surviving poliovirus was measured by plaque assays, and the ability of the different peptides to inhibit the neutralizing activity of antivirion sera was determined (Fig. 2). Peptides from four regions, 52, 66, 57, 64c, and 64d, were found to reduce the neutralizing activity found in polyclonal sera made against mature virions. All peptides that induced neutralizing antibodies were observed to inhibit the neutralizing activity of the polyclonal serum. In addition, two other peptides, 64c and 64d, were found to reduce the neutralizing activity. Peptides 64c and 64d are two peptides that overlap with and extend past the carboxyl terminus of peptide 56, completely spanning the region that by nucleic acid sequence has the most amino acid sequence variability among the three serotypes. The ability of these two peptides to inhibit the antivirion neutralization activity indicates the presence of a fourth determinant (which was not

Table 1
Neutralizing Titers of VP1 Peptide Antisera
against Different Poliovirus in Serotypes

Peptide no.	a-Type-1		a-Type-2 rabbits
	rats	rabbits	
51	—	—	n.d.
52	1/150	1/200	1/5
53	—	—	n.d.
54	—	—	n.d.
56	—	—	—
57	1/25	1/20	—
66	1/200	1/200	1/10
72	—	—	n.d.
73	—	—	n.d.
74	—	—	n.d.

n.d. indicates not determined; dash indicates no titers
observed.

observed in the peptide experiments described above) and is consistent with the
observations of other workers (Emini et al. 1983; Minor et al. 1983). Whether
these two peptides are capable of inducing a neutralizing response is currently
being tested. It is expected that they, as well as other peptides from this region,

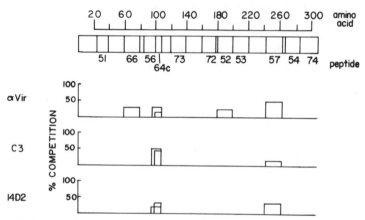

Figure 2
Inhibition of serum neutralization activity with peptides. The ability of each peptide to inhibit
the neutralizing activity of serum was tested. Peptide and sera were preincubated, and the
residual neutralizing activity was assayed. The ability of the peptide to compete away the
neutralizing activity—thereby restoring the infectivity of the input virus—is expressed as
the percent of neutralizing activity that is competed away by the preincubation of the peptide. The neutralization inhibition observed for each peptide is plotted with respect to the
peptide's location along the VP1 sequence. aVir serum is a polyclonal serum made against
mature poliovirus virions. C3 and 14D2 are neutralizing antibodies that were directed against
poliovirus virions.

will elicit a neutralizing response. Thus, it appears that for poliovirus the antipeptide antibody response in the aggregate mimics the observed immunological responses of different hosts against VP1 in the whole virion. When antivirion monoclonal antibodies are used instead of the polyclonal, only a subset of these "neutralizing peptides" will reduce the neutralizing activity. This suggests that the four peptide regions of VP1 do not in concert form a single neutralization determinant.

DISCUSSION

It is evident that there are several antigenic regions within VP1 that will induce neutralizing antibodies and that all of these regions are represented to varying extents in an animal's response to the mature virion. Thus, any development of a subunit vaccine must necessarily include all of these regions to provide an anti-VP1 antibody repertoire as complete as that found in antivirion antisera.

Because it is thought that the VP1 protein is the major neutralizing antigen in the poliovirus virion, the sole presence of anti-VP1 antibodies may protect the host from poliovirus infection. There is evidence, however, that other neutralization determinants may be present that do not reside within the VP1 protein (Emini et al. 1983), and further study will be needed to determine whether there are VP2, VP3, or VP4 peptides that will generate neutralizing antibodies, and whether these neutralizing determinants have a significant protective effect.

ACKNOWLEDGMENTS

We would like to acknowledge with appreciation the large efforts of Dr. R.A. Houghten for synthesizing the peptides. In addition, we thank Drs. R. Crainic, F. Horodniceanu, A.D.M.E. Ostergaard, and A. von Wezel for the gifts of monoclonal antibodies. Finally, we would like to thank R. Yabrov for technical assistance.

REFERENCES

Blondel, B., R. Crainic, and F. Horodniceanu. 1982. Virologie. Le polypeptide structural VP1 du poliovirus type 1 induit des anticorps neutralisants. *C.R. Acad. Sci.* **294:** 91.
Chow, M. and D. Baltimore. 1982. Isolated poliovirus capsid protein VP1 induces a neutralizing response in rats. *Proc. Natl. Acad. Sci.* **79:** 7518.
Emini, E. A., B.A. Jameson, and E. Wimmer. 1983. Priming for and induction of antipoliovirus neutralizing antibodies by synthetic peptides. *Nature* **304:** 699.
Kitamura, N., B.L. Semler, P.G. Rothberg, G.R. Larsen, C.J. Adler, C.W. Anderson, and E. Wimmer. 1981. Primary structure, gene organization and polypeptide expression of poliovirus RNA. *Nature* **291:** 547.
Minor, P.D., G.C. Schild, J. Bootman, D.M.A. Evans, M. Ferguson, P. Reeve, M. Spitz, B. Stanway, A.J. Cann, R. Hauptman, L.D. Clarke, R.C Mountford, and J. Almond. 1983. Location and primary structure of a major antigenic site for poliovirus neutralization. *Nature* **301:** 674.
Racaniello, V.R. and D. Baltimore. 1981. Molecular cloning of poliovirus cDNA and determination of the complete nucleotide sequence of the viral genome. *Proc. Natl. Acad. Sci.* **78:** 4887.

Comparison of Different Eukaryotic Vectors for the Expression of Hemagglutinin Glycoprotein of Influenza Virus

Mary-Jane Gething and Joseph F. Sambrook
Cold Spring Harbor Laboratory
Cold Spring Harbor, New York 11724

Thomas J. Braciale
Washington University School of Medicine
St. Louis, Missouri 63110

Colin M. Brand
The Wellcome Foundation, Ltd.
Beckenham, Kent BR3 3BS, England

A number of vectors have been designed and constructed that express the hemagglutinin (HA) glycoprotein of the A/Japan/305/57 strain of influenza virus in eukaryotic cells. These vectors include (1) plasmids that become integrated into the chromosome of murine cells and cause HA to be expressed constitutively during long-term culture, (2) bovine papilloma virus (BPV)-HA recombinant genomes that are maintained as episomes in continuous lines of murine cells and direct the expression of HA, and (3) SV40-HA recombinant viruses that express HA during lytic infection of simian cells. In all cases the HA is displayed at the cell surface in a form that is indistinguishable in its structural and functional properties from HA produced in cells infected with influenza virus. The amount of HA expressed reflects the number of copies of the HA gene present in the cells. The deletion mutant of HA that lacks the sequences coding for the carboxy-terminal anchoring portion of the protein has also been expressed using all these vector systems. The truncated protein is efficiently synthesized and secreted from the cells. The antigenic and immunogenic properties of the wild-type and truncated molecules are discussed below.

Continuous Expression of HA from Genes Integrated into the Chromosomes of Murine Cells

The Japan HA gene was introduced into murine LMtk⁻ cells in a recombinant plasmid containing the β-lactamase gene, the chicken thymidine kinase (*tk*) gene, and the HA gene (wild type or anchor-minus) inserted between the SV40 early promoter and SV40 early sequences containing RNA processing signals (Fig.

263

1A). *tk*+ clones were selected in HAT medium, grown into mass culture, and analyzed (1) for the presence of integrated HA DNA by Southern blotting, (2) for HA mRNA by Northern transfer, and (3) for HA protein by radioimmunoassay. Whereas all the *tk*+ clones tested had intact integrated HA genes, and some contained mRNAs corresponding in length to authentic HA mRNA from cells infected with influenza virus, the levels of mRNA expression varied widely. The production of HA protein correlated with levels of mRNA and ranged from about 5000 molecules/cell to as much as 100,000 molecules/cell. The highest levels are approximately 100-fold lower than those obtained after infection of LMtk⁻

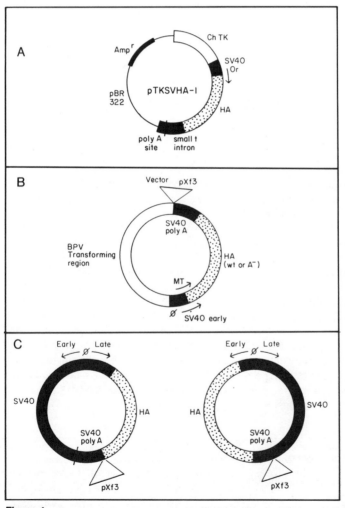

Figure 1
Vectors designed to express HA in eukaryotic cells.

cells with the A/Japan influenza virus. The HA$^+$ cell lines continued to express HA through several subclonings and continuous culture for a period of 8 months. Evidence that HA is expressed at the surfaces of these cells was provided by H2-restricted lysis of the cells by heterogeneous or cloned populations of Japan HA-specific cytotoxic T lymphocytes (CTLs) (Braciale et al. 1984). Typically, CTLs recognize the immunizing antigen with great specificity when it is displayed on the surface of a histocompatible target cell. However, CTLs that occur in both mice and humans in response to type-A influenza virus show an unusually high degree of cross-reactivity for target cells infected with serologically distinct type-A influenza virus strains. The data presented in Table 1 show that the HA molecule expressed in murine cells from an integrated cDNA copy of the HA gene (in the absence of any other influenza virus gene products) can serve as target antigen for both the subtype-specific and cross-reactive subpopulations of influenza-specific CTLs. Thus, it is possible that HAs of different subtypes of type-A influenza carry a conserved epitope (or epitopes) that is immunodominant for CTL recognition/activation but very poorly recognized by the humoral response. These findings now open the way for mapping specific CTL epitopes on the HA molecule by site-directed mutagenesis.

Continuous Expression of HA in Murine C127 Cells Transformed with BPV-HA Recombinant Vectors

To obtain cell lines that constitutively express higher levels of HA, murine C127 cells were transformed with BPV-HA vectors (Fig. 1B) in which the HA gene was under the control of either the SV40 early promoter or the murine metallothionein promoter (Pavlakis and Hamer 1983). Transformed cell lines were obtained that contained 50–200 copies of the BPV-HA genome maintained extrachromo-

Table 1
Recognition of the A/Japan/305/57 HA Gene Product by A/Japan-specific CTL

	% Specific ^{51}Cr-release from target cells[b]						
	1E2 cells (tk$^+$, HA$^+$)		pOD3 cells (tk$^+$, HA$^-$)				
Effector cells[a]	uninfected	A/Jap (H2N2)	uninfected	A/Jap (H2N2)	A/AA (H2N2)	A/PR8 (H1N1)	A/PC (H3N2)
CBA anti-A/Jap	36	78	1	46	n.d.	n.d.	n.d.
CBA anti-A/WSN	31	70	1	36	n.d.	n.d.	n.d.
CBA anti-A/Jap							
clone 36–7	65	91	8	68	9	6	4
clone 36–9	54	80	3	57	14	1	0
clone 35–6	14	88	5	85	78	90	84

[a]Heterogeneous effector cells: Spleen cells from pools of 2–3 immune CBA/J donors 3 or more weeks after inoculation with infectious A/Japan/305/57 virus were cultured with A/Japan-infected, irradiated syngeneic stimulator splenocytes. CTL effectors were used after 5–7 days of culture. Cloned effector cells: CTL clones were derived from three separate A/Japan virus-immune CBA/J donors and were maintained in continuous culture for 4–6 weeks prior to use.

[b]The ^{51}Cr-release assays were performed as described previously by Braciale et al. (1984). Effector-to-target ratios were 2:1. n.d. indicates not determined.

somally as episomes. The HA protein is expressed continuously at levels of up to approximately 10^7 molecules/cell per 24 hours. The production of HA was higher when the gene was under the control of the metallothionein promoter than when the SV40 early promoter was utilized. The addition of zinc to the medium resulted in an approximately twofold increase in expression of HA from the recombinants containing the metallothionein promoter.

In cell lines transformed with vectors containing the wild-type HA gene, cell-surface expression was demonstrated by indirect immunofluorescence and hemadsorption of guinea pig erythrocytes to the cell monolayer. The anchor-minus HA was efficiently secreted into the medium from cells transformed with vectors containing the truncated HA gene. These cell lines combine the advantage of high-level production with the convenience of constitutive and continuous expression.

High-level Expression of HA from Cells Lytically Infected with SV40-HA Recombinant Viruses

We have previously described the construction and use of SV40-HA recombinant viruses to express high levels of HA in simian cells (Gething and Sambrook 1981, 1982). CV-1 or COS-1 cells infected with recombinant SV40-HA virus vectors (see Fig. 1C) contain 10^5 to 10^6 genomes at late times after infection and synthesize approximately 5×10^8 molecules of HA per cell. Thus, up to 200 μg of wild-type HA can be produced from a 10-cm dish of cells and easily purified by detergent extraction, followed by affinity chromatography on a column of Ricin I coupled to Sepharose 4B. Alternatively, the anchor-minus HA can be obtained in almost pure form from the serum-free medium above cells infected with recombinant viruses containing the deleted HA gene.

The HA protein expressed from the wild-type HA gene has been compared with that produced in cells infected with influenza virus. The two forms were found to be essentially identical in structure, biological activity, and antigenicity (Gething and Sambrook 1981). It was thus of interest to determine whether the immunogenicities of the HAs produced from either the SV40-HA recombinants or influenza virus were also identical. Four preparations of purified HA were tested using the protocols described in Figure 2: (1) influenza-virus-derived polymer subunits purified after detergent treatment of A/Japan/305/57 virions, (2) SV40-vector-derived polymer subunits purified after detergent treatment of CV-1 cells infected with SVEHA3 virus (Gething and Sambrook 1981), (3) influenza-virus-derived monomer subunits lacking the carboxyterminal hydrophobic domain (prepared by bromelain digestion of A/Japan/305/57 virus [Brand and Skehel 1972]), and (4) SV40-vector-derived monomer subunits (anchor-minus HA) secreted from cells infected with SVEHA20-A⁻ virus (Gething and Sambrook 1982). We conclude that the HA products expressed from the SV40-HA vectors are remarkably similar in their immunogenic properties to those obtained from egg-grown influenza virus. The monomer forms resemble each other in being poor immunogens, only giving detectable responses when the mice were boosted with UV-irradiated whole virus 28 days after the initial injections. On the other hand, both types of polymer subunits show dramatically improved immunogenicities

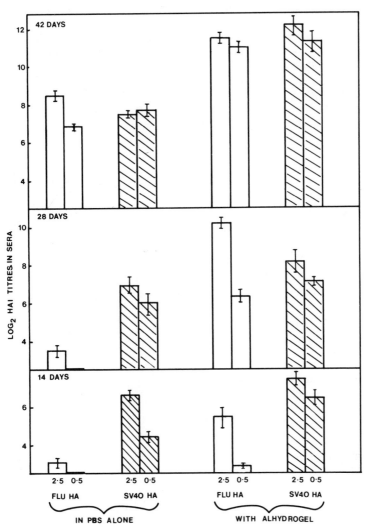

Figure 2
Immunogenicity of HA polymer subunits purified from influenza virus or from cells infected with SV40-HA recombinant virus vector. Groups of five mice were inoculated subcutaneously with 0.2 ml volumes containing 0.5 μg or 2.5 μg of the various HA preparations (with or without alhydrogel adjuvant). All mice were boosted on day 28 with a low level (0.5 μg) of UV-irradiated purified whole A/Japan/305/57 virus to detect any priming doses potent enough to have triggered memory and to determine secondary responses. Bleeds were taken on days 14, 28, and 42, and the sera were assayed for hemagglutination-inhibition (HAI) titers.

(Fig. 2). The SV40-vector-derived HA is generally more potent early on in the response than the influenza-virus-derived HA. However, the two antigen forms show very similar potencies later in the response, especially after boosting.

SUMMARY

A cDNA copy of the RNA gene coding for the HA glycoprotein from the A/Japan/ 305/57 strain of influenza virus has been expressed in eukaryotic cells using a number of different vector systems. The HA can be expressed constitutively from continuous lines of cells stably transformed by the recombinant vectors, or during the course of lytic infections by recombinant viruses. In all cases the HA produced is indistinguishable in its antigenic and immunogenic properties from that produced in cells infected with influenza virus.

REFERENCES

Braciale, T.J., V.L. Braciale, T.J. Henkel, J. Sambrook, and M.J. Gething. 1984. Cytotoxic T lymphocyte recognition of the influenza hemagglutinin gene product expressed by DNA-mediated gene transfer. *J. Exp. Med.* **159**: 341.

Brand, C. and J.J. Skehel. 1972. Crystalline antigen from the influenza virus envelope. *Nature New Biol.* **238**: 145.

Gething, M.J. and J. Sambrook. 1981. Cell surface expression of influenza haemagglutinin from a cloned DNA copy of the RNA gene. *Nature* **293**: 620.

———. 1982. Construction of influenza haemagglutinin genes that code for intracellular and secreted forms of the protein. *Nature* **300**: 598.

Pavlakis, G.N. and D.H. Hamer. 1983. Regulation of a metallothionein-growth hormone hybrid gene in bovine papilloma virus. *Proc. Natl. Acad. Sci.* **80**: 397.

Immunization Strategy: Infection-permissive Vaccines for the Modulation of Infection

Edwin D. Kilbourne
*Mount Sinai School of Medicine of
the City University of New York
New York, New York 10029*

Conventional vaccine strategy entails the prevention of disease through the prevention of infection. Immunization with living agents usually establishes effective and durable immunity sufficient to prevent infection, but potential problems of this approach (virulence reversion, overattenuation) reflect the intrinsic mutability of replicating agents. Therefore, there has been a resurgence of interest in nonreplicating antigens of minimal complexity. However, the capacity of such antigens to induce the formation of neutralizing antibody and hence prevent infection may be limited in relation to their diminished size and/or changed conformation. A case will be made that such antigens may nevertheless prove to be effective as a prelude to definitive immunization with living agents. Subsequent infection can be suppressed below the threshold required for the production of disease but must be quantitatively sufficient to induce lasting immunity. With this approach, infection is a welcome and necessary event whether initiated by a natural pathogen or by a partially attenuated living agent vaccine. Influenza virus neuraminidase (NA) vaccines will be discussed as a model of infection-permissive immunization strategy.

DISCUSSION

Although it is true that the capacity of an antigen to induce the formation of neutralizing antibody is reasonably predictive of its capacity to induce immunity, it is not necessarily true that an antigen that fails to induce neutralizing antibody demonstrable in vitro cannot immunize against disease. A case in point is the highly immunogenic NA glycoprotein of influenza virus, which does not partici-

269

pate in virus neutralization but effectively immunizes experimental animals and humans (for review, see Kilbourne et al. 1975).

Influenza Virus NA as a Prototype for Infection-permissive Immunization

The influenza virus NA is quantitatively the lesser of the two immunizing antigens of the virion envelope with respect to the proportion of total viral protein that it represents (Table 1) and the density of spikes on the virion surface (Erickson and Kilbourne 1980). The contrasting properties of the major hemagglutinin (HA) antigen and the NA protein are compared in Table 1. Notably, HA induces the formation of neutralizing antibody that prevents infection and therefore disease. In contrast, NA stimulates the formation of antibody that is neutralizing only in very high concentrations but is nevertheless protective because of its damping effect on multicycle infection under conditions where antibody is continuously present (Kilbourne et al. 1975). Thus, immunization with either antigen can prevent disease, but through different mechanisms. These different mechanisms are best illustrated by the effects of HA and NA antibodies on plaque formation, using the method of postinoculation neutralization in which antibody is incorporated into agar overlays added after viral inoculation (Jahiel and Kilbourne 1966). In this case the antibody was made to whole wild-type viruses (Table 2) but was effectively either anti-HA or anti-NA with respect to the test virus used—an antigenically hybrid reassortant of the two immunizing viruses. It is shown that over a wide range of dilutions (as in classical virus neutralization), HA antibody (anti-H1) reduces plaque *number* and at end-point dilutions has an effect on plaque size as well. NA antibody (anti-N2) has no effect on plaque number but reduces plaque *size* over a wide range of dilutions (Table 2) in proportion to antibody concentration (Jahiel and Kilbourne 1966). These results are consistent with the interpretation that NA antibody, although unable to neutralize the virus and thus prevent infection, damps successive rounds of replication in the multicycle infection through which plaques evolve. With respect to applicability to other antigens,

Table 1
HA and NA as Immunogens

Characteristics	HA	NA
Percentage of total viral protein	24	7
Induces antibody	+	+
HA-inhibiting	+	±[a]
NA-inhibiting	±[a]	+
neutralizing	+	0
protective	+	+
Prevents infection	+	0
Prevents disease	+	+[b]

[a]Variable in amount; active through steric inhibition.
[b]If level of virus replication is sufficiently diminished.

Table 2
NA Antibody Does Not Reduce Plaque Number but Reduces Plaque Size over a Wide Range of Dilutions

Antibody	Test virus	Serum dilutions leading to reduction in	
		plaque no.	plaque size
Anti-HA (*H1*N1)	H1N2	62,000–64,000[a]	8,000–64,000
Anti-NA (H2*N2*)	H1*N2*	<62	62–32,000

Data from Jahiel and Kilbourne (1966). Antigens homologous to challenge are shown in italics.
[a]Reciprocal of arithmetic dilution of serum at which 50% or greater reduction in plaque number or significant reduction in plaque size occurs.

it is important to note at this point that the effects of NA antibodies are not exclusively or necessarily dependent on inhibition of the viral enzyme but probably involve particle aggregation and binding of emerging virions to cell-associated NA as well (Kilbourne et al. 1975).

The effects of NA antibody demonstrable in in vitro virus infection have also been shown in mice (Schulman et al. 1968) and humans (Couch et al. 1974). As in cell culture, NA antibody induced in vivo is infection-permissive (Table 3), but it can reduce virus replication (challenge 1) below the threshold necessary for disease production. In this situation, replication of the partially restricted challenge virus can induce the definitive immunity characteristic of infection and resistance to subsequent challenge. In contrast, the initially superior immunity induced by the HA is only briefly sustained and vulnerability to further challenge will return.

Applicability to Other Systems

To clarify the presentation of this somewhat complex immunization strategy, the foregoing presentation has been simplistic. At reduced levels of HA antibody, infection undoubtedly can occur and disease is sometimes prevented. But even high concentrations of NA antibody are unlikely to prevent infection—a critical

Table 3
HA as Superior Immunogen Prevents Infection from Initial Challenge, but Not from Second Challenge

Immunogen[a]	Antibody induced	Challenge 1			Challenge 2	
		infection	disease	induces	infection	disease
HA	HA (neut)	0	0	0	+	+
NA	NA (non-neut)	+	0–±	HA antibody NA antibody (boost) (infection-induced durable immunity)	0	0

NA immunization is infection-permissive but disease-suppressive and allows definitive immunization from challenge 1.
[a]Isolated antigen or inactivated whole virus antigenic hybrid.

point if infection-induced immunity is the goal. The induction of large amounts of nonneutralizing but narrowly targeted infection-modulating antibodies is qualitatively different from stimulating borderline or inadequate amounts of virus-neutralizing antibody, although the effects as judged from a single challenge may appear to be similar.

Although the mechanisms of the effect may differ, antigens other than influenza virus NA can induce protection in the absence of demonstrable neutralizing antibody. Nonneutralizing monoclonal antibodies to the E_2 glycoprotein of Semliki Forest virus can protect mice from encephalitis (Boere et al. 1983). Injection of the isolated VP1 protein of foot-and-mouth disease virus is protective, although it lacks the main antigenic determinant of the intact virus (Meloen et al. 1983). Sutcliffe et al. (1983) has emphasized that many synthetic peptides induce protein-binding antibodies, which, however, are rarely neutralizing. The influence of such antibodies on virus replication in assay systems in which antibody remains present (as it does in the immunized animal) should be studied to ascertain whether such peptides have effects on virus replication not demonstrable in conventional neutralization tests. The greater sensitivity of the postinoculation neutralization (antibody-in-overlay) technique permits demonstration of plaque inhibition by certain monoclonal antibodies to influenza virus HA, which are nonreactive in hemagglutination-inhibition and conventional neutralization tests (J.L. Schulman, pers. comm.).

By analogy with influenza virus NA antibody, incorporation of antibodies to specific peptides into agar overlays in virus-plaquing systems should provide the most sensitive biological assay for the screening of potential immunogens, either singly or in combination. Antigens that induce the formation of antibody reductive of plaque size would be candidates for the induction of infection-permissive immunity.

SUMMARY AND CONCLUSIONS

Infection-restrictive immunization with the goal of inducing antibody that neutralizes virus and thereby prevents infection and disease is a time-honored objective of vaccine development. However, if effected with nonreplicating antigens, such immunity may be difficult to obtain, and transient. Living agent vaccines are subject to problems of stability and mutation to virulence or overattenuation.

As a third option, infection-permissive immunity induced with a minor antigen (e.g., influenza virus NA) is not associated with virus-neutralizing antibody and allows modified and immunizing infection to occur that can lead to lasting immunity.

Viral subunit and synthetic peptide antigens not immunogenic for neutralizing antibody should be screened for their capacity to induce antibody reactive with virus at a nonneutralizing site but suppressive to virus replication as candidates for infection-permissive vaccines.

REFERENCES

Boere, W.A.M., B.J. Benaissa-Trouw, M. Harmsen, C.A. Kraaijeveld, and H. Snippe. 1983. Neutralizing and non-neutralizing monoclonal antibodies to the E_2 glycoprotein of Semliki Forest can protect mice from lethal encephalitis. *J. Gen. Virol.* **64:** 1405.

Couch, R.B., J.A. Kasel, J.L. Gerin, J.L. Schulman, and E.D. Kilbourne. 1974. Induction of partial immunity to influenza by a neuraminidase-specific vaccine. *J. Infect. Dis.* **129:** 411.

Erickson, A.H. and E.D. Kilbourne. 1980. Mutation in the hemagglutinin of A/N-WS/33 influenza virus recombinants influencing sensitivity to trypsin and antigenic reactivity. *Virology* **107:** 320.

Jahiel, R.I. and E.D. Kilbourne. 1966. Reduction in plaque size and reduction in plaque number as differing indices of influenza virus-antibody reactions. *J. Bacteriol.* **92:** 1521.

Kilbourne, E.D., P. Palese, and J.L. Schulman. 1975. Inhibition of viral neuraminidase as a new approach to the prevention of influenza. In *Perspectives in virology* (ed. M. Pollard), vol. IX, p. 99. Academic Press, New York.

Meloen, R.H., J. Briaire, R.J. Woortmeyer, and D. Van Zaane. 1983. The main antigenic determinant detected by neutralizing monoclonal antibodies on the intact foot-and-mouth disease virus particle is absent from isolated VP1. *J. Gen. Virol.* **64:** 1193.

Schulman, J.L., M. Khakpour, and E.D. Kilbourne. 1968. Protective effects of specific immunity to viral neuraminidase on influenza virus infection of mice. *J. Virol.* **2:** 778.

Sutcliffe, J.G., T.M. Shinnick, N. Green, and R.A. Lerner. 1983. Antibodies that react with predetermined sites on proteins. *Science* **219:** 660.

Bioengineering of Herpes Simplex Virus Variants for Potential Use as Live Vaccines

Bernard Roizman
Marjorie B. Kovler Viral Oncology
Laboratories, The University of Chicago
Chicago, Illinois 60637

Bernard Meignier
Institute Merieux, Lyon, France

Bodil Norrild
Department of Medical Microbiology
The University of Copenhagen
Copenhagen, Denmark

Joseph L. Wagner
School of Medicine, University of Miami
Miami, Florida 33101

Control of herpes simplex virus (HSV) infections in humans must necessarily involve (1) antiviral chemotherapy, to reduce the amount and interval of shedding of infectious virus by patients with recurrent genital infections; (2) education, to minimize the epidemiologically significant contact between patients with genital lesions and susceptibles; and (3) immunoprophylaxis, to render susceptibles less likely to acquire severe primary and recurrent infections on contact with individuals shedding virus (for details, see Roizman et al. 1982).

The traditional venues of immunoprophylaxis are vaccines. In principle, to construct a successful vaccine, it is necessary to take into consideration the biology and epidemiology of the virus as well as the evolution of the disease in the population to be protected. With respect to HSV, two characteristics of the infectious process shape our perception of the requirements for successful immunoprophylaxis.

First, it has been long known, on clinical grounds, that patients can transmit HSV from one site to another and establish recurrent infections at the new site by autoinoculation. In recent years, molecular epidemiology based on restriction endonuclease analyses of viral DNAs firmly established that patients may become infected with more than one strain of the same serotype. The apparent failure of natural HSV infections to protect completely against superinfection is probably explained by the observations that (1) the target organ of HSV infections is also the portal of entry into the body and hence is less readily protected

275

by the immune system than in cases of infectious agents whose target organ is distal from the portal of entry, and (2) the virus becomes inaccessible to the immune system once it enters and ascends the sensory or autonomic nerve trunks innervating the portal of entry.

Second, the population most readily accessible for mass immunization consists of primary and secondary school children and college students. However, the interval of maximum risk of contracting genital infections extends to at least age 40.

These characteristics of HSV infections led us to consider live viruses, engineered to express specific properties, as the immunogens most likely to meet the requirement that the quality and duration of the protection they elicit match those induced by natural infection. This paper deals with an assessment of the currently available technology for both construction and testing of HSV variants with properties that might be desirable.

Bioengineering of Viruses with Specific Properties

The objective of our constructions is to inactivate, delete, or avoid introduction of sequences encoding properties responsible for (1) neurovirulence, (2) ability to spread from site of inoculation to distal sites, or (3) oncogenicity. An additional objective is to enhance the immunogenicity of virus strains. A prime requirement of any genetic modification is that it be stable, and this is best achieved by deletions, insertions, and gene rearrangements than by point mutations.

The scheme adopted by us for construction of site-specific gene insertions, deletions, and rearrangements is that described in a specific instance by Mocarski et al. (1980) and in more general terms by Post and Roizman (1981). As illustrated in Figure 1, the scheme utilizes the HSV thymidine kinase (*tk*) gene as a selectable marker for insertion or deletion of sequences by legitimate recombination through sequences flanking the specific site selected for gene manipulation. Figure 2 lists some of the variants constructed to date.

Testing of Variant HSV Constructs

Table 1 summarizes the tests used to assess the properties of wild-type and variant viruses with respect to their phenotypic properties relevant to live vaccine constructs. Many of the tests (e.g., oncogenicity) were not yet completed at the time this paper was written.

Virulence

The objective of the virulence tests was to assess the test systems for determining whether the variant constructs differ from wild-type viruses with respect to ability to grow in the central nervous system and ability to enter and ascend the nervous system from peripheral sites of inoculation. We have tested several of the constructs in the mouse, in Saguinus fuscicollis and Aotus trivirgatus nonhuman primates, and in guinea pigs.

As a general rule, the pfu/LD$_{50}$ ratio obtained by intracerebral (IC) inoculation of mice with wild-type viruses ranged from approximately 3×10^2 for HSV-1(F) to

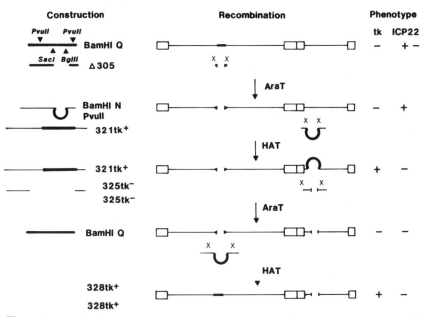

Figure 1
Diagram illustrating the procedure for the production of variants containing deletions in gene *22* (Post and Roizman 1981). Step 1 in this procedure was the isolation of a virus (Δ305) containing a deletion in the viral thymidine kinase (*tk*) gene. For this purpose, approximately 700 bp encompassing the *Sac*I-*Bgl*II cleavage sites were deleted from the *Bam*HI Q fragment (Post and Roizman 1981). The *Bam*HI Q fragment containing the deletion was then transfected into rabbit skin with intact HSV-1(F) DNA. Δ305 was selected from the progeny of the transfection by plating in the presence of thymidine arabinoside (Ara T). Step 2 was the insertion of a fragment (*Pvu*II fragment obtained by cleavage of *Bam*HI Q) containing the *tk* gene into the *Bam*HI N fragment at a site known from previous studies to be within the structural sequences of α gene *22*. In this instance the cells were transfected with the *Bam*HI N fragment carrying the insertion and intact Δ305 DNA. *tk*+ virus was selected by plating the viral progeny on *tk*- cells in the presence of HAT medium. The virus carrying the *tk* gene inserted into *Bam*HI N fragment was designated as R321. Step 3 involved construction of deletions in α gene *22*. In this instance, 100- and 700-bp deletions were constructed in the *Bam*HI N fragment, and the fragment carrying the deletions was used to transfect DNA with intact R321 DNA. *tk*- progeny containing 100-bp (R328 *tk*- virus) and 700-bp (R325 *tk*- virus) deletions were selected by plating in the presence of Ara T. The last step was to recombine the *tk* gene into the virus at its natural position by transfecting cells with the *Bam*HI Q fragment and the R325 *tk*- or R328 *tk*- DNAs. The R325 *tk*+ and R328 *tk*+ progeny were selected by plating in the presence of HAT medium. The *tk* gene is indicated by a thick line. The viral DNA is shown as consisting of two sets of unique sequences (long and short) represented by a straight line and bracketed by inverted repeats represented by open rectangles. The *tk* gene maps near the center of the long component, whereas the α gene *22* maps near the left terminus of the short component. Deletions are shown as interruptions in the line representing unique sequences.

3 for HSV-2(G). A virulent HSV-1 strain, MGH10, yielded a ratio of approximately 6 pfu/LD$_{50}$. All variant constructs tested (I358, Δ305, R328, and R325) yielded pfu/LD$_{50}$ ratios ranging from 6×10^5 (I358) to 10^7 (R325).

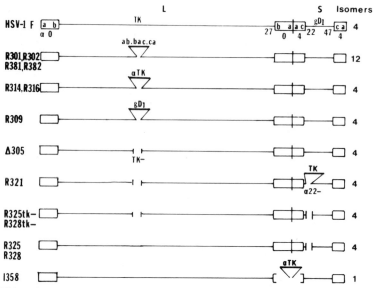

Figure 2
Variant HSV-1 constructs made according to the scheme illustrated in Fig. 1. The top line illustrates the sequence arrangement of wild-type HSV-1 DNA. The rectangles represent the inverted repeat sequences flanking the long (L) and short (S) components. TK refers to the location of the thymidine kinase gene in the prototype arrangement of HSV-1 DNA; 0, 27, 4, 22, and 47 refer to the location of the *a* genes. R301, R302, R381, and R382 contain insertions of the terminal repeat sequences (R381, R382) or junction sequences (R301, R302) into the *tk* gene. Because the insertion of the *a* sequence increased the number of DNA stretches flanked by inverted repeats of the *a* sequence, the number of isomers increased from 4 to 12 (Mocarski et al. 1980). R309 contains an insertion of a 1.8-kb *Sac* fragment into the *tk* gene; it contains the gene specifying glycoprotein D of HSV-1. Δ305, R321, R325 *tk*⁻, R328 *tk*⁻, R325 *tk*⁺(identified as R325), and R328 *tk*⁺ (identified as R328) are described in Fig. 1.

Saguinus tamarins were especially sensitive to IC inoculation but not to peripheral routes of inoculation. Most of them were severely parasitized, and death was occasionally due to parasitic infestation. Whereas 10^2 pfu of either HSV-1 (MGH10) or HSV-2(G) was uniformly lethal by the IC route, seven out of eight Saguinus tamarins survived IC inoculation with 10^6 pfu of R325. Aotus monkeys, in contrast, appeared particularly sensitive to peripheral challenge. Thus, 10^2 pfu of either HSV-1(MGH10) or HSV-2(G) was uniformly lethal when inoculated into the vagina of Aotus monkeys. However, Aotus monkeys inoculated intravaginally with 10^8 pfu of R325 shed virus for a few days but survived infection with no apparent neurologic disorders.

Genetic Stability

The objective of these studies was to determine to what extent the available test systems could detect acquisition of virulence by back mutations or by compen-

Table 1
Summary of Tests Employed for an Assessment of Vaccine Potential of Variant HSV Constructs

| Test | Mouse | Nonhuman primates | | Guinea pig |
		Saguinus	Aotus	
Virulence				
routes of inoculation	IC, IP, SQ	IC	IV	IV
Genetic stability				
route	IC	—	—	—
test	serial passage	—	—	—
Ability to establish latency				
route	eye	IC	IV	IV
ganglia	trigeminal	trigeminal	lumbosacral	lumbosacral
Antibody induction				
route	—	IC	IV	IV
test	—	immuno-precipitation	immuno-precipitation	immuno-precipitation
Protection against challenge				
route for immunization	IC, IP, SQ	IC	—	—
challenge	IC	IC	—	—
Oncogenicity				
route	IV (daily)	—	—	—
test	cytology; histopathology	—	—	—

Abbreviations: IC, intracerebral; IP, intraperitoneal; SQ, suutaneous; IV, intravaginal.
BALB/c mice were used throughout these studies. The Saguinus tamarins and the Aotus monkeys were obtained through the Pan American Health Organization. The results of the tests are discussed in the text. Procedural details will be published elsewhere.

279

satory mutations. In this series of experiments, mice were inoculated IC. At the end of 4 days, the brains were harvested and assayed for virus content, and the virus was grown in culture. The virus amplified in cell cultures was then reinoculated by the IC route into mice, and the results were shown as a plot of the ratio of virus recovered in mouse brain per amount of virus inoculated as a function of passage number. In the few instances in which this test was applied, we found that (1) R325 was stable and showed no change in ratio during nine serial IC passages; (2) a preparation of HSV-1 x HSV-2 recombinant (C7D) was contaminated with trace amounts of an unrelated wild-type virus, which became apparent between passages 5 and 8; and (3) a virulent mutant emerged between passages 6 and 9 of the HSV-1 x HSV-2 recombinant A5C; it was not a contaminant inasmuch as the mutant and A5C shared similar restriction endonuclease patterns.

Establishment of Latency

The purpose of these studies was to ascertain the relative sensitivity of the mouse models for assessment of the ability of variant HSV constructs to establish latency. Meignier et al. (1983) have shown that wild-type viruses (e.g., HSV-1[F]) readily colonized ganglia and established latent infections in mice inoculated by either the ear or eye routes. In the case of HSV-1 x HSV-2 recombinants with diminished capacity to grow in the mouse brain (Roizman et al. 1982), latent infections were established only in mice inoculated by the eye route. More recent studies have shown that none of the variant HSV constructs tested to date were able to establish latent infections by the ear route. The ability to establish latent infection by the eye route varied in frequency from approximately 50% (R325) to 10% (I358) of the animals.

It is of interest to note that R325 was able to establish latent infection of the lumbosacral ganglia in Aotus monkeys inoculated intravaginally, but it could not be recovered from the trigeminal ganglia of the Saguinus tamarins examined after immunization and subsequent challenge with HSV-1 (MGH10).

Protection Tests

Of the various tests that can be done in experimental animals, the most complex and foreign to the human situation is assessment of the capacity to induce an immune response capable of protecting against challenge. The problem stems from two considerations. First, a common end point of HSV disease in humans is morbidity caused by initial colonization of ganglia and recrudescent virus multiplication, rather than mortality due to central nervous system infections commonly seen in animals. Second, experimental animals vary considerably with respect to sensitivity to inoculation by different routes. For example, the mouse is both sensitive to IC inoculation and readily protected by IC immunization. Exemplary data are that 80 pfu of R325 protected 50% of the animals challenged IC 30 days later with 3000 LD_{50} of HSV-1(MGH10). As would be predicted for a HSV-1 virus, it took 500 pfu of R325 to confer the same level of protection against 3000 LD_{50} of HSV-2(G). The mouse, however, it not a suitable animal for assessment of the immunogenicity of live viruses administered by peripheral routes, since both wild-type and variant HSV constructs multiplied poorly under those conditions. Thus, peripheral immunization against IC challenge with 3000 LD_{50} required 10^5 to 10^8 pfu.

Preliminary studies indicate that Saguinus tamarins resembles mice with respect to both virulence and protection tests. It remains to be determined whether the extreme sensitivity of the Aotus monkeys can be utilized to design protection tests involving peripheral immunization for protection against peripheral challenge.

Immunogenicity

To date, assessments of immunogenicity were done by measuring the relative amounts of HSV-1 and HSV-2 polypeptides precipitated with sera from immunized animals and electrophoretically separated in denaturing polyacrylamide gels (Roizman et al. 1982). The accumulated data indicate that variant HSV constructs that protect against challenge with virulent viruses generally induce significant amounts of antibody reactive with viral membrane proteins.

CONCLUSIONS

The technology is now available for rapid construction of variant HSV genomes containing insertions, deletions, gene rearrangements, etc. This technology permits rapid development of variant HSV constructs suitable for identification of the genes involved in virulence, latency, immunogenicity, and manifestations of HSV infections. Less readily available are the experimental models that mimic the manifestations of human disease. Studies on variant HSV constructs and of experimental models are continuing and hopefully will contribute to the understanding of the molecular basis of pathogenesis of HSV infections and to vaccines designed to prevent them.

REFERENCES

Meignier, B., B. Norrild, and B. Roizman. 1983. Colonization of murine ganglia by a super-infecting strain of herpes simplex virus. *Infect. Immun.* **41:** 702.

Mocarski, E.S., L.E. Post, and B. Roizman. 1980. Molecular engineering of the herpes simplex virus genome. Insertion of a second L-S junction into the genome causes additional genome inversions. *Cell* **22:** 243.

Post, L.E. and B. Roizman. 1981. A generalized technique for deletion of specific genes in large genomes: *a* Gene 22 of herpes simplex virus 1 is not essential for growth. *Cell* **25:** 227.

Roizman, B., J. Warren, C.A. Thuning, M.S. Fanshaw, B. Norrild, and B. Meignier. 1982. Application of molecular genetics to the design of live herpes simplex virus vaccines. *Dev. Biol. Stand.* **52:** 287.

Reoviral Hemagglutinin: Specific Attenuation and Antigenic Mimicry as Approaches for Immunization

Bernard N. Fields, Arlene H. Sharpe, Dale R. Spriggs, and Mark I. Greene
Departments of Microbiology and Pathology Harvard Medical School, and Department of Medicine (Infectious Disease), Brigham and Women's Hospital, Boston, Massachusetts 02115

Mammalian reoviruses are segmented double-stranded RNA viruses. The segmentation of the genomic RNA has allowed us to generate a large number of reassortant viruses consisting of combinations of genes derived from the two parents following mixed infection of cells in tissue culture. Segmentation of genes has also allowed us to perform a genetic analysis that has facilitated understanding the function of each of the capsid proteins in viral pathogenesis. It is now clear that reovirus type 3 is tropic to neurons, spares ependymal cells, and produces destructive encephalitis following intracerebral inoculation of young mice. In contrast, reovirus type 1 binds to ependymal cells and produces a benign ependymitis while sparing neurons. Reovirus type-3 infection similarly spares ependymal cells. Reassortant viruses containing nine genes from type 3 and the gene encoding the viral hemagglutinin (HA) of type 1 (designated 3.HA1) are tropic for ependymal cells in a manner identical to that of type-1 reovirus. In contrast, reassortant viruses containing nine genes of type 1 and the HA gene of type 3 (designated as 1.HA3) are neurotropic, producing destructive encephalitis in a fashion identical to that of the type-3 parental virus.

Other aspects of virulence have been analyzed similarly and have provided insight into the function of each of the outer capsid proteins. Following entry into the gastrointestinal tract (the natural portal of entry), the *M2* gene (encoding the μ1C protein) is digested by host-cell proteases. This digestion, in part, influences subsequent cellular immune responses. The σ1 protein, the viral HA, which is the product of the *S1* gene, interacts with immunological and nonimmunological receptors on the surfaces of cells of the immune system (lymphocytes) and neurons and in this way determines cell and tissue tropism. The viral HA is thus the

283

major antigen that determines specific antiviral humoral or cellular immune response. The $o3$ protein, the product of the *S4* gene, is responsible for inhibiting host-cell RNA and protein synthesis and plays a critical role in allowing reovirus to initiate persistent infection of cultured cells. The parental viruses are normally cytocidal. Thus, each of the three outer capsid polypeptides displays different functions, and it may be possible to manipulate and attenuate virus virulence by separately mutating each of the genes encoding outer capsid polypeptides. Because of its critical role in cell and tissue specificity, we have focused our studies on attempting to define the function and structure of the $o1$ protein (Fields 1982).

Monoclonal Antibodies Directed against the Reovirus Type-3 HA

We have isolated 13 hybridoma-secreting antibodies directed against type-3 $o1$ proteins. When tested against the serologic properties of the HA, two of the monoclonal antibodies, A2 and G5, were efficient in neutralizing infectivity. A second series of monoclonal antibodies, represented by antibodies B6, C1, and A4, displayed little or no neutralizing activity but inhibited viral HA. A third group of antibodies, such as B2, had neither neutralizing nor hemagglutination-inhibition (HI) activity against any of the reovirus type-3 isolates tested. Thus, these initial studies clearly show that reovirus type-3 HA is organized into discrete functional regions, one of which displays the critical property of virus neutralization. Having defined these functionally distinct antigenic domains, we next analyzed the topography of the antigenic sites on the reovirus type-3 HA using a competitive radioimmunoassay. Unlabeled monoclonal antibodies were used to compete with ^{125}I-labeled antibodies for binding to the HA. In this manner, we were able to show that the antibodies fell into three groups. The first group comprised the previously identified neutralization-specific monoclonal antibodies A2 and G5 in addition to a monoclonal antibody D2 that weakly neutralized infectivity but competed efficiently with the other monoclonal antibodies. A second group comprised those antibodies with predominant HI activity; these antibodies competed reciprocally with each other, but their binding was not blocked by antibodies of the first group. A third group was identified by the monclonal antibody B2 and was distinct from the two other groups. Thus, the functionally discrete antigenic domains are also topographically distinct (Fields and Greene 1982).

Attenuated Reovirus Type-3 Variants Generated by Immunoselection with Monoclonal Antibody

Infection of suckling mice with reovirus type 3 results in fatal encephalitis associated with marked destruction of neurons. Having identified discrete domains of the reoviral HA, we were interested in isolating mutants to determine whether specific alterations in the HA would change neurovirulence. Reovirus type-3 viruses with antigenically altered HA proteins were immunoselected by incubating the neurovirulent virus stock (Dearing strain) with the G5 neutralizing monoclonal antibody. Three variant viruses, designated A, F, and K, that were isolated in this manner were resistant to neutralization by monoclonal G5 parental virus.

The three variants encode an HA protein that is antigenically altered as detected by the monoclonal antibodies but can be recognized with a standard hyperimmune antiserum. To determine whether the variants were altered in terms of virulence, we compared them with regard to their relative capacity to cause neurological disease in suckling mice. Our results indicated that all the variants are at least 10^4 times less virulent than the Dearing strain from which they were derived. The three variants also differed significantly from the Dearing strain in that they had a reduced ability to grow in mouse brain during the acute infection, particularly after the fifth day postinoculation. In contrast to this defective capacity to grow in mouse brain, all variants grew well in tissue culture. Thus, the pattern of restricted growth of these viruses in the brain is not due simply to a general defect in the ability of the three variant viruses to replicate, but appears to be due to growth in restricted sites in the brain (Fields and Greene 1982). The three variant viruses are also altered in their capacity to spread to various organs, including the central nervous system, following extraneural inoculation. Most of the mice inoculated intraperitoneally with the Dearing strain are dead by day 14. Variant viruses inoculated intraperitoneally did not grow in the brain of the infected animal, indicating that they are restricted in their capacity to enter and replicate in the central nervous system.

To define the basis for the reduced neurovirulence of the reovirus type-3 variants following direct intracerebral inoculation, we analyzed the anatomic distribution of variants as compared with the parental type-3 virus. These studies showed that, whereas Dearing virus shows a broad tropism infecting neurons and several regions of the brain including the cerebral cortex, thalamus, and medulla, the variant viruses infected a subset of neurons restricted to the limbic system of the brain, which includes the hippocampus, hypothalamus, mammillary bodies, and septum. Therefore, selective alterations in one antigenic domain of reovirus type-3 HA can change the extent and distribution of virus in the brain after intracerebral inoculation and can even alter the capacity of virus to enter the brain after peripheral inoculation. These observations suggest that certain variant viruses might be useful as "vaccines." The variants are stable, and we have been unable to isolate revertants from infected animals (Fields and Greene 1982).

Anti-idiotypes as Vaccines

Antibodies can act as antigens and provoke the synthesis of anti-antibodies. These features of antigenic uniqueness of the antibody molecule result from the conformational structures in the antigen-combining site and are referred to as idiotopes or, collectively, as idiotypes. Antibodies that recognize such determinants are called anti-idiotype antibodies or anti-idiotypes. The anti-HA antibody response to reoviral HA is of limited heterogeneity. Most anti-HA antibodies of BALB/c mice fall within a narrow pI range (6.9–7.1) as determined by isoelectric focusing. It was also shown that BALB/c anti-HA antibodies share structural idiotypes identified by rabbit anti-idiotypes (Nepom et al. 1982).

To prepare the rabbit anti-idiotypic antiserum, anti-reovirus 3 antibodies were used as an immunogen. The rabbit antiserum (anti-idiotype) was purified by passage over a normal mouse immunoglobulin immunosorbent. We next demonstrated that the mouse anti-reovirus 3 antibody could bind ^{125}I-labeled type-3 σ1 protein and that anti-idiotype inhibited this interaction. These experiments showed that the idiotype-anti-idiotype interactions are antigen–combining-site-determined. A series of monoclonal antibodies specific to the σ1 were examined for their ability to inhibit the idiotype-anti-idiotype interaction. We reasoned that inhibition would occur if a significant amount of the rabbit antiserum recognized the major determinant shared between the monoclonal antibody and the anti-σ1 antibody. One monoclonal antibody, G5, was found to greatly inhibit the binding of the rabbit antiserum to the anti-type-3 immunoglobulin. Thus, the G5 immunoglobulin appeared to have the idiotypic determinants recognized by the rabbit serum (Nepom et al. 1982).

The reoviral HA, as noted above, is the viral attachment protein. It thus interacts with receptors on somatic cells in the host. The lymphoid cellular receptor has the same discriminating capacity as anti-HA antibody. For example, the functionally important region of the reoviral HA is defined by its binding to the G5 neutralizing monoclonal antibody as well as to lymphoid cell receptors. We reasoned that if antibody (i.e., G5) and the somatic-cell receptor are structurally similar and bind to the same portion of the HA, anti-idiotypic antibody to the G5 idiotype might bind to the cell-surface receptor.

The test of the hypothesis that such anti-idiotypic antibody would recognize similar idiotypelike conformations on cellular receptors was validated by the staining of reovirus-receptor-bearing lymphoid lines and neuronal cells with the anti-idiotypic antibody. More recently, anti-idiotypic monoclonal reagents have been developed that identify the same cellular receptors for reovirus as the virus itself. This monoclonal antibody, made by syngeneic immunization to the G5 antibody, binds to the G5 idiotype but has only one specificity, since it is derived from a cloned hybridoma cell line. Adsorption of this monoclonal antibody on lymphoid cells with specific receptivity for type 3 removed 97% of the G5-binding activity as measured by radioimmunoassay. In addition, we have recently shown that anti-idiotypes are capable of "priming" for adoptively transferable T-cell-dependent immune reactivity to the virus. Thus, monoclonal anti-idiotypic antibody resembles the virus in that it can associate with reoviral receptors on cells such as neurons and can also interact with reovirus-specific immune cells. We have used such monoclonal antibodies to block binding of virus (Kauffman et al. 1983) and to inhibit infection of susceptible tissues. Thus, the anti-idiotypic antibody can identify cell-surface determinants on cells, including lymphocytes, and occupy those sites preempting viral binding. Our data suggest that the structure of the anti-idiotypic antibody resembles the structure of the HA polypeptide responsible for interacting with cell-surface receptors. Monoclonal anti-idiotype mimics the reoviral HA both immunologically and in its interactions with cellular receptors.

CONCLUDING REMARKS

In this review of certain general features of the reoviruses and specific features of the reoviral HA, we have attempted to illustrate how the mammalian reoviruses have permitted the study of viral pathogenesis. The genetic analysis of reoviruses has provided a means for identifying the role of individual virus components in the production of virulence, making the study of viral host interactions more amenable to direct experimentation. In particular, our studies have revealed that the outer capsid proteins play a critical role in virulence. The σ1 protein, the protein responsible for determining cell and tissue tropism and for binding to cell-surface receptors, has provided insights into specific ways to attenuate and immunologically manipulate viruses. These studies may facilitate the development of new vaccines.

REFERENCES

Fields, B.N. 1982. Molecular basis of reovirus virulence. *Arch. Virol.* **71:** 95.

Fields, B.N. and M.I. Greene. 1982. Genetic and molecular mechanisms of viral pathogenesis: Implications for prevention and treatment. *Nature* **300:** 12.

Kauffman, R., J.H. Noseworthy, J. Nepom, R. Finberg, B.N. Fields, and M.I. Greene. 1983. Cell receptors for the mammalian reovirus. I. Syngeneic monoclonal antiidiotypic antibody identifies the cell surface receptor for reovirus. *J. Immunol.* **131:** 2539.

Nepom, J.T., H.L. Weiner, M.A. Dichter, D.R. Spriggs, C.F. Gramm, M.L. Powers, B.N. Fields, and M.I. Greene. 1982. Identification of a hemagglutinin specific idiotype associated with reovirus recognition shared by lymphoid and neural cells. *J. Exp. Med.* **155:** 155.

Spriggs, D.R. and B.N. Fields. 1982. Generation of attenuated reovirus type 3 strains by selection of hemagglutinin antigenic variants. *Nature* **297:** 68.

Immunogenic and Protective Power of Avirulent Mutants of Rabies Virus Selected with Neutralizing Monoclonal Antibodies

Anne Flamand and Patrice Coulon
Laboratoire de Génétique des Virus
91190 Gif-Sur-Yvette, France

Michel Pepin and Jean Blancou
Centre National d'Etudes sur la Rage
BP n° 9, 54220 Malzeville, France

Pierre Rollin and Denis Portnoi
Institut Pasteur, 75724 Paris, France

It has been demonstrated that most mutants of the CVS strain of rabies virus that are resistant to neutralization by monoclonal antibodies 194-2 *and* 248-8 exhibit a markedly reduced pathogenicity. Virulence seems to be associated with the presence of an arginine residue at position 333 of the glycoprotein. Theoretically, it should be possible to select avirulent mutants from any strain of rabies virus that would be neutralized by both monoclonal antibodies. Such mutants have already been isolated by this method from the CVS and ERA strains of rabies virus (Coulon et al. 1982,1983; Dietzschold et al. 1983).

To find a suitable live vaccine for oral vaccination of foxes, the pathogenic, immunogenic, and protective powers of one hypovirulent mutant (AvO$_1$) of the CVS strain have been tested in mice and foxes. Pathogenic power was also studied in eight nontarget species.

Isolation of Avirulent Mutants

Nine neutralizing monoclonal antibodies that recognize three antigenic sites on the glycoprotein (Lafon et al. 1983) were used to select mutants resistant to neutralization. A total of 278 mutants were selected from a 5-fluorouracil (5-FU)-mutagenized CVS stock, and 56 spontaneous mutants were isolated from 7 cloned preparations of the same virus strain.

One hundred and twelve 5-FU-induced mutants were injected intracerebrally into five adult mice. Like CVS, most mutants were fully pathogenic and killed the animals between day 7 and day 9. Nine mutants had an altered pathogenicity; all were resistant to both monoclonal antibodies 194-2 and 248-8. Some of these

289

mutants were totally avirulent in adult mice whatever the inoculation route, whereas others were attenuated: They produced transient symptoms, leading eventually to death. They were called, respectively, AvO and AtO mutants (Av, avirulent; At, attenuated; O, Orsay).

Virulence seemed to be associated with a special configuration of the antigenic site(s) recognized by these two monoclonal antibodies. To verify this hypothesis, 17 spontaneous mutants resistant to neutralization by both monoclonal antibodies were injected intracerebrally into adult mice. Thirteen were found attenuated or avirulent, whereas four were still virulent, indicating that correlation between avirulence and resistance to specific anti-G monoclonal antibodies was not absolute.

The AvO and AtO mutants were not functionally affected in cell cultures. They grew efficiently in BHK-21, CER, and neuroblastoma (NS 20) cells and were not thermosensitive. Why are they avirulent? Previous results indicated that intervention of the immune response is probably necessary for the survival of animals, since nude and suckling mice died after inoculation of the mutants, although with different symptoms and after a longer incubation period. Preliminary experiments indeed demonstrated that the immune response was efficiently stimulated after infection with avirulent or attenuated viruses. It was therefore tempting to investigate the possibility that avirulent mutants could be used as an innocuous and efficient live vaccine. AvO_1, a 5-FU-induced mutant, was chosen as the prototype and used in further studies in comparison with the CVS parental strain. Residual pathogenicity of AvO_1 for mice, foxes, and other species was carefully investigated, as well as immunogenic and protective power of the virus.

Residual Pathogenicity of AvO_1

In addition to nude and suckling mice, cyclophosphamide-treated animals died after AvO_1 inoculation. Residual pathogenicity of the mutant for 3- and 4-week-old mice has been observed; males were more sensitive than females. In a few cases, virulent virus was isolated from the brains of dying animals, indicating that AvO_1 could revert to a wild-type phenotype. Adult mice always survived the inoculation and no virus could be isolated from the brains of inoculated animals.

All CVS-infected animals died after a dose equal to less than 1 pfu per animal in the case of intracerebral inoculation and 1000 pfu per animal in the case of intramuscular inoculation.

Fifteen foxes and 226 animals from 8 nontarget species (Microtidae, Muridae, and Mustelidae) resisted intramuscular or oral administration of AvO_1. Only one, *Arvicola terrestris,* was found susceptible to AvO_1 ingestion. We conclude that almost complete attenuation of the virus was observed for adult animals of all species studied.

Comparison of the Immune Response of Animals Inoculated with AvO_1 or CVS

Various parameters of the immune response were investigated after intramuscular injection of 10^5 pfu of AvO_1 or CVS into BALB/c adult mice.

Production of Circulating Antibodies

Until day 7, when CVS-inoculated animals died, no difference could be detected in the titer of circulating antibodies which rose to 200 or 2000 units, depending on the experiment (titers are expressed as the dilution of sera that reduces to 50% the pfu in CER cells). The antibody titer continued to increase in AvO_1-infected animals and usually reached a plateau at 10,000 units.

Production of Interferon

The production of interferon was assayed in the serum and in the brain. The injection of CVS and AvO_1 was followed by early production of interferon in the serum within the first 8 hours. This initial production lasted longer with AvO_1 than with CVS (Fig. 1). With CVS, a second period of production was detected between day 4 and day 7, whereas there was none with AvO_1. At that time, there was also a peak of interferon in the brains of animals inoculated with CVS, and to a lesser extent with AvO_1.

Cytotoxic Activity of Splenocytes

"Natural Killer" Cell-mediated Cytotoxicity of Splenocytes. Assays of natural killer (NK) activity of splenocytes gave results similar to those for interferon production. In the first 24 hours after intramuscular inoculation, an important NK activity was observed with AvO_1. Again, this activity persisted longer than with CVS. Correlatively with the second production of interferon, another period of increased NK activity was detected on days 4 and 5 in the CVS-injected mice.

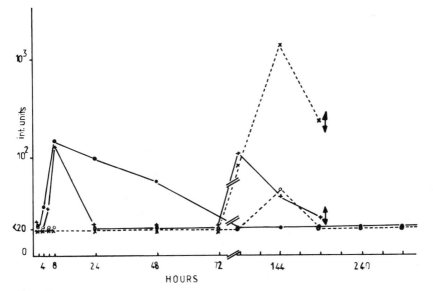

Figure 1
Interferon production. Interferon was titrated in BALB/c serum and brain extracts by inhibition of VSV cytopathic effect on L 929 cells. (+) CVS-inoculated mice (serum); (×) CVS-inoculated mice (brain); (●) AvO_1-inoculated mice (serum); (○) AvO_1-inoculated mice (brain).

T Cytotoxic Activity of Splenocytes.   In preliminary experiments, susceptibility of normal and CVS-infected mouse (H.2[a]) neuroblastoma cells (MNB) to NK activity was determined. MNB cells were susceptible to NK activity, and the virus infection enhanced this susceptibility, leading to a situation where NK activity could be confused with T cytotoxic activity of splenocytes. In A/J mice, syngeneic to MNB cells, a lytic activity of the splenocytes of AvO_1-inoculated mice was found. It was maximum at days 6 and 7, when no NK activity could be detected. The results obtained with splenocytes from CVS-inoculated animals were extremely variable, probably because of the poor condition of the animals.

Protective Power of AvO_1

The protective power of AvO_1 was evaluated in mice and foxes. Mice surviving decreasing doses of AvO_1 were challenged by cerebral or muscular routes with $10^{4.3}$ mouse intracerebral lethal doses 50 (MICLD50) of the wild fox strain (salivary glands, SG) of rabies virus (Fig. 2). Resistance appears to be directly correlated with dose of AvO_1 previously inoculated.

Oral vaccination of foxes with increasing doses of AvO_1 was also attempted. Animals were challenged 90 days later with $10^{3.5}$ MICLD50 of the SG strain of rabies virus. Their antibody titers were determined as well. The results of this experiment are shown in Table 1. Resistance appears to be closely related to the dose of virus ingested, but not always to the antibody titers, an observation that has been previously reported with other live vaccines.

DISCUSSION

Our results demonstrate that efficient protection against rabies virus could be obtained through immunization with one hypovirulent mutant of the CVS strain.

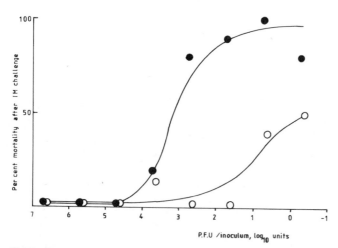

Figure 2
Protective power of the AvO_1 strain after injection of decreasing doses of the virus via muscular (●) or cerebral (○) route. Mice were challenged with $10^{4.3}$ MICLD50 of wild rabies virus.

Table 1
Efficiency of Oral Vaccination of Foxes

Amount of virus vaccine (log₁₀) (MICLD50)	Fox no.	Neutralizing antibody titer (day 30) in final dilution (or IU)	Result of challenge (10³·⁵ MICLD50) at day 90	Day of death	Mean day of death
8.1 ± 0.6	10	1/12 (0.05)	surviving	—	
	27	1/113 (0.5)	surviving	—	
	29	undetectable	surviving	—	
	38	undetectable	dead	19	
	48	undetectable	surviving	—	
	57	1/790 (3.42)	surviving	—	
	25	undetectable	surviving	—	
	39	1/12 (0.05)	dead	22	
	13	undetectable	dead	28	
	64	1/300 (1.3)	surviving	—	$22.8 (\pm 4.6)$
7.15 ± 0.6	06	1/156 (0.68)	surviving	—	
	03	1/50 (0.22)	surviving	—	
	05	undetectable	surviving	—	
6.15 ± 0.6	04	undetectable	dead	23	
	09	1/50 (0.22)	dead	20	
	12	undetectable	dead	31	
	14	1/43 (0.18)	surviving	—	
	53	undetectable	dead	17	
Control	258		dead	18	
	259		dead	18	
	271		dead	22	$22.0 (\pm 4.0)$
	294		dead	23	
	285		dead	29	

Production of circulating antibodies, interferon, and cytotoxic T cells has been measured in mice inoculated intramuscularly with 10^5 pfu of AvO₁ or CVS. After day 7, when CVS-inoculated animals died, the titer of circulating antibodies was similar. It continued to increase in AvO₁-inoculated animals, reaching values as high as 10,000 units per milliliter of serum. AvO₁ was a remarkable inducer of early interferon, an observation that could be correlated with its lack of pathogenicity for adult mice. Natural killer and cytotoxic-T-cell activities were also strongly stimulated. Why a mutation in site III of the glycoprotein changed the potentiality of the virus to stimulate the production of early interferon and cytotoxic cells is under investigation.

Potentiation of the immune response is not the only effect of the mutation leading to loss of virulence for adult animals. We also found that the host-range spectrum of the virus toward neuronal cells is modified; for instance, the virus loses its capability to invade the parasympathetic terminal endings. The brain of nude mice is never totally invaded as it is in the case of CVS infection even when the animals are moribund. Further studies are necessary to delineate the multiple aspects of this problem in order to understand virus virulence.

As far as the use of hypovirulent mutants in vaccination is concerned, our results demonstrate that they could be powerful live vaccines, although their residual pathogenicity for young animals should always be kept in mind. In fact, we consider this study a model for situations where better protection than that offered by an inactivated virus is necessary. Practically, it is advisable to select avirulent mutants of strains already used as live vaccines, since they are undoubtedly potentially less dangerous. Avirulent mutants of the SAD strain of rabies virus are presently under isolation and characterization.

ACKNOWLEDGMENTS

Part of this work was supported by the Centre National de la Recherche Scientifique through LA-040086 and by the Ministère de la Recherche et de l'Industrie through ATP 83V0085. We thank P. Vigier for helpful discussions and J. Benejean, C. Thiers, J. Gagnat, and J. Alexandre for excellent technical assistance. Monoclonal antibodies 194-2 and 248-8 were a generous gift from T. Wiktor.

REFERENCES

Coulon, P., P.E. Rollin, and A. Flamand. 1983. Molecular basis of rabies virus virulence. II. Identification of a site on the CVS glycoprotein associated with virulence. *J. Gen. Virol.* **64:** 693.

Coulon, P., P. Rollin, M. Aubert, and A. Flamand. 1982. Molecular basis of rabies virus virulence. I. Selection of avirulent mutants of the CVS strain with anti-G monoclonal antibodies. *J. Gen. Virol.* **61:** 97.

Dietzschold, B., W.H. Wunner, T.J. Wiktor, A.D. Lopes, M. Lafon, C.L. Smith, and H. Koprowski. 1983. Characterization of an antigenic determinant of the glycoprotein that correlates with pathogenicity of rabies virus. *Proc. Natl. Acad. Sci.* **80:** 70.

Lafon, M., T.J. Wiktor, and R.I. Macfarlan. 1983. Antigenic sites on the CVS rabies virus glycoprotein: Analysis with monoclonal antibodies. *J. Gen. Virol.* **64:** 843.

Construction of Live Recombinant Vaccines Using Genetically Engineered Poxviruses

Enzo Paoletti, Dennis Panicali,
Bernard R. Lipinskas, Susan Mercer,
Marilyn Wright, and Carol Samsonoff
Laboratory of Immunology
Center for Laboratories and Research
New York State Department of Health
Albany, New York 12201

The successful reinsertion of unique endogenous viral sequences into infectious virus by in vivo recombination (Nakano et al. 1982) suggested a protocol for the introduction of foreign genes into the DNA of infectious vaccinia virus. This basic protocol, wherein the appropriately engineered foreign DNA sequence is located in a nonessential genetic locus flanked by contiguous viral DNA sequences, was used to insert the herpes simplex virus (HSV) gene encoding thymidine kinase into the DNA of infectious vaccinia virus, thus establishing poxviruses as eukaryotic expression vectors (Panicali and Paoletti 1982). The efficacy of using vaccinia virus as a live vaccine against smallpox is attested to by the recent declaration of the World Health Organization that this disease has been eradicated from the world. We have considered that genetically engineered poxviruses might be useful as live recombinant vaccines for the control of a variety of infectious diseases. This strategy involves the introduction of appropriate genes from pathogenic organisms into the poxviral genome by in vivo recombination. Inoculation of animals or humans with this live recombinant vaccinia virus would elicit antibodies not only to its own endogenous antigens, but also to the antigen specified by the foreign DNA sequences, thus immunizing the recipient to the heterologous pathogen.

As examples of this approach, we have genetically engineered vaccinia virus to contain and express in vitro and in vivo genes coding for the influenza hemagglutinin (HA), the hepatitis-B virus surface antigen (HBsAg), and the glycoprotein D (gD) from HSV. In each example, the foreign gene was expressed in vitro under vaccinia virus regulation, and the gene product was shown to be antigenic by virtue of its reactivity with authentic homologous antiserum. Significantly, when

295

expressed in vivo after inoculation of the animal with the recombinant vaccinia viruses, the foreign genes elicited the production of antibodies specific for those antigens demonstrating their immunogenic potential. Some results and the significance of these studies are reported here.

DISCUSSION

Expression of the Influenza HA Gene in Recombinant Vaccinia Virus

A 1.8-kb cDNA of the influenza RNA segment encoding the HA was inserted proximal to an early vaccinia virus promoter such that the translational start site was localized approximately 30 bp from the insertion site. The influenza HA gene was expressed as an early viral function and was shown to be antigenic when probed with homologous antiserum in radioimmunoassays. Moreover, when animals were inoculated with the live vaccinia recombinant expressing the influenza HA gene, specific anti-HA antibodies were produced. The antiserum was shown to be reactive with authentic influenza HA by radioimmunoassay, to neutralize influenza infectivity as demonstrated by plaque-reduction assays, and to inhibit the hemagglutination of guinea pig erythrocytes by authentic influenza HA (for details, see Panicali et al. 1983). An example of antibody levels present in rabbits after inoculation with recombinant vaccinia virus expressing the gene for the influenza HA is shown in Table 1. Measurable levels of anti-HA antibodies are detected 1 week after inoculation, reaching a peak 3–6 weeks postinoculation. The lower levels and the slower rise in hemagglutination-inhibition (HI) titers in the rabbits inoculated through skin abrasions are compatible with the lower level of inoculum introduced through this route and the slower dissemination and replication of the virus. In contrast, those rabbits inoculated intravenously show a more rapid appearance and higher HI peak titers.

Expression and Immunogenicity of HBsAg
Synthesized by Vaccinia Virus Recombinants

A 1.1-kb DNA fragment derived from a cloned HBV (subtype *ayw)* encoding HBsAg was inserted such that the translational start site was approximately 20

Table 1
Induction of HI Antibodies in Rabbits Inoculated with a Vaccinia Virus Recombinant Expressing the Influenza Virus HA

Rabbit	Route of inoculation	Weeks postinoculation					
		1	2	3	4	5	6
449	intravenous	40	640	≥5120	≥5120	2560	640
450	intravenous	40	160	1280	2560	5120	640
458	skin abrasion	20	40	80	160	320	320
459	skin abrasion	40	80	80	160	320	320

The reciprocal of the serum dilution inhibiting 4 HA units is shown. Preimmune sera or sera prepared against standard vaccinia virus showed HI titers of less than 10.

bp from an endogenous vaccinia promoter. This vaccinia recombinant was shown to express HBsAg in a variety of tissue-culture cells (Paoletti et al. 1984). Approximately 200 ng of the HBsAg was synthesized in an overnight infection of 10^6 cells at a multiplicity of infection of 1–2 pfu/cell. Approximately 75% of the HBsAg synthesized in tissue-culture cells infected with the recombinant vaccinia virus was localized extracellularly. This secreted HBsAg material had a characteristic density of 1.2 g/cc on CsCl gradients, similar to the HBsAg secreted from cells transformed with HBV or the HBsAg found in the sera of carriers. Electron micrographs of the secreted HBsAg banding at 1.2 g/cc on CsCl gradients demonstrated typical morphological structures averaging about 22 nm (Fig. 1). To determine whether this recombinant vaccinia virus would elicit antibodies reactive with authentic HBsAg, rabbits were inoculated and serum was collected at weekly intervals. Table 2 demonstrates that significant levels of anti-HBsAg antibodies are produced in rabbits on inoculation with the recombinant vaccinia virus expressing HBsAg. Intradermal inoculation gives a slower rise in antibody levels than that observed with intravenous inoculation. However, similar levels of antibody are observed by 6 weeks postinoculation regardless of the route of inoculation and the 20-fold difference in inoculum tested (see Table 2). The expression of HBsAg in vaccinia virus recombinants has also been recently reported by Smith et al. (1983).

Vaccinia Virus Recombinants Expressing HSV gD

HSV gD is considered to be important in the infectivity and dissemination of HSV. gD is localized on the surface of virus-infected cells. Antibodies directed

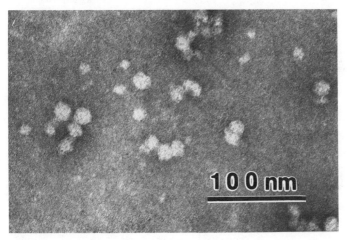

Figure 1
Electron micrograph of HBsAg secreted from cells infected with the vaccinia recombinant expressing the HBsAg coding sequences. Particles banding at 1.2 g/cc in CsCl gradients were negatively stained with 1% uranyl acetate. Magnification, 250,000 ×. Bar, 100 nm. Electron micrograph was kindly provided by W.A. Samsonoff (New York State Department of Health).

Table 2
Production of Antibodies against HBsAg in Rabbits Inoculated with a Vaccinia Virus Recombinant
Expressing HBsAg

Rabbit	Route of inoculation	Weeks postinoculation					
		1	2	3	4	5	6
472	intravenous	1.6×10^{3a}	5.2×10^5	n.d.[b]	1.2×10^6	1.3×10^6	1.4×10^6
488	intradermal	2.7×10^2	5.0×10^3	1.8×10^4	2.1×10^5	9.0×10^5	1.3×10^6

[a]Antibody levels are expressed in radioimmunoassay units per milliliter of rabbit serum as assayed by the AUSAB detection kit (Abbott). Rabbits were inoculated using 3.6×10^8 (472) or 1.8×10^7 (488) pfu of the recombinant vaccinia virus as titered on CV-1 cells. Backgrounds obtained from preimmune sera have been subtracted.
[b]n.d. indicates not done.

against gD neutralize the infectivity of HSV and are considered important in immunity. gD has been localized by a number of studies to genome map unit 0.9–0.945. A 2.5-kb restriction fragment encoding the HSV gD was inserted into vaccinia virus. This recombinant was shown to express HSV gD in vitro (Paoletti et al. 1984). Furthermore, when this live recombinant vaccinia virus was injected into rabbits, antibodies reactive with authentic HSV gD were produced. This antiserum was also shown to neutralize the infectivity of HSV as assayed by plaque-reduction tests. To determine whether this recombinant vaccinia virus would confer immunity to an animal, the following experiment was performed. Mice were inoculated intraperitoneally with saline, wild-type vaccinia virus, or the vaccinia virus recombinant expressing the HSV gD. Three weeks after inoculation, the mice were challenged with an intraperitoneal injection of infectious HSV. In mice inoculated with either saline or wild-type vaccinia virus, only 10–15% survived the infection with HSV. Significantly, all of the mice challenged with HSV, but previously immunized with the recombinant vaccinia virus expressing the HSV gD, survived infection (Table 3).

SUMMARY AND CONCLUSION

Recombinant vaccinia viruses have been constructed that express the genes encoding influenza HA, HBsAg, and HSV gD. Each of these recombinant vaccinia viruses was shown to elicit antibodies to the product of the foreign gene

Table 3
Protection against HSV by Immunization with a Live Recombinant Vaccinia
Virus Expressing HSV gD

Inoculum	No. of mice in test group	No. of survivors	% survival
Saline	20	3	15
Wild-type vaccinia	10	1	10
Recombinant vaccinia	10	10	100

Mice were inoculated intraperitoneally with saline or 9×10^7 pfu of either wild-type vaccinia virus or a recombinant vaccinia virus expressing the gD gene from HSV and challenged 3 weeks later with 2.5×10^5 pfu of HSV (type 1) strain AA.

carried within the vaccinia DNA. Examples of potential live recombinant vaccines utilizing genetically engineered vaccinia viruses and directed against respiratory, enteric, and neurotropic and dermotropic infectious agents have been presented. One of these recombinants was used to demonstrate protection in mice against a lethal challenge with infectious HSV, thus demonstrating the feasibility of immunizing against a heterologous agent using a live recombinant poxvirus. It would appear that many, if not all, infectious disease processes whether they be viral, bacterial, or parasitic might be amenable to control by appropriately engineered poxviruses, thus providing a universal approach toward the control of infectious diseases.

REFERENCES

Nakano, E., D. Panicali, and E. Paoletti. 1982. Molecular genetics of vaccinia virus: Demonstration of marker rescue. *Proc. Natl. Acad. Sci.* **79:** 1593.

Panicali, D. and E. Paoletti. 1982. Construction of poxviruses as cloning vectors: Insertion of the thymidine kinase gene from herpes simplex virus into the DNA of infectious vaccinia virus. *Proc. Natl. Acad. Sci.* **79:** 4927.

Panicali, D., S.W. Davis, R.L. Weinberg, and E. Paoletti. 1983. Construction of live vaccines using genetically engineered poxviruses: Biological activity of recombinant vaccinia virus expressing the influenza virus hemagglutinin. *Proc. Natl. Acad. Sci.* **80:** 5364.

Paoletti, E., B.R. Lipinskas, C. Samsonoff, S. Mercer, and D. Panicali. 1984. Construction of live vaccines using genetically engineered poxviruses: Biological activity of vaccinia virus recombinants expressing the hepatitis B virus surface antigen and the herpes simplex virus glycoprotein D. *Proc. Natl. Acad. Sci.* **81:** 193.

Smith, G.L., M. Mackett, and B. Moss. 1983. Infectious vaccinia virus recombinants that express hepatitis B virus surface antigen. *Nature* **302:** 490.

A General Method for the Production and Selection of Vaccinia Virus Recombinants Expressing Foreign Genes

**Michael Mackett, Geoffrey L. Smith,
and Bernard Moss**
*Laboratory of Biology of Viruses, National
Institute of Allergy and Infectious Diseases
National Institutes of Health
Bethesda, Maryland 20205*

Application of recombinant DNA technology to the development of vaccines has been primarily directed toward the preparation of protein subunits. One alternative is the genetic engineering of hybrid viruses. Although a variety of viruses have been used as vectors, they generally have a restricted capacity for foreign DNA and are defective, requiring helper virus or special cell lines for replication. In contrast, initial experiments indicate that vaccinia virus vectors retain infectivity (Panicali and Paoletti 1982; Mackett et al. 1982) and can accommodate at least 25,000 bp of additional DNA equivalent to about 20 average genes (Smith and Moss 1983). Moreover, the successful use of vaccinia virus for the eradication of smallpox suggests that recombinants expressing genes of unrelated pathogens might be useful as live-virus vaccines. In support of this possibility, experimental animals that have been vaccinated with recombinants containing the hepatitis-B virus surface antigen and the influenza virus hemagglutinin genes produce high levels of antibody (Smith et al. 1983a,b).

DISCUSSION

Design of Plasmid Insertion Vectors

The strategy we use to insert and express foreign DNA in vaccinia virus takes into account the large 187,000-bp size of the genome, the noninfectious nature of isolated DNA, and evidence that unique transcriptional regulatory sequences are recognized by the viral RNA polymerase. Basically, a chimeric gene containing vaccinia virus transcriptional regulatory sequences and foreign protein cod-

301

ing sequences is constructed in vitro and inserted into a nonessential region of the vaccinia genome by homologous recombination in infected cells (Mackett et al. 1982). To facilitate this process, special plasmid insertion vectors were constructed. These plasmids contain a segment of vaccinia virus DNA that includes the thymidine kinase (*tk*) gene (Weir and Moss 1983), with unique restriction endonuclease sites for insertion of foreign DNA engineered next to the *tk* transcriptional start site (e.g., pMM4) or next to another vaccinia virus transcriptional regulatory sequence (e.g., pGS20, pGS21) translocated into the body of the *tk* gene (Fig. 1). The translocated segment was derived from an early gene that encodes a 7.5K polypeptide (Venkatesan et al. 1981). The various plasmids described in Figure 1 differ with regard to the available unique restriction endonuclease sites or to the orientation of the promoter relative to the surrounding DNA. Significantly, these plasmids do not contain an ATG triplet between the RNA start site and the site used for insertion of foreign DNA. Consequently, the transcribed ATG of the foreign gene will be used for initiation of translation, thereby avoiding problems associated with improper phasing of reading frames or with fusion proteins. Since the plasmid insertion vectors contain a variety of unique restriction endonuclease sites, insertion of a foreign gene coding sequence is usually straightforward. In particular, the blunt end generated by *Sma*I can be used in virtually all situations by removing the 5' or 3' nucleotide extensions at the ends of the foreign DNA segment. The next step is to transfect cells that have already been infected with vaccinia virus so that homologous recombination occurs between the *tk* sequences flanking the chimeric gene in the plasmid and the *tk* sequences in the viral genome. The *tk*⁻ recombinant virus is then selected in the presence of 5-bromodeoxyuridine, and isolated plaques are checked by dot-blot hybridization for foreign DNA sequences and by enzymatic or immunological methods for gene expression.

Construction of Vaccinia Virus Recombinants That Express *cat*

To characterize and optimize the use of vaccinia virus as a vector, the prokaryotic chloramphenicol acetyltransferase (*cat*) gene was employed. Previous studies with SV40 vectors demonstrated the absence of background activity in eukaryotic cells and the sensitive and quantitative nature of the enzyme assay (Gorman et al. 1982). A DNA segment containing the *cat* coding sequence was excised from pBR328 and inserted into the vectors pMM4, pGS20, and pGS21, and the resulting plasmids were precipitated with calcium phosphate and used to transfect cells infected with wild-type vaccinia virus. *tk*⁻ recombinants were selected as described above and screened for the presence of *cat* DNA by a dot-blot hybridization procedure (Mackett et al. 1982). Structures of four recombinants shown in Figure 2 were confirmed by Southern blot hybridizations. Recombinant vC1 contains the *cat* gene adjacent to the vaccinia virus *tk* promoter; vC24 and vC30 contain the *cat* gene correctly oriented next to the 7.5K polypeptide gene promoter but differ in their polarities with respect to flanking DNA. vC31 contains the 7.5K polypeptide gene promoter at the distal end of the *cat* gene in order to provide a control for expression experiments.

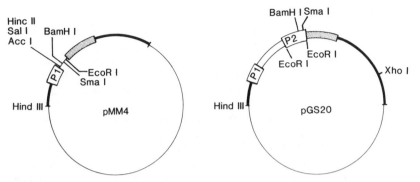

Figure 1
Insertion vectors. P1 refers to the *tk* promoter, and P2 refers to the transcriptional regulatory sequences and RNA start site of the early 7.5K polypeptide gene (Venkatesan et al. 1981). Stippled box indicates vaccinia virus *tk*-gene sequences distal to the unique *Eco*RI site. Bold lines indicate flanking vaccinia virus sequences. pGS20 and pGS21 (not shown) are identical except for the orientation of the promoter with respect to the flanking DNA. pMM4 contains unique *Hinc*II, *Sal*I, *Acc*I, *Bam*HI, *Sma*I, and *Eco*RI sites, and pGS20 and pGS21 contain *Bam*HI and *Sma*I sites for cloning foreign protein coding sequences.

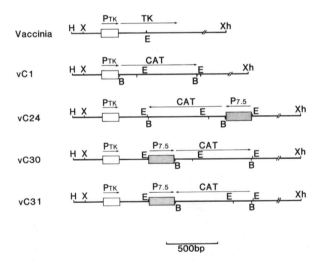

Figure 2
Structures of chimeric *cat* genes in vaccinia virus recombinants. A 2-kb segment from the left side of the *Hind*III J fragment of vaccinia virus is shown in the first line. Lines below that contain chimeric *cat* genes inserted into the body of the *tk* gene. The *tk* and 7.5K polypeptide gene promoters are indicated by the letter P over an open or stippled box, respectively. For construction of vC1, a 780-bp *cat Bam*HI fragment was inserted into the *Bam*HI site of pMM4. For construction of vC24, the same *Bam*HI fragment was inserted into pGS21. vC30 and vC31 were both constructed by insertion of the *Bam*HI *cat* fragment in opposite orientations in pGS20. (H) *Hind*III; (B) *Bam*HI; (E) *Eco*RI; (X) *Xba*I; (Xh) *Xho*I.

Expression of *cat* by Vaccinia Virus Recombinants

The time course of CAT synthesis in cells infected with the four recombinants is shown in Figure 3. CAT was detected within 2 hours after vC1 infection and peaked at 6 hours, reflecting the "early" character of the *tk*-gene promoter. As expected, addition of cytosine arabinoside (Ara C), an inhibitor of DNA replication, had little effect on CAT synthesis. Nearly identical levels of CAT were made in cells infected with vC24 or vC30, which differ only in the orientation of the chimeric gene within the virus. Approximately 30 times more CAT was made using the 7.5K polypeptide gene promoter constructs compared with the *tk* promoter construct and synthesis was partially inhibited by Ara C, suggesting that it functions before and after DNA replication. A very low but significant level of CAT was made in cells infected with vC31, a recombinant that lacks correctly positioned transcriptional regulatory sequences adjacent to the *cat* gene.

CONCLUSIONS

Procedures and specific plasmid vectors have been developed for the construction of vaccinia virus recombinants that express foreign genes. Defined vaccinia

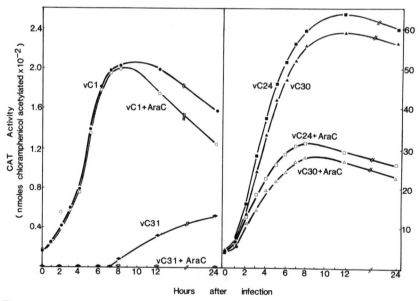

Figure 3
Time course of CAT synthesis in cells infected with recombinant viruses. HeLa S3 cells in suspension culture were infected with 30 pfu/cell of vC1 (●), vC24 (■), vC30 (▲), or vC31 (♦) in the presence (open symbols) or absence (closed symbols) of 40 μg/ml of Ara C. At the indicated times after infection, 5-ml samples (2.5 × 10⁶ cells) were removed and assayed for CAT at appropriate dilutions. CAT activity is expressed as nmoles of chloramphenicol acetylated per 2.5 × 10⁶ cells. The scales used in the left and right panels differ by a factor of 25. To ensure that Ara C inhibited virus replication, plaque assays were performed. In each case, the 24-hr virus titers were considerably lower than the virus input.

virus transcriptional regulatory sequences were used to achieve high levels of expression. The *cat* gene was used as a model because of the sensitive and quantitative nature of the enzyme assay. However, the general usefulness of the system has been demonstrated by expressing genes from DNA and RNA viruses as well as prokaryotes and eukaryotes.

REFERENCES

Gorman, C.M., L.F. Moffat, and B.H. Howard. 1982. Recombinant genomes which express chloramphenicol acetyltransferase in mammalian cells. *J. Mol. Cell. Biol.* **2:** 1044.

Mackett, M., G.L. Smith, and B. Moss. 1982. Vaccinia virus: A selectable eukaryotic cloning and expression vector. *Proc. Natl. Acad. Sci.* **79:** 7415.

Panicali, D. and E. Paoletti. 1982. Construction of poxviruses as cloning vectors: Insertion of the thymidine kinase from herpes simplex virus into the DNA of infectious vaccinia virus. *Proc. Natl. Acad. Sci.* **79:** 4927.

Smith, G.L. and B. Moss. 1983. Infectious poxvirus vectors have capacity for at least 25,000 base pairs of foreign DNA. *Gene* **25:** 21.

Smith, G.L., M. Mackett, and B. Moss. 1983a. Infectious vaccinia virus recombinants that express hepatitis B virus surface antigen. *Nature* **302:** 490.

Smith, G.L., B.R. Murphy, and B. Moss. 1983b. Construction and characterization of an infectious vaccinia virus recombinant that expresses the influenza hemagglutinin gene and induces resistance to influenza virus infection in hamsters. *Proc. Natl. Acad. Sci.* **80:** 7155.

Venkatesan, S., B.M. Baroudy, and B. Moss. 1981. Distinctive nucleotide sequences adjacent to multiple initiation and termination sites of an early vaccinia virus gene. *Cell* **25:** 805.

Weir, J.P. and B. Moss. 1983. Nucleotide sequence of vaccinia virus thymidine kinase gene and the nature of spontaneous frameshift mutants. *J. Virol.* **46:** 530.

Vaccination with Live Attenuated Human Cytomegalovirus

Stanley A. Plotkin
The Children's Hospital of Philadelphia
The University of Pennsylvania
and The Wistar Institute
Philadelphia, Pennsylvania 19104

Although human cytomegalovirus (CMV) is a typical virus of the herpes group and therefore shares characteristics of latency and reactivation, it also has singular attributes that make vaccination against it a formidable task. A review of these singularities is therefore a necessary prelude to a discussion of prevention.

First, some definitions are necessary. Infection and disease are not synonymous. In the case of CMV, most acquired infection manifested by virus excretion and antibody response is subclinical. However, a small percentage of normal individuals and a high proportion of the immunodeficient will show disease, which typically is expressed as hepatitis, thrombocytopenia, leukopenia, pneumonia, and increased susceptibility to bacteria and fungi. The immunodeficient include the fetus and immature newborn, the recipient of a transplant, the patient treated for cancer, and the victim of AIDS (Plotkin 1982).

An additional critical set of definitions pertains to the source of the virus. Primary infection means infection by exogenous virus transmitted transplacentally, by organ transplant, by blood, or by infected excretions. Reactivated infection means the recrudescence of endogenous virus probably latent in white blood cells or kidney epithelium. Reactivation is difficult to distinguish from reinfection, which implies infection of a previously infected host by a new CMV virus. Note that under certain conditions both exogenous and endogenous viruses can infect nominally immune hosts.

Finally, immunity itself must be defined. It is a cliché that antibody is unimportant in herpesvirus infections. This is, of course, untrue if the infection in question is a primary infection where the agent must get through the blood stream to infect the target organs. However, it is true that cellular rather than humoral immunity

307

protects the host against reactivation. The identity of the cellular functions that are important is the subject of debate. It is fair to say that both natural killer cell activity and HLA-restricted T-cell cytotoxic lymphocyte activity against CMV-infected targets are important functions for suppression of active CMV replication and that lymphocyte proliferation is a simple way of measuring cellular sensitization (Rook et al. 1984). T-cell helper/suppressor ratios are also reduced in acute CMV infection.

This rather complex situation is portrayed in Figure 1, which emphasizes the interplay of the variables of age, immune status, and route of infection. Two points should be emphasized: (1) Transplacental infection of the immune fetus is usually not attended by sequelae, whereas in the nonimmune fetus whose mother is undergoing a primary infection, CMV may cause central nervous system damage. (2) Organs carrying CMV pose a great hazard for the nonimmune recipient. Immune transplant recipients, because they are immunosuppressed, may also suffer disease but are three to four times less likely to do so. Thus, the goal of a CMV vaccine becomes clear: to convert a potential primary infection to no infection, or at most to reinfection, by inducing a status of immunity.

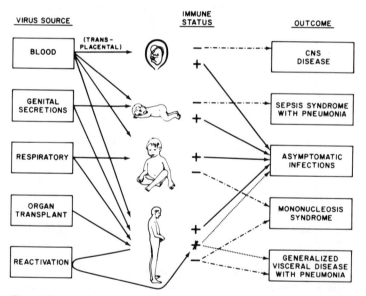

Figure 1
Pathogenesis of CMV is represented diagrammatically. The virus may be acquired from blood (infected white blood cells), respiratory and genital secretions, or a transplanted organ. Virus may also reactivate in previously infected individuals if their immune status is compromised. The result of infection will depend on the age and immune status of the host. Nonimmune hosts will, in general, suffer symptomatic disease, whereas previously immune hosts will tend to develop symptomatic illness, the severity of which will be inversely proportional to the competence of the immune system. Thus, an adult organ transplant recipient who is seronegative is likely to develop mild or severe CMV illness. A seropositive adult organ transplant recipient will likely remain asymptomatic, but in the presence of sufficient compromise may also sustain illness.

Vaccination with Herpes CMV

Elek and Stern (1974), in England, provided the initial data that CMV could be modified to give an immunogenic stimulus without producing disease. Our own work was based on the suppositions that variants of CMV could be selected that would immunize without inducing latency and that the protection afforded by vaccine would prevent transplacental infection in pregnant women. Although, initially, attempts were made to develop cold-adapted mutants, eventually it was decided to minimize defectiveness by passage at normal temperatures and by selection with cloning.

The resultant virus, called Towne for the name of the infant from whom it was isolated, was tested for its biological properties at 125 passages (Plotkin et al. 1975, 1976).

Vaccination of Normal Volunteers

The results of studies of vaccination in normal volunteers may be summarized as follows (Fig. 2):

1. Serologic responses typical for primary infection appeared by the fourth week postvaccination, including anticomplement immunofluorescence, complement fixation, and neutralizing antibodies.
2. Specific in vitro lymphocyte proliferation responses to CMV antigen developed in all vaccinees. These responses were not strain-specific; i.e., antigens prepared from all laboratory and wild strains tested stimulated proliferation of lymphocytes.
3. No CMV was isolated from urine, throat secretions, buffy coat, semen, or cervical secretions after vaccination of any normal subject.
4. The only clinical reaction was a local erythema and induration at the injection site that developed during the second week postvaccination and then disappeared.
5. In collaboration with Dr. M. Hirsch (Harvard Medical School), we studied the lymphocyte subsets after vaccination of normal volunteers. Altered T-cell helper/suppressor ratios or diminished concanavalin-A responses, which occur commonly in natural CMV infection, did not develop.

Renal Transplant Trial

A controlled trial involving renal transplant recipients was organized to test the safety and efficacy of Towne vaccine. Transplant recipients received on a random basis either vaccine or placebo 8 weeks or more prior to transplantation.

Ninety-one patients, who had the transplant for at least 6 months, were analyzed with respect to the original serological status of donors and recipients prior to vaccination, and whether the recipients received vaccine or placebo. CMV infections and diseases were almost absent in the donor-negative, recipient-negative group, the only exception being a single placebo recipient who may have been infected through blood transfusion. The overall infection rate was almost 100% in the recipients who had received a kidney from a seropositive donor, regardless of the recipients' vaccination status. However, infected placebo pa-

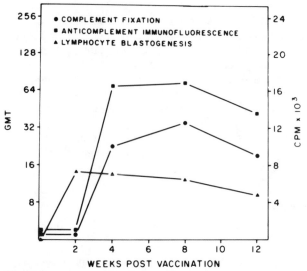

Figure 2
Serological and CMV-specific lymphocyte proliferation responses in normal volunteers who received Towne live attenuated CMV by subcutaneous injection.

tients were almost always ill (91%), compared with 60% illness in vaccinees ($p = 0.07$ by chi-square). Examination of the viruses isolated from vaccinees after transplantation by restriction endonuclease methodology substantiated the idea that they were nonvaccine strains coming in with the transplant, rather than the vaccine virus.

If the patients in the donor-positive, recipient-negative group are divided into those who were asymptomatic after transplant, those who had mild or moderate illnesses scoring 1–6, and those who had more severe illnesses with scores of 7 or greater, we see (Table 1) a significantly ($p < 0.05$) different distribution in the vaccinees and placebo recipients. Whereas about half of the placebo recipients had scores of 7 or greater, only 1 of the vaccinees fell into this group. The mean scores for the placebo group revealed an average of more than twice the clinical

Table 1
Clinical Scores in Recipients Who Received Kidneys from Seropositive Donors According to Prior Vaccine Status

	Score		
	0	1–6	≥7
Vaccine	7	9	1
Placebo	4	4	7

Recipients were seronegative before receiving vaccine or placebo.

severity compared with the vaccine group (5.67 vs. 2.70, respectively). Thus, Towne vaccine did not prevent infection with CMV but did mitigate the disease that resulted from the infection.

ACKNOWLEDGMENT

This work was supported in part by National Institutes of Health grant AI-14927 and the Hassel Foundation.

REFERENCES

Elek, S.D. and H. Stern. 1974. Development of a vaccine against mental retardation caused by cytomegalovirus infection in utero. *Lancet* **1:** 1.

Plotkin, S.A. 1982. Immunology of cytomegalovirus. In *Comprehensive immunology. Immunology of human infection* (ed. A.J. Nahmias and R.J. O'Reilly), p. 89. Plenum Medical Book Company, New York.

Plotkin, S.A., J. Farquhar, and E. Hornberger. 1976. Clinical trials of immunization with the Towne 125 strain of human cytomegalovirus. *J. Infect. Dis.* **134:** 470.

Plotkin, S.A., T. Furukawa, N. Zygraich, and C. Huygelen. 1975. Candidate cytomegalovirus strain for human vaccination. *Infect. Immun.* **12:** 521.

Rook, A.H., W.J.R. Frederick, J.F. Manischewitz, L. Jackson, B.B. Lee, C.B. Currier, and G.V. Quinnan. 1984. Correlation of clinical outcome of cytomegalovirus infection and immunosuppression with virus specific cytotoxic lymphocyte responses in renal transplant recipients. In *CMV: Pathogenesis and prevention of human infection* (ed. S.A. Plotkin et al.), vol. 20. Alan R. Liss, New York.

Vaccinia Virus Recombinants Expressing Genes from Pathogenic Agents Have Potential as Live Vaccines

Geoffrey L. Smith, Michael Mackett,
Brian R. Murphy,* and Bernard Moss
Laboratory of Biology of Viruses and
*Laboratory of Infectious Diseases, National
Institute of Allergy and Infectious Diseases
National Institutes of Health
Bethesda, Maryland 20205

Genetic engineering of infectious hybrid viruses provides a novel approach to vaccine development. In this volume (Mackett et al.) and elsewhere (Mackett et al. 1982; Moss et al. 1983), we have described a facile procedure for the insertion of any continuous foreign protein-coding sequence into the vaccinia virus genome under control of defined vaccinia virus promoters. Here, we describe the properties and possible usefulness of vaccinia virus recombinants that express the hepatitis-B virus surface antigen (HBsAg) and influenza-A virus hemagglutinin (HA) genes.

Vaccinia Virus Recombinants That Express HBsAg

As described previously (Smith et al. 1983a), a 1.3-kb *Bam*HI restriction fragment from hepatitis-B virus (HBV) strain *adw* was inserted into the plasmid vector pGS20 to form a chimeric gene with the transcriptional regulatory sequences of an early vaccinia virus gene adjacent to the coding sequence for HBsAg. The chimeric gene, flanked by sequences from the vaccinia virus thymidine kinase (*tk*) gene, was then introduced into the genome of vaccinia virus by homologous recombination, and infectious *tk*⁻ recombinants expressing HBsAg were isolated and plaque-purified. Restriction endonuclease analysis of the recombinant viral DNA indicated that the HBsAg gene was stably integrated at the correct location and no compensatory deletions or other genomic rearrangements had occurred. When the recombinant virus was used to infect tissue-culture cells, HBsAg was synthesized within 1 hour of infection and subsequently released into the culture medium over a 24-hour period. Since 90% of the progeny virus remained cell-associated, the presence of HBsAg in the medium was evidently due to its secretion through the cell membrane. We calculated that approximately 1.4×10^8 molecules of HBsAg were produced per cell. The biophysical properties of the secreted particles were indistinguishable from those of HBsAg released by hepatoma cells. An electron micrograph of purified 22-nm particles produced by cells infected with the vaccinia virus recombinant is shown in Figure 1A. The polypeptide composition of these particles is compared with that of authentic HBsAg particles derived from human serum in Figure 1B. Both preparations contain polypeptide P1 and its glycosylated derivative P2, as well as two minor higher-molecular-weight polypeptides.

To evaluate the potential of this vaccinia virus recombinant as a live vaccine against HBV, animals were inoculated intradermally. Typical local vaccination reactions developed within 5–10 days and subsequently healed completely; no HBsAg or vaccinia virus was detected in blood samples. The time course of antibody production in two rabbits following vaccination with recombinant virus on day 0 is shown in Figure 2. Significantly, the antibody response was rapid, high, and sustained. The classical biphasic response was presumably due to successive synthesis of IgM and IgG antibodies. Subtyping of the anti-HBsAg demonstrated that it recognized the a determinant, an important result, since such antibodies can neutralize infectivity of all HBV strains. Currently, we are investigating whether the vaccinia virus recombinant can protect chimpanzees against challenge with HBV.

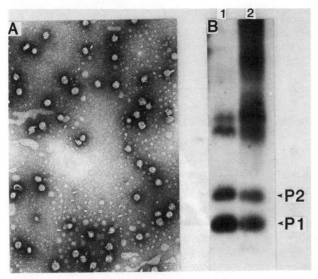

Figure 1
HBsAg particles synthesized in CV-1 cells infected with vaccinia virus recombinant. (A) Electron micrograph showing HBsAg particles purified by CsCl and sucrose density gradient centrifugation. Average particle size is 21.4 nm. (B) Western blot of HBsAg polypeptides. (1) HBsAg particles shown in A; (2) HBsAg particles purified from sera of infected humans. Polypeptides were resolved on a 15% polyacrylamide gel and transferred electrophoretically to nitrocellulose, which was subsequently incubated with anti-HBsAg followed by ^{125}I-labeled Staph-A protein. An autoradiograph is shown.

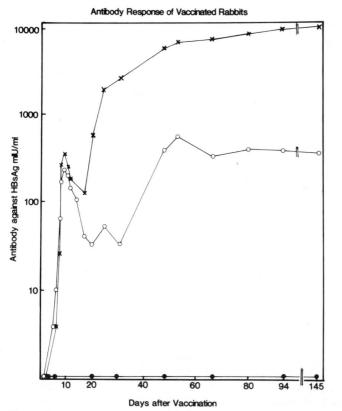

Figure 2
Anti-HBsAg response of vaccinated rabbits. Rabbits were infected intradermally with 10^8 pfu of either wild-type vaccinia (●) or vaccinia virus recombinant expressing HBsAg at one site (x – x) or four sites (○). Serum was tested for anti-HBsAg by radioimmunoassay (Abbott Laboratories).

Vaccinia Virus Recombinants That Express Influenza HA

The gene encoding HA from several influenza-A subtypes has been cloned, sequenced, and expressed in defective SV40 vectors. As described recently (Smith et al. 1983b), infectious vaccinia virus recombinants expressing the HA gene from influenza A/Jap/305/57 have also been constructed. A 1.7-kb *Bam*HI DNA fragment containing the entire HA coding sequence was inserted into vaccinia virus under control of a defined early promoter. The stability and location of the inserted DNA were checked by restriction endonuclease analysis and hybridization procedures. Initial evidence for expression of HA was obtained by the specific binding of antibodies against influenza HA to plaques formed by recombinant virus (Fig. 3A). The nature of the HA polypeptide synthesized by cells infected with the vaccinia virus recombinant was investigated by immunoprecipitation followed by polyacrylamide gel electrophoresis (Fig. 3B). [^{35}S]Methionine- and [^{3}H]glucosamine-labeled polypeptides with molecular weights of 75,000 were

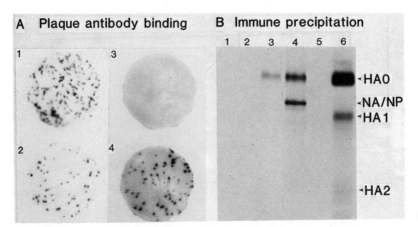

Figure 3
Expression of influenza HA in cells infected with vaccinia virus recombinant. (*A*) Binding of anti-vaccinia (*1,2*) or anti-influenza (*3,4*) antibodies to plaques formed on CV-1 cell mono-layers by wild-type vaccinia (*1,3*) or recombinant vaccinia (*2,4*). Bound antibody was detected by incubation with ¹²⁵I-labeled Staph-A protein. (*B*) Immunoprecipitation of [³⁵S]methionine-labeled (*1–4*) or [³H]glucosamine-labeled (*5,6*) cell extracts with anti-influenza A/Jap/305/57 serum. Polypeptides were resolved on a 15% polyacrylamide gel. (*1*) Uninfected; (*2,5*) wild-type vaccinia; (*3,6*) vaccinia recombinant expressing HA; (*4*) influenza A/Jap/305/57.

present in extracts of cells infected with recombinant virus (Fig. 3B, lanes 3 and 6), and these comigrated with authentic HA from influenza-infected cells (Fig. 3B, lane 4). Immunofluorescence studies also demonstrated that the HA molecule is located on the cell surface (not shown).

Both rabbits and hamsters inoculated intradermally on their backs with recombinant vaccinia virus developed antibodies to influenza HA. Moreover, the antibody levels achieved were similar to or higher than those occurring after infection of hamsters with influenza virus (Table 1). When the hamsters were challenged intranasally with influenza virus at 40 days after vaccination, protection was obtained, as indicated by a significant decrease in both the number of animals yielding virus and the amount of virus recovered.

CONCLUSIONS

Infectious vaccinia virus recombinants expressing HBsAg and influenza HA were constructed. In each case, synthesis of authentic polypeptides was demonstrated by polyacrylamide gel electrophoresis of immunoprecipitates, and vaccination of animals led to the production of specific antibodies. Vaccination with recombinant virus expressing influenza HA protected hamsters against challenge with influenza virus, and similar protection experiments with recombinants expressing HBsAg are in progress in chimpanzees. Experience with smallpox vaccination suggests that hybrid vaccinia virus vaccines should be cheap to produce, easy to administer, and particularly useful for mass immunizations to pre-

Table 1
Antibody Responses of Hamsters Inoculated with Wild-type Vaccinia, Vaccinia Recombinant Expressing HA, and Influenza A/Jap/305/57 and Their Response to Challenge with Influenza Virus A/Jap/305/57

Hamsters inoculated with	No. of animals	Mean HI serum antibody titer on day 40[a]	No. of animals yielding virus $> 10^{3.0}$ TCID$_{50}$/g[b]	Mean log$_{10}$ virus titer TCID$_{50}$/g lung on day 1[c]
Wild-type vaccinia	10	0	7	4.4 ± 0.6
Vaccinia recombinant	10	104	0	2.6 ± 0.1
Influenza A/Jap/305/57	10	47	0	2.6 ± 0.1

[a]Antibody titers are reciprocals. HI denotes hemagglutination-inhibiting.
[b]Lungs and nasal turbinates were removed 1 or 2 days after challenge (5 animals/group/day) and assayed for infectious influenza virus on MDCK cells. Lowest level of detectable virus was $10^{3.0}$ TCID$_{50}$/g.
[c]For calculation of mean titers, animals from which virus was not recovered were assigned maximum possible values of $10^{2.5}$ TCID$_{50}$/g.

vent human and animal disease. Moreover, as stable vaccinia virus recombinants containing at least 25,000 bp of foreign DNA have been constructed (Smith and Moss 1983), polyvalent vaccines may be created.

ACKNOWLEDGMENTS

We thank Joe Sambrook and Mary-Jane Gething for supplying cloned influenza HA gene, John Gerin for supplying cloned HBV DNA and for electron microscopy, D. Djurikovic for vaccinating rabbits and collecting serum, and Mike Roth for immunofluorescence studies.

REFERENCES

Mackett, M., G.L. Smith, and B. Moss. 1982. Vaccinia virus: A selectable eukaryotic cloning and expression vector. *Proc. Natl. Acad. Sci.* **79**: 7415.
Moss, B., G.L. Smith, and M. Mackett. 1983. Use of vaccinia virus as an infectious molecular cloning and expression vector. In *Gene amplification and analysis* (ed. T. Papas et al.), vol. 3, p. 201. Elsevier, North Holland.
Smith, G.L. and B. Moss. 1983. Infectious poxvirus vectors have capacity for at least 25,000 base pairs of foreign DNA. *Gene* **25**: 21.
Smith, G.L., M. Mackett, and B. Moss. 1983a. Infectious vaccinia virus recombinants that express hepatitis B virus surface antigen. *Nature* **302**: 490.
Smith, G.L., B.R. Murphy, and B. Moss. 1983b. Construction and characterization of an infectious vaccinia virus recombinant that expresses the influenza hemagglutinin gene and induced resistance to influenza virus infection in hamsters. *Proc. Natl. Acad. Sci.* **80**: 7155.

Use of Reassortant Rotaviruses and Monoclonal Antibodies to Make Gene-coding Assignments and Construct Rotavirus Vaccine Candidates

Harry Greenberg, Karen Midthun,
Richard Wyatt, Jorge Flores,
Yasutaka Hoshino, Robert M. Chanock,
and Albert Kapikian
*Laboratory of Infectious Diseases, National
Institute of Allergy and Infectious Diseases
National Institutes of Health
Bethesda, Maryland 20205*

Rotaviruses, newly classified members of the Reoviridae family, are an important cause of infantile diarrhea in a wide variety of mammalian species including man. Because they have a segmented genome, rotaviruses undergo genetic reassortment at high frequency during mixed infection (Greenberg et al. 1981). We used a genetic approach that took advantage of this high frequency of reassortment to isolate a series of rotavirus reassortants that were used to establish gene-coding assignments for several major antigenic specificities and functional activities of these viruses.

DISCUSSION

Gene-coding Assignments Determined by Analysis of Rotavirus Reassortants

Temperature-sensitive (*ts*) mutants of UK bovine rotavirus and rhesus rotavirus (RRV) were isolated after in vivo mutagenesis with 5' azacytidine. The *ts* mutants of the UK strain of bovine rotavirus were used to produce reassortants with three separate strains of noncultivatable human rotavirus, W, Wa, and DS-1. The W and Wa strains of human rotavirus both belong to serotype 1. The DS-1 strain of human rotavirus belongs to serotype 2 and is distinct from W and Wa rotaviruses by neutralization assay. Forty-nine reassortants were isolated from African green monkey kidney (AGMK) or MA104 cells coinfected with a *ts* mutant of the UK bovine rotavirus and one of the three noncultivatable human strains. Selection of reassortants was accomplished by plaquing the growth yield of the coinfected

319

culture at restrictive temperature. In addition, the growth yield was incubated with high-titered neutralizing antiserum to bovine rotavirus in order to select for reassortants with human rotavirus neutralization specificity. Of note, the antiserum used in these experiments was directed at the NCDV strain of bovine rotavirus and not at the homologous UK strain. This antiserum contained a high concentration of antibody reactive with VP7 of UK rotavirus but did not contain neutralizing activity directed at the fourth gene product, VP3, of this bovine rotavirus.

The genotype of the 49 reassortants was determined by coelectrophoresis of reassortant and parental virion RNAs and by hybridization of ^{32}P-labeled parental mRNA to reassortant double-stranded RNA (Fig. 1). By comparing the serotype, as determined by plaque-reduction assay, with the genotype of each reassortant, we were able to establish coding assignments for proteins responsible for serotype specificity. The neutralization antigen of both W and Wa viruses was coded for by the ninth RNA segment, in order of electrophoretic mobility, and the neutralization antigen of the serotypically distinct DS-1 strain of human rotavirus was coded for by the eighth RNA segment (Table 1) (Kalica et al. 1981; Greenberg et al. 1983a).

Under the conditions of in vitro cultivation employed in these studies, none of the three human rotavirus parents (W, Wa, and DS-1) produced detectable infectious progeny when injected singly into tissue culture. On the other hand, each of the 49 reassortants grew efficiently in tissue culture. Interestingly, none of the 49 cultivatable reassortants derived its fourth gene from the noncultivatable human rotavirus parent, whereas all other genes of the noncultivatable human parents were represented in at least one cultivatable reassortant. This observation

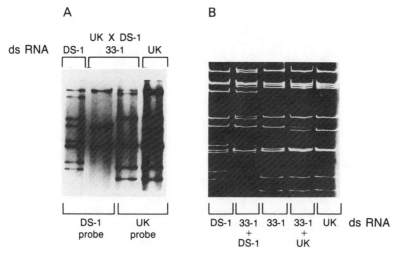

Figure 1
Analysis of the genotype of UK × DS-1 reassortant 33-1 hybridization using ^{32}P-labeled single-stranded RNA (*A*) and coelectrophoresis of reassortant and parental virion RNAs (*B*). Electrophoresis was carried out on 7.5% PAGE. Genes *3, 6,* and *8* of reassortant 33-1 were derived from DS-1, and the remainder, from UK bovine rotavirus.

Table 1
Genotype and Phenotype of Reassortant Viruses Derived from the Cross of Cultivatable *ts* Bovine Rotavirus (UK Strain) and Noncultivatable Human Rotavirus (DS-1 Strain)

Rotavirus gene segment	Reassortants[a]							
	41-2	*33-1*	*8-2*	*17-1*	*10-2*	*11-2a*	*5-2a*	*7-1a*
1	■	□	■	■	■	■	■	■
2	■	□	■	■	■	■	■	■
3	□	■	■	■	■	□	□	■
4	□	□	□	□	□	□	□	□
5	■	□	■	□	□	□	■	□
6	■	■	□	■	■	■	□	□
7	□	□	■	■	□	□	□	□
8	■	■	■	■	■	□	□	□
9	□	□	□	□	■	■	■	□
10	■	□	■	■	■	■	■	■
11	□10	□	□10	■	□10	□10	□10	□10
Neutralization serotype	DS-1	DS-1	DS-1	DS-1	DS-1	UK	UK	UK

[a](■) Segment derived from human rotavirus (DS-1); (□) segment derived from bovine rotavirus (UK). Subscript number indicates gene origin in parental virus.

suggests that the fourth gene of fastidious human rotaviruses is responsible for restriction of growth in tissue culture.

Some rotaviruses, such as RRV, possess a viral hemagglutinin, and others, such as the UK bovine rotavirus, do not. In addition, exogenous protease increases the infectivity of many rotaviruses in tissue culture and is absolutely required for growth of other strains, especially human and murine rotaviruses. In the absence of exogenous trypsin, the UK bovine rotavirus produces plaques with low efficiency in MA104 cells. In contrast, RRV does not require exogenous trypsin to produce plaques efficiently in these cells. To establish gene-coding assignments for the rotaviral hemagglutinin and for protease-enhanced plaque formation, we took advantage of the phenotypic differences between RRV and UK rotaviruses with respect to these two properties. Seventeen reassortants from cells coinfected with a *ts* mutant of bovine rotavirus (UK strain) and a *ts* mutant of RRV (MMU18006 strain) were isolated and studied. Analysis of the genotypes and phenotypes of the 17 individual reassortants disclosed that the viral hemagglutinin and neutralization specificities segregated independently (Table 2). Interestingly, protease-enhanced plaque formation cosegregated with the viral hemagglutinin (Table 2). Genetic analysis of the 17 reassortants disclosed that only the fourth gene of RRV was invariably associated with hemagglutination (Kalica et al. 1983). Conversely, if a reassortant derived its fourth gene from the UK bovine rotavirus, it did not hemagglutinate. In addition, the fourth gene of the UK rotavirus appeared to code for protease-enhanced plaque formation. As expected, the neutralization specificity of both the UK bovine and rhesus rotaviruses was coded for by either the eight or ninth gene.

Table 2
Genotype of UK × RRV Reassortants

Reassortant virus	Phenotype (serotype/HA)	Parental origin of indicated RNA segment by PAGE[a]											Titer (pfu/ml) of reassortant grown in MA104 cells	
		1	2	3	4	5	6	7	8	9	10	11	with trypsin	without trypsin
81-2	bovine/−	□	■	□	□	□	□	□	□	□	□	■	1.5 × 10^6	<10^2
85-2	bovine/+	□	■	■	■	□	■	■	[−	−]^b	■	■	1 × 10^7	1 × 10^6
37-1	rhesus/+	■	■	□	■	□	□	■	■	■	■	■	6 × 10^7	2 × 10^7
19-1	rhesus/−	□	■	■	□	□	□	■	■	■	■	■	1.6 × 10^6	<10^2

[a](□) UK segment; (■) rhesus segment.
[b]The comigrating eighth and ninth segment complex contained one gene from each parent. The order could not be determined.

Monoclonal Antibodies Directed at the Surface Proteins of Rotavirus

To increase our efficiency of selecting monoclonal antibodies directed at surface proteins of RRV, we used a hemagglutination-inhibition (HI) assay as well as a solid-phase radioimmunoassay (RIA) to screen hybridomas. Over 40 monoclones with HI activity were isolated and cloned. Most of these (38) immunoprecipitated a major RRV surface protein (VP3) of approximately 82,000 daltons from [^{35}S]-methionine-labeled RRV-infected cell lysates (Fig. 2). These monoclonal antibodies and a series of reassortants derived from mating rhesus rotavirus and the nonhemagglutinating UK bovine rotavirus were assayed by RIA to determine the gene that coded for the 82K RRV hemagglutinin. These selected monoclonal antibodies with HI activity reacted only with reassortants whose fourth gene was derived from the RRV parent, demonstrating that the 82K protein was the product of gene *4*. This is consistent with evidence from our previous genetic studies

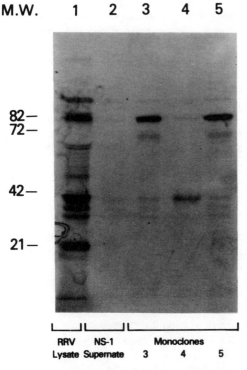

(3= 954/145/55; 4= 954/96/18; 5= 954/177/14)

Figure 2
Immunoprecipitation of ^{35}S-labeled RRV-infected cell lysate by monoclonal antibodies directed at the fourth (lanes *3* and *5*) or the eighth or ninth (lane *4*) gene products of RRV. (*1*) RRV-infected cell lysate; (*2*) NS-1 cell supernatant; (*3*) monoclone 954/145/55; (*4*) monoclone 954/96/18; (*5*) monoclone 954/177/14. Molecular weights (× 10^3) are shown at the left.

which showed that the fourth gene product of RRV was the viral hemagglutinin. It is of interest that rotavirus-neutralizing activity was detected when selected monoclonal antibodies directed at VP3 were amplified in ascites fluid and then assayed by plaque reduction. The neutralizing activity was not, however, as high titered as that demonstrated by monoclonal antibodies directed at VP7 (see below).

Three monoclonal antibodies with HI activity did not precipitate the 82K RRV protein. Instead, they immunoprecipitated a 38K glycosylated protein (VP7). When studied by RIA, the three monoclonal antibodies reacted only with UK × RRV reassortants that were serotypically rhesus rotavirus. After analyzing the genotype of the UK × RRV reassortants, it became clear that the reactive monoclonal antibodies were directed at the eighth or ninth gene product, the primary neutralization protein. Plaque-reduction neutralization assay with the three monoclonal antibodies disclosed that they had high-level neutralizing activity against the homologous RRV. In addition, each neutralized the canine rotavirus (CU-1), a serotypically related strain.

Since previous genetic analysis demonstrated that the RRV hemagglutinin was coded for by the fourth gene segment, it was surprising that monoclonal antibodies directed against the eighth or ninth gene product had considerable HI activity. To study this question in more detail, we assayed selected UK × RRV reassortants by HI assay, using monoclonal antibodies directed at either the fourth, eighth, or ninth gene product of RRV. Monoclonal antibodies directed at the 82-kD protein had HI activity against each reassortant irrespective of its serotype (i.e., UK or RRV). On the other hand, monoclonal antibodies directed at VP7 exhibited HI activity only against UK × RRV reassortants that were serotypically RRV. This suggests that these neutralizing monoclonal antibodies inhibit hemagglutination sterically by binding to the surface protein, VP7, that is in close proximity to the viral hemagglutinin, VP3 (Greenberg et al. 1983b).

Use of Monospecific Neutralizing Antisera to Isolate Reassortants That Are Candidate Vaccine Strains

We isolated a series of reassortants produced by coinfection with wild-type animal rotavirus and noncultivatable human rotavirus. The wild-type animal rotaviruses, UK and RRV, had been plaque-purified and passaged in primary AGMK cells, and in the case of RRV, the final passage was in DBS-FRhL-2 cells. The D and DS-1 human rotaviruses, originally derived from the stool of ill children, were passaged in gnotobiotic calves, and a filtrate of stool from an infected calf was used in the mating. Filtered stool from an ill patient was used for coinfection with the P strain. The D strain was chosen because it represents the most prevalent human serotype. In addition, this strain had been shown to produce illness in volunteers (Kapikan et al. 1983a,b). Wild-type UK bovine rotavirus was reassorted with human strains D, DS-1, and P that represent human serotypes 1, 2, and 3, respectively. Wild-type RRV was reassorted with human strains D and DS-1 but not with P, since RRV and P are serotypically related. AGMK cells were coinfected with an animal rotavirus and a noncultivatable human rotavirus.

Selection of the desired viral reassortants was achieved by exposing the progeny of coinfected cultures to monoclonal antibodies or antiserum that specifically neutralized the animal rotavirus parent. Under the culture conditions employed in these studies, the human rotaviruses did not grow. Hyperimmune antiserum directed at the NCDV strain of bovine rotavirus was used to neutralize the UK animal parent. As noted earlier, this antiserum is highly cross-reactive with VP7 of UK rotavirus but does not have neutralizing activity directed at the fourth gene product, VP3, of the UK rotavirus. A pool of three monoclonal antibodies directed at the neutralizing protein, VP7, of RRV was used to select against the RRV animal parent. These monoclonal antibodies immunoprecipitate the 38,000-dalton glycoprotein, VP7, and neutralize viruses that contain the RRV neutralizing protein, but they do not neutralize either human rotavirus serotype 1 or 2.

Many reassortants were isolated from the various coinfections, but only a small proportion have been genotyped by hybridization of ^{32}P-labeled parental mRNA to reassortant double-stranded RNA. Of the first six reassortants characterized from the human rotavirus strain D (serotype 1)–UK bovine rotavirus coinfection, three contained only the ninth gene segment from the human rotavirus parent, whereas the other three contained the ninth gene segment and one other gene segment (3, 6, and 7 or 8) from the human rotavirus parent. The only reassortant characterized from a cross between human strain D and animal strain RRV received only the ninth gene segment from the human rotavirus parent (Fig. 3). The first four reassortants characterized from the human rotavirus strain P (serotype 3)–UK bovine rotavirus coinfection derived only the eighth or ninth gene segment from their human rotavirus parent (Fig. 4). The eighth and ninth genes of the P strain of human rotavirus cannot be separated by gel electrophoresis, but these reassortants were neutralized specifically by antiserum to the P strain, indicating that the only gene derived from the human rotavirus parent was the

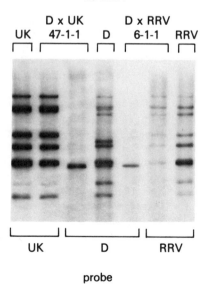

Figure 3
Analysis of genotype of D × UK and D × RRV reassortants 47-1-1 and 6-1-1, respectively. In both reassortants, only the ninth gene is derived from the human rotavirus parent (D).

ds RNA

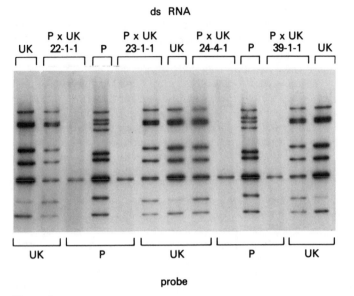

Figure 4
Analysis of genotype of P × UK reassortants 22-1-1, 23-1-1, 24-4-1, and 39-1-1. In each of these reassortants, only the eighth or ninth gene is derived from the human rotavirus parent (P).

one that coded for the major neutralization protein. The only reassortant from the cross between the human DS-1 rotavirus and bovine UK rotavirus that has been genotyped received gene segments 6 and 8 from the human rotavirus parent. Two reassortants from the cross between DS-1 and RRV have been genotyped; one contains gene segments 5 and 8 and the other contains segments 1, 5, 6, and 8 from the human rotavirus parent.

These preliminary data suggest that the distribution of genotypes of these reassortants differs from that observed when one of the parents was a *ts* mutant. In the latter situation, the non-*ts* parent contributed three or more genes to each reassortant. In contrast, reassortants derived from the crosses between a wild-type animal rotavirus and a noncultivatable human rotavirus frequently received only one or two genes from the human rotavirus parent. When a *ts* animal rotavirus was used for production of reassortants, there was selection by antibody against its neutralization antigen and by high temperature against its *ts* genes, whereas when both rotavirus parents were non-*ts*, selection was only against the gene coding for the neutralization protein of the animal rotavirus parent. In addition, silent mutations in other genes of the mutagenized, *ts* animal rotavirus parent may have been responsible for selection against these genes during coinfection.

One benefit of using wild-type animal rotavirus instead of a *ts* animal rotavirus mutant in preparing reassortants for vaccine purposes is that the former was not exposed to chemical mutagenesis. Thus, silent point mutations, which are often genetically unstable, would be minimized in reassortants derived from wild-type animal rotaviruses. The advantage of relying exclusively on monospecific neutralizing antiserum or monoclonal antibodies directed against the animal rotavirus parent to favor the desired phenotype is that selection is exerted only against the major neutralization protein of this parent. In contrast, the other genes of the animal rotavirus parent are allowed to outcompete their noncultivatable human rotavirus counterparts, and in this manner, reassortants derive all or most of their genes, except for the gene coding for the major neutralization protein, from a nonhuman rotavirus.

In summary, reassortants were prepared by coinfection with a wild-type animal rotavirus and a noncultivatable human rotavirus and were selected with monospecific neutralizing antiserum or monoclonal antibodies. In general, these reassortants grow to high titer in tissue culture, produce plaques with high efficiency, possess the major neutralizing protein of the human rotavirus parent, and receive almost all of their genes from the animal rotavirus parent. Because of the host specificity exhibited by bovine and human rotaviruses (J. Flores, pers. comm.), bovine-human rotavirus reassortants with a single human rotavirus gene substitution represent promising candidate live-vaccine strains. Single gene substitution reassortants of this sort should retain the growth restriction of bovine rotavirus for human tissues and hence be attenuated for man. On the other hand, the major protective antigen would be derived from the human rotavirus parent.

ACKNOWLEDGMENT

We gratefully acknowledge the assistance of Mr. Ronald Jones, Mr. José Valdesuso, and Ms. Linda Jordan.

REFERENCES

Greenberg, H.B., J. Flores, A.R. Kalica, R.G. Wyatt, and R. Jones. 1983a. Gene coding assignments for growth restriction, neutralization and subgroup specificities of the W and DS-1 strains of human rotavirus. *J. Gen. Virol.* **64:** 313.

Greenberg, H.B., A.R. Kalica, R.G. Wyatt, R.W. Jones, A.Z. Kapikian, and R.M. Chanock. 1981. Rescue of noncultivatable human rotavirus by gene reassortment during mixed infection with *ts* mutants of a cultivatable bovine rotavirus. *Proc. Natl. Acad. Sci.* **78:** 420.

Greenberg, H.B., J. Valdesuso, K. van Wyke, K. Midthun, M. Walsh, V. McAuliffe, R.G. Wyatt, A.R. Kalica, J. Flores, and Y. Hoshino. 1983b. Production and preliminary characterization of monoclonal antibodies directed at two surface proteins of rhesus rotavirus. *J. Virol.* **47:** 267.

Kalica, A.R., J. Flores, and H.B. Greenberg. 1983. Identification of the rotaviral gene that codes for hemagglutination and protease-enhanced plaque formation. *Virology* **125:** 194.

Kalica, A.R., H.B. Greenberg, R.G. Wyatt, J. Flores, M.M. Sereno, A.Z. Kapikian, and R.M. Chanock. 1981. Genes of human (strain Wa) and bovine (strain UK) rotaviruses that code for neutralization and subgroup antigens. *Virology* **112:** 385.

Kapikian, A.Z., R.G. Wyatt, M.M. Levine, R.H. Yolken, D.H. VanKirk, R. Dolin, H.B. Greenberg, and R.M. Chanock. 1983a. Oral administration of human rotavirus to volunteers: Induction of illness and correlates of resistance. *J. Infect. Dis.* **147:** 95.

Kapikian, A.Z., R.G. Wyatt, M.M. Levine, R.E. Black, H.B. Greenberg, J. Flores, A.R. Kalica, Y. Hoshino, and R.M. Chanock. 1983b. Studies in volunteers with human rotaviruses. *Dev. Biol. Stand.* **53:** 209.

Attenuation of Wild-type Influenza-A Viruses for Man by Genetic Reassortment with Attenuated Donor Viruses

Brian R. Murphy, Alicia J. Buckler-White,
Shu-fang Tian, and Robert M. Chanock
Laboratory of Infectious Diseases, National
Institute of Allergy and Infectious Diseases
National Institutes of Health
Bethesda, Maryland 20205
Mary Lou Clements
Center for Vaccine Development, Department of
Medicine, University of Maryland
School of Medicine, Baltimore, Maryland 21218
Hunein F. Maassab
Department of Epidemiology
School of Public Health, University of
Michigan, Ann Arbor, Michigan 48109
William T. London
National Institute of Neurological and
Communicative Disorders and Stroke, National
Institutes of Health, Bethesda, Maryland 20205

Influenza-A viruses are unique among viruses that infect the respiratory tract in that they undergo significant antigenic variation. This antigenic change takes two forms. The first, which is called antigenic drift, involves the accumulation of point mutations in one or more epitopes of the hemagglutinin (HA) and neuraminidase (NA) glycoproteins as the virus spreads from person to person. The second is called antigenic shift, and this involves the sudden introduction into the human population of a virus that bears an antigenically distinct HA and/or NA. Both of these forms of antigenic variation allow the new variant virus to spread more efficiently in individuals who are immune to previous influenza viruses. The strategy for developing a live-virus vaccine must take this continuous process of antigenic variation into account. Since it is not feasible to rapidly and predictably attenuate each new variant of influenza virus that appears in nature by multiple passages of the virus in tissue culture or eggs, an alternative strategy has been developed in which attenuation is effected in a single step. This is achieved by transfer of genes that confer attenuation from an attenuated donor virus to each new epidemic or pandemic virulent virus. This process of gene exchange between influenza viruses is readily achieved because the viral genome exists as eight RNA segments that undergo independent reassortment following coinfection of a susceptible cell. Since resistance to influenza-A virus is mediated by the development of an immune response to the HA and NA glycoproteins, live attenuated reassortant viruses must contain the genes coding for the surface antigens of the epidemic virus, while deriving the attenuating genes that code for nonsurface viral proteins from the attenuated parent. Henceforth, we refer to these as internal genes. In this approach, it is necessary that the genes responsible for attenuation not code for surface antigens, since these genes cannot be transferred to new epidemic or pandemic viruses. Ideally, attenuated reassortant vaccine virus should receive each of the internal genes from the attenuated donor virus, because this gene constellation would be expected to yield the most predictable level of attenuation each time a new virus is constructed. Reassortant viruses containing mixed internal genes have on occasion exhibited greater virulence than either parent (Vallbracht et al. 1980). The generation of such undesirable reassortants would be minimized by isolating reassortant viruses that derived each of their internal genes from their attenuated parent.

If this strategy is to be effective, the attenuated donor virus must reproducibly confer on wild-type viruses the following set of properties: (1) satisfactory attenuation, (2) sufficient immunogenicity to induce resistance to infection with wild-type virus, (3) stability of the attenuation phenotype after replication in man, and (4) greatly diminished transmissibility.

Temperature-sensitive (ts) mutants and viruses such as A/PR/8/34 (H1N1), which has been passaged many times in a heterologous host, did not reproducibly confer these desired properties on reassortant viruses (Florent 1980; Tolpin et al. 1982). ts viruses bearing missense mutations were not sufficiently stable phenotypically after replication in fully susceptible children. Reassortant viruses bearing the six internal PR-8 genes were not fully attenuated, and satisfactory attenuation of PR-8 reassortant viruses for man required a specific mixed constellation of PR-8 and wild-type human influenza H3N2 polymerase genes. This requirement for a mixture of genes from the attenuated donor virus and the virulent H3N2 parent virus may prove a limiting factor in the use of the PR-8 donor virus, since it is not certain that the polymerase genes of future epidemic viruses will interact with the PR-8 polymerase genes to bring about satisfactory attenuation of reassortant viruses for man.

A promising donor virus now being actively studied is the A/Ann Arbor/6/60 (H2N2) cold-adapted (ca) virus (La Montagne 1983). This virus was adapted to grow well at the suboptimal temperature of 25°C by serial passage at successively lower temperatures in primary chick kidney cell culture. This temperature is restrictive for wild-type human influenza viruses. During this process of cold adaptation, the virus sustained one or more ts mutations and acquired a ts phenotype, as indicated by an in vitro shutoff temperature for plaque formation of 38°C. The A/Ann Arbor/6/60 virus sustained mutations in each of its polymerase genes (Cox et al. 1981). The PB2 and PB1 genes appear to be important in functional properties related to the ts phenotype. A reassortant virus possessing the internal genes of the ca donor virus except for the PB1 gene was as attenuated for man as one possessing all six *ca* internal genes. This suggested that the PB1 gene was not the primary determinant of attenuation of this virus in man. Biochemical and/or genetic evidence also indicates that the NP, M, and NS genes have sustained mutations. Two reassortant viruses possessing the internal genes of the *ca* donor virus except for the M or NS gene were as attenuated for man as reassortants possessing all six internal genes. Thus, the PB1, M, and NS genes do not appear to be primary determinants of attenuation of the *ca* donor virus for man.

The genetic basis for the attenuation of the *ca* virus remains unclear. It appears from studies of *ca* viruses in ferrets and man that the level of temperature sensitivity of the virus in vitro is not the primary determinant of attenuation, as was shown to be the case for *ts* viruses whose mutations were induced by chemical mutagenesis (La Montagne 1983). This suggests that the A/Ann Arbor/6/60 virus sustained host-range mutations during its passage at low temperature in heterologous avian kidney tissue culture. These host-range mutations permit efficient replication of virus in the avian cells but not in the respiratory tract of man.

As previously indicated, new reassortant viruses derived from the *ca* donor virus should ideally receive all of their internal genes from the *ca* donor virus and the surface glycoprotein genes from the new influenza variant. This is readily achieved by mating the *ca* donor and the wild-type human virus at 25°C and selecting reassortant progeny at this temperature. Of the *ca* reassortants produced in this manner, 66% have the desired gene constellation (Cox et al. 1981). Four of these viruses have been extensively studied in man (Fig. 1). In each case,

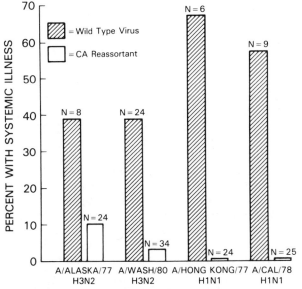

Figure 1
Response of susceptible (serum HI ≤1:8) adult volunteers to four *ca* influenza-A reassortant viruses.

the acquisition of the six internal genes from the *ca* donor viruses resulted in the attenuation of the resulting reassortant for man. The few systemic illnesses observed were generally less than 24 hours duration and were less severe than that seen following infection with wild-type virus. The human infectious dose 50 (HID_{50}) of the four *ca* reassortants was approximately $10^{5.5}$ to $10^{6.1}$ $TCID_{50}$. Since these viruses grow in eggs to a titer of $10^{8.0}$ to $10^{8.5}$ $TCID_{50}$ per milliliter of allantoic fluid, it is possible to produce enough virus to administer doses greater than 50 HID_{50} to vaccinees. Drs. P. Wright and R. Belshe (pers. comm.) estimate the HID_{50} for completely susceptible children to be about $10^{4.0}$ $TCID_{50}$. At doses of 50–100 HID_{50}, the *ca* reassortant viruses are satisfactorily immunogenic in adults and children. Furthermore, the viruses appear to be stable with regard to *ca* and *ts* phenotypes even in susceptible young children studied by Wright and Belshe and to be nontransmissible in adults and children.

The influenza A/Washington/80 (H3N2) *ca* reassortant with six internal genes from the *ca* parent was recently compared with commercially available inactivated vaccine with regard to protective efficacy against experimental challenge with homologous wild-type virus. The live-virus vaccinees exhibited greater resistance than the vaccinees who received inactivated vaccine parenterally. The *ca* vaccinees had a significantly lower rate of infection and shed significantly less virus. The live-virus vaccinees failed to develop systemic illness, but this was not statistically different from the low frequency of illness in the recipients of inactivated vaccine. Thus, in this experimental setting, the *ca* reassortant virus induced greater resistance to infection than did inactivated vaccine.

From these observations, the six internal genes of the *ca* donor virus reproducibly confer a satisfactory level of attenuation and antigenicity on virulent H3N2 and H1N1 viruses. For this reason, the A/Ann Arbor/6/60 *ca* virus represents a promising donor of genes for attenuation of new epidemic or pandemic influenza-A viruses.

Avian Influenza Viruses as Donors

An alternate approach to constructing attenuated influenza viruses involves the use of an avian influenza-A donor virus that is restricted in its replication in primate cells (Murphy et al. 1982). In this situation, restriction manifested by avian–human reassortant viruses is effected by naturally occurring avian influenza virus genes, rather than by mutant genes selected by limited passage of virus in an unnatural host. Many of the influenza-A-virus genes that have evolved over a long period in birds differ significantly in nucleotide sequence from the corresponding genes of human influenza-A virus. Because of these marked differences, we would expect some avian influenza viruses to replicate inefficiently in primate cells and thereby be attenuated, and this is indeed the case. Avian viruses exhibit a spectrum of replication in the lower respiratory tract of primates. Several avian influenza-A viruses replicate at least 1000 times less efficiently than human influenza-A viruses. Furthermore, in tissue culture, avian influenza-A viruses replicate efficiently at 42°C, a temperature restrictive for human influenza-A viruses. One avian influenza-A virus, the A/Mallard/6750/78 (H2N2) strain, which was markedly restricted in replication in the trachea of monkeys, was evaluated as a donor of its internal genes for attenuation of virulent human influenza-

A viruses. Avian–human influenza reassortant viruses were produced by mating the avian influenza virus and a virulent human virus at 37°C and selecting progeny at 42°C in the presence of antibodies to the surface antigens of the avian parent virus. In three such matings, each reassortant virus isolated had the desired genotype; i.e., the surface antigen genes were derived from the human influenza virus, whereas the internal genes came from the avian influenza parent. Like their avian influenza parent, each of the avian–human influenza reassortant viruses produced plaques efficiently at 42°C, indicating that one or more avian influenza genes that code for nonsurface proteins specify growth at 42°C.

The level of replication of two avian–human influenza reassortant viruses in the lower respiratory tract of the squirrel monkey was compared with that of their parental virus. The two avian–human influenza reassortant viruses were as restricted in growth in the monkey's trachea as their avian influenza parental virus. In each instance, the reassortant viruses were shed in lower titer and for a shorter period than the human influenza virus parent. These findings indicate that restriction of replication of the avian influenza virus is a function of one or more of its internal genes. To investigate which avian gene(s) was responsible for the restriction of replication in primates, reassortant viruses were produced that contained the human influenza virus surface antigens from the influenza A/Udorn/72 (H3N2) virus and one or more internal genes derived from the avian influenza virus parent (Table 1). Avian–human reassortant viruses that contained only an RNA 1, RNA 3, or NS RNA segment of avian influenza origin did not exhibit restricted replication; i.e., they grew to the same level as their human influenza A/Udorn/72 parent. In contrast, avian–human influenza reassortants that contained only the avian NP or M gene were as restricted in their growth as their avian influenza parent. Avian–human influenza reassortant viruses containing two or more genes derived from their avian influenza parent virus were restricted in replication if they possessed an NP or M gene from the avian parent. Thus, the avian NP and M genes appear to play a major role in the host-range restriction exhibited by the avian influenza virus and their six internal gene reassortants. Since the NP or M gene is able to effect restriction by itself, restoration of virulence of six-gene avian-human reassortants for man would require appropriate genetic changes in both genes. Dr. W.J. Bean (pers. comm.) has recently demonstrated by hybridization analysis that all avian influenza-A-virus NP genes, including those of the mallard strain we have studied, belong in one of two groups, whereas human influenza-A-virus NP genes fall into a third group. Thus, restriction of virus replication in primate respiratory epithelium specified by the mallard NP gene would appear to be a function of significant sequence differences between avian and human NP genes. The nature and extent of nucleotide differences between the avian NP and M genes and the corresponding human genes are currently under investigation.

Significant resistance to challenge with wild-type human influenza virus was observed in monkeys previously infected with the avian–human influenza reassortant viruses. Thus, despite restricted replication of the avian–human influenza reassortant viruses, significant resistance was induced to challenge with virulent virus. An avian–human influenza reassortant virus (A/Washington/80 [H3N2]) was examined for stability of phenotype, transmissibility, and safety in squirrel monkeys. This virus was passaged alternately five times in monkeys and eggs. Alter-

Table 1
Effect of Substitution of a Single Avian Influenza Virus Gene on Growth of Human Influenza-A Virus in Monkeys

Influenza virus[a]	Parental origin of genes in avian–human influenza reassortant viruses[b]								Virus replication in trachea	
	RNA1	RNA2	RNA3	HA	NA	NP	M	NS	average duration of virus shedding (days)	mean peak titer ($\log_{10}$ TCID$_{50}$/ml) of tracheal lavage fluid
Human	□	□	□	□	□	□	□	□	5.3	5.1
Avian-human reassortant six internal avian virus genes	■	■	■	□	□	■	■	■	0.3[c]	0.7[c]
single substitution of an avian virus gene	■	□	□	□	□	□	□	□	6.0	5.2
	□	□	■	□	□	□	□	□	5.0	5.4
	□	□	□	□	□	■	□	□	0.0[c]	0.5[c]
	□	□	□	□	□	□	■	□	3.3[c], 2.0[c,d]	2.6[c], 1.6[c,d]
	□	□	□	□	□	□	□	■	5.0	4.4

aAvian virus was A/Mallard/New York/6750/78 (H2N2), and human virus was A/Udorn/307/72 (H3N2). Each virus was tested in at least four squirrel monkeys.
b(□) Gene derived from human virus; (■) gene derived from avian virus.
cStatistically significant difference from wild-type human influenza virus.
dTwo independently derived reassortants with this gene constellation.

Table 2
Response of Seronegative Adults to Influenza A/Washington/80 (H3N2) Avian–Human Reassortant or Wild-type Virus

Influenza-A virus administered	Dose of virus ($TCID_{50}$)	No. in group	% Infected	Virus shedding (nasal wash)		Percent with immunological response		Percent with indicated illness	
				% shedding	peak mean[a] log_{10} titer ($TCID_{50}/ml$)	serum HI, NI, and/or IgG ELISA antibody	nasal wash ELISA IgA HA antibody	febrile, systemic or both	any ill-ness[b]
Avian-human reassortant									
	$10^{5.0}$	12	17	17	1.0	8	8	0	0
	$10^{6.0}$	13	67	8	0.6	46	25	0	0
	$10^{7.0}$	19	84	11	0.6	74	37	0	0
	$10^{7.5}$	20	80	10	0.5	79	47	0	0
	$10^{8.0}$	19	100	49	0.7	89	74	11[c]	11
Wild type	$10^{6.0}$	24	96	88	3.6	91	93	38	46

Transmission of reassortant virus to six contact controls was not observed. Virus was not recovered from blood or rectal swabs. HI, hemagglutination-inhibiting; NI, neuraminidase-inhibiting; ELISA, enzyme-linked immunosorbent assay.
[a] Data from each infected volunteer were used for calculations.
[b] This category also includes upper respiratory tract illnesses.
[c] Afebrile illness of less than 24 hr duration.

nate passages in eggs were required because the amount of virus recovered from infected monkeys was not sufficient to infect other monkeys. Following this alternate passages series, the reassortant retained its restriction of growth in the monkey's respiratory tract. Furthermore, the virus was not transmitted to susceptible monkeys housed in the same cage.

Since avian influenza-A viruses can cause enteric and systemic infections in their natural hosts, it was important that we define the pathogenesis of an avian–human reassortant virus in primates. Monkeys were sacrificed on days 2, 4, and 8 after administration of the avian–human A/Washington/80 influenza reassortant, and 26 tissues were removed and assayed for virus. Virus was recovered only from the respiratory tract of the monkeys. This indicated that the transfer of the six internal RNA segments did not lead to systemic spread or enterotropism. Instead the internal avian influenza genes imposed a reduction in the level of virus replication in primate respiratory tissue.

Two additional avian–human reassortant viruses were produced by mating the A/Mallard/Alberta/573/78 (H1N1) or A/Pintail/Alberta/121/79 (H7N8) avian virus with the human influenza A/Udorn/72 (H3N2) virus. Reassortant viruses containing the HA and NA genes from the human virus and the other six RNA segments from the avian parent were evaluated for their level of replication in the upper and lower respiratory tracts of squirrel monkeys. Each reassortant virus was as restricted in the lower respiratory tract as its avian influenza parent. Thus, with three successive avian influenza viruses tested, the internal genes of the avian parental virus constituted the primary determinants of restriction of replication in squirrel monkey respiratory epithelium. By evaluating a large series of avian influenza viruses that differ in their levels of replication in primates, it should be possible to identify one whose internal genes reproducibly confer an acceptable balance of attenuation and immunogenicity on avian–human influenza reassortants.

Considered together, these findings have implications for the production of influenza-A vaccine viruses that are attenuated for man. A preliminary evaluation of the six-gene avian–human A/Washington/80 influenza reassortant virus in man indicates that it is attenuated and immunogenic but not transmissible (Table 2). The reassortant virus grows poorly in the human respiratory tract. This is consistent with its satisfactory level of attenuation. The HID_{50} of the avian-human reassortant is similar to that of the influenza A/Washington/80 ca reassortant virus. Neither viremia nor growth of reassortant virus in the intestinal tract was detected. A continued evaluation of the avian–human influenza reassortant viruses should identify an avian donor that will reproducibly confer on each new epidemic human virus a satisfactory level of attenuation, phenotypic stability, immunogenicity, and lack of, or greatly diminished, transmissibility.

REFERENCES

Cox, N.J., I. Konnecke, A.P. Kendal, and H.F. Maassab. 1981. Genetic and biochemical analysis of the A/Ann Arbor/6/60 cold-adapted mutant. In *Genetic variation among influenza viruses* (ed. D. Nayak), p. 639. Academic Press, New York.

Florent, G. 1980. Gene constellation of live influenza A vaccines. *Arch. Virol.* **64:** 171.

La Montagne, J.R., P.F. Wright, M.L. Clements, H.F. Maassab, and B.R. Murphy. 1983. Prospects for live, attenuated influenza vaccines using reassortants derived from the A/Ann Arbor/6/60 (H2N2) cold-adapted (*ca*) donor virus. In *The origin of pandemic influenza viruses* (ed. W.G. Laver), p. 243. Elsevier Science Publishing Co., New York.

Murphy, B.R., V.S. Hinshaw, D.L. Sly, W.T. London, N.T. Hosier, F.T. Wood, R.G. Webster, and R.M. Chanock. 1982. Virulence of avian influenza A viruses for squirrel monkeys. *Infect. Immun.* **37:** 1119.

Tolpin, M.D., M.L. Clements, M.M. Levine, R.E. Black, A.J. Saah, W.C. Anthony, L. Cisneros, R.M. Chanock, and B.R. Murphy. 1982. Evaluation of a phenotypic revertant of the A/Alaska/77-ts-1A2 reassortant virus in hamsters and in seronegative adult volunteers: Further evidence that the temperature-sensitive phenotype is responsible for attenuation of ts-1A2 reassortant viruses. *Infect. Immun.* **36:** 645.

Vallbracht, A.C., B. Scholtissek, B. Flehmig, and H.J. Gerth. 1980. Recombination of influenza A strains with fowl plague virus can change pneumotropism for mice to a generalized infection with involvement of the central nervous system. *Virology* **107:** 452.

Engineering the Genome of Influenza Viruses for Immunoprophylaxis: Progress and Obstacles

Ching-Juh Lai, Lewis J. Markoff,
Bor-Chian Lin, and Robert M. Chanock

*Molecular Viral Biology Section, Laboratory of
Infectious Diseases, National Institute of
Allergy and Infectious Diseases
National Institutes of Health
Bethesda, Maryland 20205*

Influenza differs from other viral diseases because the viral pathogen undergoes frequent major or progressive minor antigenic variations that render previous immunity ineffective. Observations made during a recent epidemiologic study showed that immunity which developed after natural infection was far more effective than that afforded by vaccination with inactivated whole virus. Several attempts have been made to attenuate influenza virus with the intent of developing a live influenza virus vaccine. These include isolation of temperature-sensitive mutants, cold-adapted mutants, and host-range mutants. Although there has been considerable success, there is still some concern for the possibility of reversion to wild-type virulence. This problem could be solved if it were possible to use recombinant DNA techniques to construct viable deletion mutants, since these mutants would be unlikely to revert and therefore should be stable phenotypically. In this approach, one would select an internal gene or a combination of several internal genes to engineer deletions so that the resulting mutant virus remained viable but did not exhibit virulence. Such mutant genes could then be transferred by reassortment to new epidemic and pandemic viruses as they emerged. In this manner, attenuation could be achieved rapidly and reproducibly.

Cloning Full-length Influenza Virus DNA Sequences

Two approaches have been taken to obtain full-length cloned DNA sequences of influenza virus gene segments. In the first approach, negative-strand virion RNA was reverse-transcribed using a synthetic DNA primer complementary to the

339

conserved 3'-terminal sequence, yielding positive-strand cDNA. Poly(A)-containing influenza mRNA from infected cells was also reverse-transcribed using oligo(dT) as a primer to generate negative-strand cDNA. Duplex DNAs were formed from the corresponding cDNA strands and cloned at the *Pst*I site of pBR322 DNA using oligo(dG-dC) as linker sequences (Lai et al. 1980). In the second approach, the positive cDNA strand, produced as described above, was converted to double-stranded DNA using a second synthetic DNA primer that corresponds to the common 5'-terminal sequences of virion RNA. The double-stranded DNA fragments were cloned in pBR322 DNA using *Bam*HI linker sequences. Thus far, we have cloned and characterized six full-length genes; the remaining two genes, PB1 and PA, have not been cloned in complete form. Analysis of the terminal nucleotide sequences showed that the six full-length DNA clones contained the conserved 3'- and 5'-terminal nucleotides; thus, the viral terminal sequences were fully represented. In addition, flanking sequences of either the dG-dC linker or the *Bam*HI linker added during cloning were present. Potentially, these full-length DNA clones could produce corresponding RNA transcripts that contain the control sequences needed for replication of viral genes.

Expression of Cloned Influenza Virus DNA

We used SV40 DNA as a vector to facilitate introduction and subsequent transcription of influenza virus DNA in mammalian cells. African green monkey kidney (AGMK) cells were chosen because they are permissive for influenza virus as well as for SV40 and thus offer a system in which coinfection might lead to gene reassortment. A series of recombinants were constructed by inserting each cloned influenza virus DNA into the SV40 late region, replacing the SV40 structural genes. In primate cells infected with such recombinants, transcription of influenza virus DNA is placed under the control of SV40 initiation and termination sequences. Depending on the orientation of insertion with respect to the SV40 signals, these recombinants produce either positive-strand or negative-strand influenza virus RNA transcripts. AGMK cells infected with recombinant DNA bearing an insert from which positive-strand RNA is transcribed produced a full-length functional influenza virus polypeptide, as demonstrated in studies with cloned DNA coding for hemagglutinin (H3), neuraminidase (N2), matrix protein, or nucleoprotein (Sveda and Lai 1981). Functional expression of cloned influenza virus DNA in an SV40 vector made it possible to construct further a number of mutants that exhibited altered functional properties (Fig. 1A). For example, mutants specifying a hemagglutinin (HA) that failed to anchor on the outer membrane and was secreted extracellularly were constructed by removing the DNA sequences encoding the hydrophobic carboxyl terminus that is responsible for insertion into the membrane. Functionally defective, unglycosylated HA that accumulated intracellularly was synthesized from a deletion mutant of HA DNA that lacked the signal peptide coding sequences. Modification of HA DNA by site-specific mutagenesis resulted in the production of HAs that contained amino acid substitutions in strategic regions such as the signal sequences. As shown in Figure 1B, many of these variant HAs were defective for cell-surface expression, whereas others were apparently normal. In this manner, molecular dissection and modification of the HA enabled us to analyze functional specificities of var-

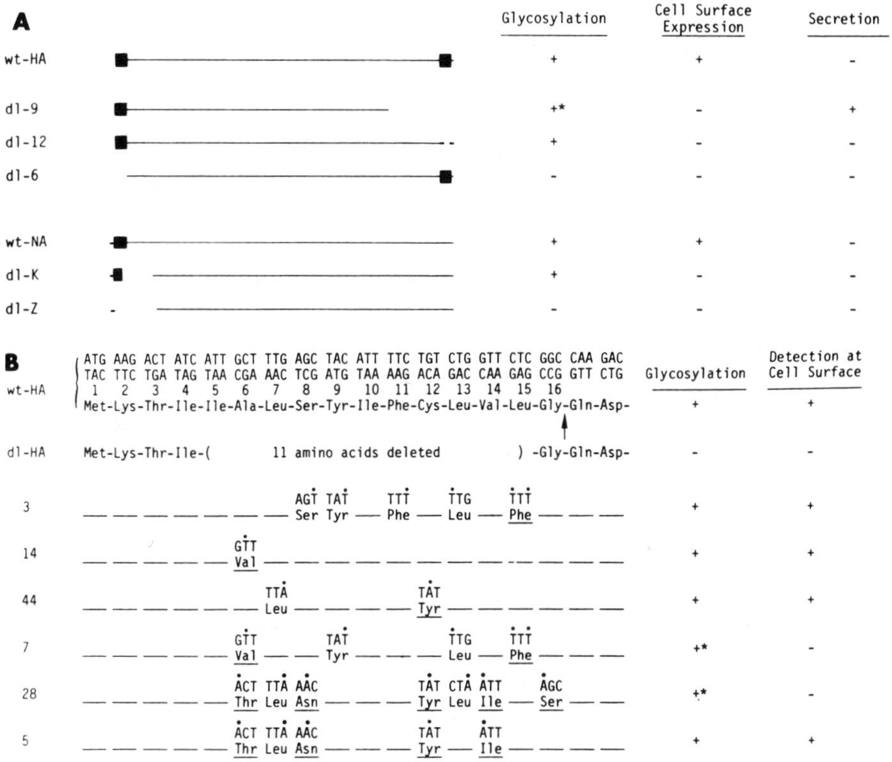

A

	Glycosylation	Cell Surface Expression	Secretion
wt-HA	+	+	-
dl-9	+*	-	+
dl-12	+	-	-
dl-6	-	-	-
wt-NA	+	+	-
dl-K	+	-	-
dl-Z	-	-	-

B

```
         ATG AAG ACT ATC ATT GCT TTG AGC TAC ATT TTC TGT CTG GTT CTC GGC CAA GAC                Detection at
         TAC TTC TGA TAG TAA CGA AAC TCG ATG TAA AAG ACA GAC CAA GAG CCG GTT CTG   Glycosylation   Cell Surface
wt-HA     1   2   3   4   5   6   7   8   9  10  11  12  13  14  15  16
         Met-Lys-Thr-Ile-Ile-Ala-Leu-Ser-Tyr-Ile-Phe-Cys-Leu-Val-Leu-Gly-Gln-Asp-      +              +
                                                                    ↑
dl-HA    Met-Lys-Thr-Ile-(        11 amino acids deleted       ) -Gly-Gln-Asp-           -              -

                          AGT TAT    TTT    TTG    TTT
  3      — — — — — — — — — Ser Tyr — Phe — Leu — Phe — — —                               +              +

                          GTT
 14      — — — — — — — — — Val — — — — — — — — — — — — —                                  +              +

                          TTA           TAT
 44      — — — — — — — — — Leu — — — — — Tyr — — — — — —                                  +              +

                          GTT    TAT        TTG    TTT
  7      — — — — — — — — — Val — Tyr — — — — Leu — Phe — — —                              +*             -

                          ACT TTA AAC    TAT CTA ATT    AGC
 28      — — — — — — — — — Thr Leu Asn — Tyr Leu Ile — Ser — —                           +*             -

                          ACT TTA AAC    TAT    ATT
  5      — — — — — — — — — Thr Leu Asn — Tyr — Ile — — — —                                +              +
```

Figure 1

Properties of altered influenza surface antigens. (*A*) Schematic representation of HA, NA, and their derived deletions (dl). (■) Hydrophobic terminal sequences are indicated on the left (amino terminus) and on the right (carboxyl terminus). Deletion mutants were constructed from their respective DNA in the SV40 vector. Polypeptide products from recombinant-infected AGMK cells were characterized for glycosylation, detection at the cell surface, and extracellular secretion. (*B*) Characterization of HAs containing amino acid substitutions in the signal sequences. The aminoterminal sequences cleaved (arrow) from the wild-type HA are presented. Altered HAs from a deletion mutant and several substitution mutants were analyzed as described.

ious sequences. Similar construction and isolation of mutants of cloned neuraminidase (NA) DNA were also performed, and their polypeptide products were characterized. In this study, deletion of sequences within the amino terminus of the NA gene affected insertion of NA into the outer cell membrane, as well as its pattern of glycosylation. This series of experiments illustrate that a wide range of mutants exhibiting different biochemical and functional properties can be generated by genetic surgery of cloned DNA derived from a specific gene segment.

Allele Replacement

For recombinant DNA techniques to prove useful in immunoprophylaxis of influenza, it is essential that mutations generated in cloned influenza DNA be transferred into the influenza virus so that the mutant viruses can be characterized and evaluated for their usefulness in vaccination. This requires that the cloned DNA be converted back to virion RNA packaged in the virion. To test this possibility, we performed influenza gene rescue experiments, so-called allele replacement, using recombinants of HA-SV40 and NA-SV40 because of the ease of detection of these two surface antigens. Also, specific antisera that effectively neutralized virus bearing HA or NA of the coinfecting virus could be used to facilitate detection of reassortant virus that had undergone replacement of a surface glycoprotein allele.

Permissive AGMK cells were infected sequentially with an HA-SV40 or NA-SV40 recombinant and influenza A/WSN/33 (H1N1), which bears surface antigens of another subtype. Infected cell lysates were passaged once and neutralized with antiserum to remove parental virus. This protocol should allow us to detect reassortants that had acquired an RNA segment derived from a recombinant transcript that replaced the corresponding WSN gene. When HA-SV40 that produced positive-strand influenza transcripts was tested in this manner, rescued virus could not be identified. Using NA-SV40 recombinants that produced either a positive-strand or negative-strand NA RNA transcript, it was also not possible to detect rescued virus.

In view of the evidence that positive full-length influenza virus RNA transcripts produced by an M-SV40 recombinant are flanked by SV40 control sequences (Fig. 2) (Lamb and Lai 1982), it is possible that the viral replicase provided by influenza virus coinfection did not recognize 3'-terminal influenza virus sequences and initiate virion RNA synthesis. On the other hand, assuming that negative RNA transcripts were produced in a similar manner from the recombinant DNA with the influenza DNA insert in the other orientation, failure of rescue would suggest that the transcripts containing flanking sequences were neither replicated nor encapsidated and packaged in virions. Precise terminal sequences may be a prerequisite for transcription, replication, and encapsidation.

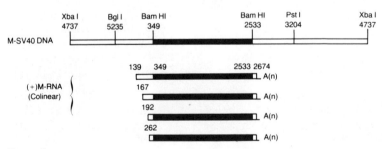

Figure 2
Transcription of cloned full-length M DNA in an SV40 vector. Full-length cloned DNA coding for the influenza virus matrix protein (M) was inserted into the SV40 late region (between SV40 nucleotides 349 and 2533) of an expression vector using *Bam*HI linkers. Transcription from the late SV40 promoter yielded positive-strand M RNA transcripts from the recombinant that contained the insert in the sense orientation. Colinear M RNA products from AGMK cells were flanked by SV40 sequences at both termini. Several M RNA species that varied at their 5' ends and terminated at the common poly(A) site are shown.

Persistent Expression of Cloned Influenza Virus DNA

Although the SV40-AGMK cell system readily produced influenza virus RNA transcripts and in turn the encoded polypeptides from a cloned influenza DNA segment, the cytolytic effect of SV40 infection might limit the use of such expressed functions for biological studies such as gene rescue and functional complementation of defective mutants. To circumvent this difficulty, we have initiated a collaborative effort with Drs. P. Howley and M.F. Law (National Cancer Institute) to obtain expression of cloned genes in persistently infected, stably transformed cells using a bovine papilloma virus DNA vector. Recombinants of BPV-NP (see legend to Fig. 3) were constructed for transformation of a suitable mouse cell line (C127). Transformed cells produced what appeared to be functional NP as indicated by its molecular size, specific immunoprecipitation, localization in the nucleus, and phosphorylation (Fig. 3). To extend this approach to a cell system that is permissive for influenza virus infection and hence can be employed for gene rescue or functional complementation, we also succeeded in obtaining persistent expression of NP in a primate-derived CV-1 cell line using the neomycin coselection procedure developed by Southern and Berg (Stanford University). Using indirect immunofluorescence for detection of antigen, it was observed that NP was synthesized in 2–3% of neomycin-resistant cells. Single cells are being cloned

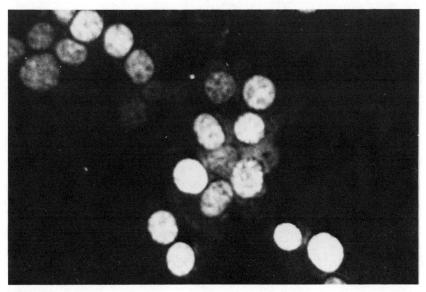

Figure 3
Immunofluorescence detection of influenza nucleoprotein in mouse cells persistently infected with cloned DNA. Recombinant DNA was constructed between bovine papilloma virus (BPV) DNA and cloned DNA specifying the influenza nucleoprotein (NP). Metallothionine promoter and SV40 poly(A)-addition sequences were also inserted for active transcription of the NP gene. Mouse cells (line C127) were transformed with the BPV-NP DNA recombinant. Transformed cells produced NP in the nucleus as detected by an immunofluorescence assay.

to obtain persistent expression of NP at a higher frequency. Cell lines persistently expressing a cloned influenza gene should be suitable for the growth of naturally occurring viral mutants bearing a defect such as a deletion mutation in that gene. This type of complementation should enable us to select for such mutants that can be further assessed for restriction of growth and attenuation. In this manner, it may be possible to identify stable, naturally occurring deletion mutations that can be used to confer attenuation on epidemic or pandemic viruses by gene reassortment.

SUMMARY

Deletion mutants of influenza virus offer an attractive alternative for stabilization of the attenuation phenotype. Construction of such mutants requires that genetic manipulation be performed at the cloned influenza DNA level and that the modified DNA must be converted to RNA and transferred to an infectious influenza virion. Gene-rescue experiments indicate that transcripts of either the positive-strand or the negative-strand influenza RNA synthesized from cloned SV40 recombinants failed to reassort with the corresponding gene of a coinfecting influenza virus. It is possible the 5'- and 3'-flanking SV40 sequences contained in the recombinant DNA transcripts may have impaired the rescue event. To provide a specific terminal sequence in the RNA transcripts, further removal of flanking sequences in the recombinant will be required. This will entail the design of a new vector for introduction and specific transcription of cloned DNA in suitable host cells. In this manner, recombinant DNA transcripts would be chemically as well as genetically similar to the viral RNA species and therefore functionally active. Alternatively, deletion mutants that can be used to confer attenuation might be selected from naturally occurring or laboratory-passaged strains using a cell system permissive for growth of these viral mutants. We have had some success in the development of persistently transfected stable cell lines for functional expression of cloned influenza DNA. In this manner, it may be possible to isolate defined viral mutants or eventually strategically engineer influenza virus genes.

ACKNOWLEDGMENTS

We thank Ms. Jo Ann Berndt and Ms. Salome Kruger for their technical assistance. We are also grateful to Drs. Brian Murphy, Robert Lamb, Michael Sveda, Kenji Sekikawa, and Joanna Hansen for their helpful discussions and valuable contributions during the course of this work.

REFERENCES

Lai, C.-J., L.J. Markoff, S. Zimmerman, B. Cohen, J.A. Berndt, and R.M. Chanock. 1980. Cloning DNA sequences from influenza viral RNA segments. *Proc. Natl. Acad. Sci.* **77:** 210.

Lamb, R.A. and C.-J. Lai. 1982. Spliced and unspliced mRNAs synthesized from cloned influenza virus M DNA in an SV40 vector: Expression of the influenza virus membrane protein (M1). *Virology* **123:** 237.

Sveda, M.M. and C.-J. Lai. 1981. Functional expression in primate cells of cloned DNA coding for the hemagglutinin surface glycoprotein of influenza virus. *Proc. Natl. Acad. Sci.* **78:** 5499.

Alterations in Pathogenicity
of Influenza Virus
through Reassortment

Rudolf Rott, Christoph Scholtissek,
and Hans-Dieter Klenk
Institut für Virologie
Justus-Liebig-Universität Giessen
D-6300 Giessen, West Germany

One important consequence of the particular genomic organization of influenza viruses is that the eight separate RNA segments that code for specific gene products can be reassorted freely when a single host cell is infected by two different viruses (for references, see Palese 1977; Scholtissek 1978). Taking advantage of the fact that through reassortment, biological properties of the virus are changed, reassortment seems to offer a significant advantage over all other techniques for rapid and efficient production of live vaccine viruses. The deliberate mating of two or more viruses, each bearing a desired trait, can easily be carried out and an appropriate progeny virus can be selected (Kilbourne et al. 1967). Such a procedure obviates tedious adaptation until appropriate mutants, if any, become manifest. Candidates for live vaccine strains would be reassortants containing the hemagglutinin (HA) and neuraminidase of the current epidemic virus that were still infectious and immunogenic, having appropriate capacity for replication, but not causing clinical disease. Of course, all these characteristics would have to be stable.

There are some technical problems in the construction of such reassortants that can be overcome by application of appropriate methods. One of the difficulties encountered in producing reassortants is that owing to intrinsic interference between some parent strains, simultaneous double infection might not be possible. This difficulty can be obviated by ensuring optimal growth conditions (Rott et al. 1981). Another complication is that because of the existence of heterozygotes, the reassortants must be carried through several plaque passages in order to obtain a homogeneous virus population. Furthermore, our experience has been that in a given cell system, for unknown reasons not all the expected possibilities of reassortment can be realized (Rott et al. 1976).

It is predictable that reassortment of genes will reduce the probability of expression of any polygenic characteristics such as pathogenicity. However, the opposite possibility cannot be excluded, since new phenotypes with increased pathogenicity might appear by reassortment. Therefore, it is highly desirable to have a reliable test system available to examine the correlation between the gene constellation and pathogenicity in the laboratory.

In the last few years, our group has concentrated mainly on the question of whether a certain gene combination of an influenza virus will reflect its pathogenic properties (Rott 1979). Pathogenicity in this context means the clear manifestation of a clinically overt disease. This easily detectable and reliable clinical marker may be readily studied in the avian system.

The avian system offers the advantages that one can work in the natural host of the virus and that naturally occurring avian influenza viruses are available that differ in pathogenicity. Highly pathogenic strains exist among the H7 and H5 subtypes. As far as we know, virus strains of all the other subtypes are nonpathogenic for chickens (Easterday 1975; Bosch et al. 1979).

One must be cautious, however, not to generalize the findings obtained in the avian system. The overall clinical manifestations of the organ system involved are not identical in fowl and in mammals. The disease in mammals is virtually always a result of localized infection of the respiratory tract epithelium, whereas the disease in fowl infected with pathogenic viruses is commonly associated with a systemic infection and death. Even if the course of infection in fowl is similar to that in mammals, the host specificity might be retained, and a given virus pathogenic for one species will not cause clinical manifestations in another host.

HA as a Determinant for Pathogenicity

The course of the disease in fowl depends to a large extent on the spread of infection in the organism. It was found that pathogenicity of the avian viruses correlates with the susceptibility of the precursor HA polypeptide to proteolytic cleavage into the subunits HA_1 and HA_2, which is essential for the formation of infectious virus. The HA of the nonpathogenic strains is cleaved only in a few types of host cells. Therefore, in most cell types, noninfectious virus is formed and, in this way, spread of infection in the organism is inhibited. On the other hand, the HA of the pathogenic strains is cleaved in a wide range of cell types in different tissues, thus allowing rapid spread. In this way, HA has been shown to be the major determinant of pathogenicity of naturally occurring avian influenza viruses (for references, see Klenk and Rott 1980; Rott 1982).

Gene Constellation and Pathogenicity

Studies with reassortants obtained after double infection in vitro revealed that in viruses constructed artificially in this way, pathogenicity is due not only to the structure of the HA cleavage site, but is of polygenic nature (McCahon and Schild 1972; Mayer et al. 1973; Rott et al. 1976). In these cases, the HA gene of a pathogenic virus is a necessary, but not sufficient, condition for pathogenicity.

This conclusion was reinforced by genetic analysis of a large number of reassortants obtained from fowl plague virus (FPV), highly pathogenic for chickens, and other nonpathogenic influenza virus prototype strains from birds and mammals. It was shown that the acquisition of single genes from different influenza viruses might attenuate FPV for chickens (Scholtissek et al. 1977). The pathogenic properties of the reassortants are found to be determined by the particular gene that was exchanged as well as by the virus strain from which this gene was derived. For example (Table 1), if the gene coding for PB2 of FPV is replaced by the allelic gene of the influenza virus strain PR8, pathogenicity is lost, whereas the PB2 gene transferred from swine influenza virus yielded reassortants as pathogenic as the wild-type FPV. On the other hand, if the gene coding for PB1 originates from swine influenza virus and the other seven genes from FPV, pathogenicity is lost again, whereas replacement of the PB1 gene by yet another influenza virus yields highly pathogenic reassortants. These findings confirmed earlier conclusions of other investigators that pathogenicity cannot be confined to a particular gene (for references, see Burnet 1959; Kilbourne 1963).

With multiple gene exchanges, the chance for attenuation of FPV corresponded, in principle, with the number of genes derived from other influenza viruses (Rott et al. 1978). This was not the case, however, when related genes were exchanged. It is our experience that the closer the genes of parent viruses are genetically related, the better the replacements of particular genes are tolerated. Furthermore, when the complete set of genes coding for the polymerase complex was derived from one or the other parent virus, the reassortants were, in general, pathogenic. In contrast, all nonpathogenic reassortants had a mixed RNA polymerase complex (Rott and Scholtissek 1982). This was the case whether these genes ultimately came from either nonpathogenic or pathogenic strains. Reassortment, even between highly pathogenic parent strains, may lead to pathogenic as well as nonpathogenic isolates. As shown in Table 2, loss of pathogenicity seems to be again dependent on the genes involved in viral RNA synthesis (Rott et al. 1979).

These data indicate that a certain gene constellation specifies pathogenicity or lack of pathogenicity irrespective of the character of the individual parent virus. Therefore, it does not seem necessary to use an attenuated master strain for reassortment so that the reassortant can acquire attenuation.

Table 1
Influence of Single Gene Exchanges on Pathogenicity of FPV for Chickens

| FPV gene exchanged | Genes derived from | | | |
	PR8	A2 Singapore	swine influenza	virus N
PB2	○	◑	●	◑
PB1	◑	●	○	●
PA	◑	◑	◑	●

Chickens were inoculated intramuscularly with 1 ml of infectious allantoic fluid containing 128 HA units. (●) Highly pathogenic; (◑) weakly pathogenic; (○) nonpathogenic. (For details, see Scholtissek et al. 1977.)

Table 2
Correlation between Gene Constellation and Pathogenicity of Recombinants between FPV (H7N1) and Avian Influenza Virus A/Turkey/England/63 (H7N3)

Isolate no.	Pathogenic for chicken	Derivation of genes from either FPV (●) or turkey (○)							
		PB2	PB1	PA	HA	NP	NA	M	NS
2	+	○	○	○	○	○	○	○	○
21	+	○	○	○	○	○	○	○	○
8	+	○	○	○	○	○	○	●	○
18	+	○	○	○	○	○	○	●	○
12	+	○	○	○	●	○	●	●	○
14	+	○	○	○	●	○	●	●	○
13	+	○	●	●	●	●	●	●	○
9	−	●	○	○	○	○	●	○	○
19	−	●	○	○	○	○	●	○	○
22	−	●	○	○	○	○	●	○	○
1	−	○	○	●	●	○	○	○	●
17	−	○	○	●	●	○	○	○	●
15	−	●	○	●	●	○	○	○	○
3	−	●	○	○	●	●	○	●	○
10	−	●	○	●	●	○	○	●	○
16	−	●	●	●	●	○	○	●	○
23	−	●	●	○	●	●	●	●	●
24	−	●	○	●	●	●	●	●	●

For details, see Rott et al. (1979).

Increase of Pathogenicity by Reassortment

Reassortment can also lead to increase in pathogenicity. This cannot, however, be detected in the fowl system. As mentioned above, the pathogenic property of avian influenza viruses with a cleavable HA is extremely high and cannot be further increased, whereas nonpathogenic virus strains with noncleavable HA can never induce clinical disease. Therefore, we used neurovirulence for mice as a pathogenicity marker.

It could be demonstrated by reassortment of FPV (A/FPV/Rostock [H7N1]) and A/England/1/61 (H2N2) or FPV and A/PR/8/34 (H1N1), which by themselves are nonneurovirulent for mice, that reassortants can be isolated that are neurovirulent after intracerebral inoculation (Vallbracht et al. 1979). Analysis of the gene composition of the neurovirulent isolates revealed that all of these reassortants possessed an avian virus HA that could be shown to be activated by proteolytic cleavage in a broad spectrum of host cells. The composition of the other genes involved in neurovirulence depended on the parent virus strains used as donor for reassortment. It seems, however, that again the genes coding for viral RNA synthesis are important in this context (Scholtissek et al. 1979). Most interestingly, virus isolates with a combination of the HA and M genes from FPV and certain polymerase genes from the human influenza viruses produced systemic infection in the mouse with involvement of the central nervous system after intraperitoneal infection (Vallbracht et al. 1980; Bonin and Scholtissek 1983).

Changes in the Host Range by Reassortment

The studies on neurovirulence obtained by reassortment showed that neurotropic reassortants acquire a new host range in vitro that might be an essential property of the virus in the establishment of a systemic infection in vivo (Vallbracht et al. 1979, 1980). A strict correlation could be demonstrated between the ability of an isolate to propagate in mouse embryo fibroblasts in vitro and induction of a systemic infection in the mouse. These properties could not be segregated, even by backcrosses or crosses between reassortants. Since none of the parent viruses infected mouse embryo fibroblasts productively, the highly neurovirulent reassortants exhibited a new broadened host range in cell culture.

That changes in host-cell range resulting from reassortment might be paralleled by changes in pathogenicity is also suggested by the following finding. It could be shown that after mixed infection of an FPV mutant and A/Hong Kong/68, isolates containing the HA gene of FPV and the NP gene of Hong Kong virus were nonpathogenic and failed to plaque on chick embryo cells, although they could still do so in MDCK cells. When one of the reassortants was mated with another avian influenza virus (A/Chick/Germany/N/49 [H10N7]) or A/Equine/Miami/1/63 (H3N8), some of the progeny could once again produce plaques on chicken cells and were pathogenic for chicken (Scholtissek et al. 1978).

It is tempting to speculate that such a complete change in host range and pathogenicity by one round of gene assortment could be a possible explanation for the epidemiological disappearance and reappearance of influenza viruses. An example for this proposal could be the reappearance of H1N1 viruses 27 years after this subtype had been displaced by the H2N2 virus.

Genetic Stability of Reassortants

In nonpathogenic reassortants, reversion to pathogenic properties by mutation is, in principle, something to be reckoned with. This was shown in experiments in which pathogenicity for the chicken of a number of nonpathogenic reassortants obtained from different parent influenza viruses could be reactivated by passaging serially under von Magnus conditions at the nonpermissive temperature (see below) for such isolates at 41°C (Rott et al. 1983). As shown in Figure 1, the infectivity of nonpathogenic reassortants declined rapidly as expected under these conditions. However, with most reassortants tested, the infectivity thereafter increased with further passages, the number of which depended on the reassortants used, and varied from experiment to experiment. This means that nonpathogenic reassortants have lost their temperature sensitivity under this selection pressure of undiluted passages at 41°C. Most interestingly, all isolates obtained in this way had regained pathogenic properties, although the degree of pathogenicity varied. After intramuscular inoculation, some isolates killed the chickens 2–3 days after infection, like the highly pathogenic wild-type viruses, whereas with other isolates, chickens died only after a prolonged incubation or became sick, but did not die, during a 14-day observation (Table 3). The pathogenicity-reactivated reassortants showed no change in gene constellation (Table 4). Thus, the reappearance of pathogenicity must have occurred by mutation. The fact that in repeated experiments the time of appearance of highly

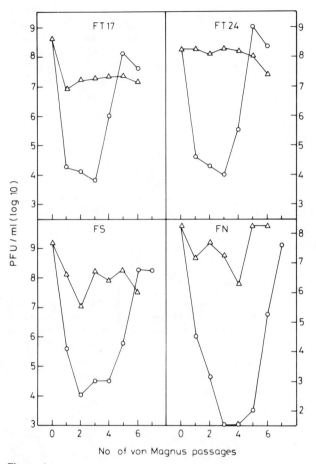

Figure 1
Behavior of infectivity of different influenza virus reassortants during undiluted passages at 37°C (△) or 41°C (○). (For details, see Rott et al. 1983.)

pathogenic reassortants varied indicates that this is a random event and possibly more than one mutation is required for this change. It is not yet known by which mechanism of mutagenesis pathogenic viruses can be generated from nonpathogenic reassortants, or how high the reactivation rate is. To estimate the implications of this phenomenon for a possible live vaccine generated by reassortments, additional data will be needed.

Suppressor Recombination

Unfortunately, restoration of pathogenicity is also possible as a result of extragenic suppression of temperature-sensitive (*ts*) defects in viral genes by mutation or reassortment (Murphy et al. 1980; Tolpin et al. 1981; Scholtissek and Spring 1982). It has been shown that a *ts* defect can be phenotypically reverted by replacement of a different influenza virus gene. For instance, a *ts* defect in

Table 3
Pathogenicity for Chicken of Influenza Virus Reassortants before and after von Magnus Passages

		Pathogenicity[c]		
			after von Magnus passages at	
Reassortants[a]	*Gene constellation*[b]	*before*	*37°C*	*41°C*
FT1	TTFFTTTF	−	−	+ (4)
FT3	FTTFFTFT	−	−	±
FT15	FTFFTTTT	−	−	±
FT17	TTFFTTTF	−	−	+ (6)
FT22	FTTTTFTT	−	−	+ (2)
FT23	FFTFFFFF	−	+ (7)	+ (2)
FT24	FFTFFFFF	−	−	+ (3)
FS	FSFFFSFF	−	−	+ (5)
FE	FFFFEEFF	−	−	+ (7)
FN	FFNFFNNN	−	−	±

For details, see Rott et al. (1983).
[a]Reassortants were obtained after mixed infections with the parent viruses. F, A/Fowl Plague/Rostock/34 (H7N1); T, A/Turkey/England/63 (H7N3); N, A/Chick/Germany/N/49 (H10N7); S, A/Swine/1976/31 (H1N1); E, A/Equine/1/63 (H3N8).
[b]Letters indicate the parental source of the genes and are arranged according to the electrophoretic migration rates of the RNA of A/Fowl/Plague/Rostock. The order designates the genes in the following sequence: PB2, PB1, PA, HA, NP, NA, M, and NS.
[c]Chickens die (+) after infection (no. of days), or become sick (±), or showed no signs of illness (−) during a 14-day observation period.

the NS gene of FPV mutants could be rescued by reassortment by the PR8 strain. The gene of the *ts* mutants that was replaced was, however, not the NS gene as might have been expected, but the PB1 gene. By backcrosses with the parental strain, it could be shown that all of these reassortants still contained the defect in the NS gene, in spite of the wild-type phenotype (Scholtissek and Spring 1982).

In such suppressor recombinations, it is expected that the defective gene or gene product in some way can cooperate with the gene product of the replaced gene. Thus, it is not sufficient to introduce by reassortment a gene with a defect into another virus strain and then expect this new reassortant to exhibit the corresponding phenotype. Within a new gene constellation, this defect might be suppressed.

Selection for Optimal Genomic Composition

There is hardly any doubt that new human and especially avian influenza viruses can arise in nature by segmented genomic reassortment (for references, see Beare 1982; Hinshaw and Webster 1982). It can be assumed that these viruses would have an optimally functioning genome, which is necessary for optimal growth in their hosts. This appears to be the case for all naturally occurring avian virus strains because, in contrast to the reassortants obtained in vitro, in the avian viruses only the HA decides whether or not these viruses are pathogenic.

Table 4
Gene Constellation of Reassortants before and after Undiluted Passages at 41°C

Reassortants[a]	von Magnus passages at 41°C	Pathogenic for chicken[b]	PB2	PB1	PA	HA	NP	NA	M	NS
FT1	−	−	T	T	F	F	T	T	T	F
	+	+	T	T	F	F	T	T	T	F
FT22	−	−	F	T	T	T	T	F	T	T
	+	+	F	T	T	T	T	F	T	T
FT23	−	−	F	F	T	F	F	F	F	F
	+	+	F	F	T	F	F	F	F	F
FT24	−	−	F	T	F	F	F	F	F	F
	+	+	F	T	F	F	F	F	F	F

[a]Designations correspond to that of virus reassortants between FPV and Turkey/England (FT) described by Rott et al. (1979).
[b]Chickens died between 2 and 4 days after infection (+) or survived an observation period of 14 days without showing signs of disease (−).

This implies that the selection for optimal genomic composition must have taken place in the infected avian organism.

The question arises as to what selective pressure determines this outcome. We were able to show in a series of experiments that the body temperature of the bird at 41°C represents the selective barrier for the formation of reassortants pathogenic for the chicken (Rott et al. 1982). Pathogenic reassortants grow equally well at 37°C and 41°C, whereas the nonpathogenic reassortants have a significantly lower growth rate at 41°C (Fig. 2). As a consequence of double infection in vitro with two different influenza viruses at the elevated temperature, reassortants are selected that are exclusively pathogenic for chickens. On the other hand, when mixed infection is performed at 37°C, the progeny are non-pathogenic.

The results of these experiments, which were performed to permit mutual reassortment of all viral genes, argue again for the genes coding for viral RNA synthesis as being significant for pathogenicity. Hybridization studies with reassortants derived from FPV and A/Turkey/England/63 revealed that at 41°C, such reassortants are selected that possess all the four genes coding for the polymerase complex from one wild-type parent virus (Table 5). The behavior of reassortants at 41°C is therefore a useful marker for rapid in vitro selection of pathogenic or nonpathogenic reassortants that should be helpful in preparing live vaccine viruses very rapidly after the occurrence of a new pathogenic influenza virus in birds.

CONCLUSIONS

The following are implications of our observations with reassortant avian influenza viruses for pathogenicity:

1. To be pathogenic for the chicken, a virus must possess an HA that is activated by proteolytic cleavage in a broad range of different host cells; hence, virus is spread in the organism, leading to a systemic infection.

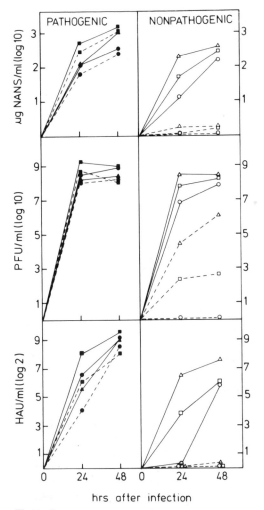

hrs after infection

Figure 2
Growth at 37°C or 41°C of representative influenza virus reassortants pathogenic or non-pathogenic for chicken. Chick embryo cells were infected with a multiplicity of about 3×10^4 and kept at 37°C (———) or 41°C (— — —). (▲, ■, ●) Yields of different pathogenic reassortants; (△, □, ○) different nonpathogenic reassortants. (For details, see Rott et al. 1982.)

2. In each reassortment, a specific gene constellation responsible for the pathogenic properties might be achieved, which is dependent on the parent virus strains used. Therefore, there is no general rule which gene or genes have to be replaced in order to increase or attenuate pathogenicity.
3. The composition of genes coding for the polymerase complex, nonetheless, seems to be especially important for pathogenic properties.
4. An alteration in pathogenicity through reassortment can be paralleled by changes in host range.

Table 5
Correlation among Gene Constellation, Growth at 41°C, and Pathogenicity for Chicken of Influenza Virus Reassortants

Reassortants[a]	Gene constellation[b]	Virus growth at 41°C	Pathogenic for chicken
FT8	TTTTTTFT	+	+
FT12	TTTFTFFT	+	+
FT13	FFFFFFFT	+	+
FT14	TTTFTFFT	+	+
FT1	TTFFTTTF	−	−
FT3	FTTFFTFT	−	−
FT9	FTTTTFTT	−	−
FT10	FTFFTTFT	−	−
FT15	FTFFTTTT	−	−
FT17	TTFFTTTF	−	−
FT22	FTTTTFTT	−	−
FT23	FFTFFFFF	−	−

For details, see Rott et al. (1982).
[a]FT are reassortants between FPV (F) and A/Turkey/England/63 (T) (Rott et al. 1979).
[b]Genes were ordered according to the electrophoretic migration rates of the RNA segments of FPV (Scholtissek 1978).

5. An increase in pathogenicity following reassortment between nonpathogenic parents is possible.
6. Initially nonpathogenic reassortants can mutate into pathogenic ones under von Magnus conditions.
7. Reassortants pathogenic for chickens are selected by the body temperature of the bird.

These findings will have consequences for the development of live vaccines from human influenza virus. With the techniques currently available, it should not be difficult to obtain by reassortment attenuated viruses for the various subtypes of human influenza strains. The possibility that an attenuated master strain may not be needed for the production of live vaccine reassortants has widened the scope for obtaining viruses with optimal biological and antigenic properties.

Since reassortants that have increased pathogenicity can also be produced, one must always consider the hazard that might be associated with reassortants that could develop or retain pathogenicity for man. Reassortants deriving the HA of pathogenic avian influenza viruses are of particular concern. Such reassortants are predestined to produce a systemic infection even in mammals.

Although there is a certain amount of evidence that, with human viruses also, the genes coding for the polymerase complex have a particular significance for pathogenicity, the current information on human influenza reassortants (like that found in other virus-host systems) does not allow us to deduce any rules by which gene replacement ultimately will lead to attenuation (for references, see Beare 1982). This indeed is not to be expected. We have learned that replacement of genetically highly related allelic genes might be without any consequence for biological properties of corresponding reassortants. On the other hand, there is evidence that certain biological properties might be determined by two or more genes. The cooperative interplay between such genes or gene products might be severely affected when one or the other gene is replaced. In this context, the phenomenon of suppressor recombination and pathogenicity reactivation under certain selection pressure must be remembered.

Altogether, there seems little chance of finding a specific genetic marker for pathogenicity with influenza viruses. This is especially true for human influenza viruses for which no laboratory system is available to test pathogenicity. Since change in host range could be shown to be paralleled with alterations in pathogenicity, it is questionable whether experimental animals can replace experiments on human volunteers. Because of all of these difficulties, one has to ask whether the production of reassortants for use as live vaccines has fulfilled the goals expected of them. This question can be extended to ask whether, in view of the plasticity of the influenza virus genome, a live vaccine can even be completely safe. Much more work will be needed in order to show what the probability of undesirable genetic events in an influenza-virus-immunized human population might be.

ACKNOWLEDGMENTS

Original work was done in collaboration with our co-workers identified in the respective publications and was supported by the Deutsche Forschungsgemeinschaft (Sonderforschungsbereich 47).

REFERENCES

Beare, A.S. 1982. Research into the immunization of humans against influenza by means of living viruses. In *Basic and applied influenza research* (ed. A.S. Beare), p. 211. CSR Press, Boca Raton, Florida.

Bonin, J. and C. Scholtissek. 1983. Mouse neurotropic recombinants of influenza A viruses. *Arch. Virol.* **75:** 255.

Bosch, F.X., M. Orlich, H.-D. Klenk, and R. Rott. 1979. The structure of the hemagglutinin, a determinant for the pathogenicity of influenza virus. *Virology* **95:** 197.

Burnet, F.M. 1959. Genetic interaction between animal viruses. In *The viruses* (ed. F.M. Burnet and W.M. Stanley), vol. 3, p. 275. Academic Press, New York.

Easterday, B.C. 1975. Animal influenza. In *Influenza viruses and influenza* (ed. E.D. Kilbourne), p. 449. Academic Press, New York.

Hinshaw, V.C. and R.G. Webster. 1982. The natural history of influenza A viruses. In *Basic and applied influenza research* (ed. A.S. Beare), p. 79. CSR Press, Boca Raton, Florida.

Kilbourne, E.D. 1963. Influenza virus genetics. *Prog. Med. Virol.* **5:** 79.

Kilbourne, E.D., F.S. Lief, J.L. Schulman, R.I. Jahiel, and W.G. Laver. 1967. Antigenic hybrids of influenza viruses and their implication. *Perspect. Virol.* **5:** 87.

Klenk, H.-D. and R. Rott. 1980. Cotranslational and posttranslational processing of viral glycoproteins. *Curr. Top. Microbiol. Immunol.* **90:** 19.

Mayer, V., J.L. Schulman, and E.D. Kilbourne. 1973. Nonlinkage of neurovirulence exclusively to viral hemagglutinin or neuraminidase in genetic recombinants of A/NWS (H0N1) influenza virus. *J. Virol.* **11:** 272.

McCahon, D. and G.C. Schild. 1972. Segregation of antigenic and biological characteristics during influenza virus recombination. *J. Gen. Virol.* **15:** 73.

Murphy, B.R., M.D. Tolpin, J.G. Massicot, H.W. Kim, R.H. Parrott, and R.M. Chanock. 1980. Escape of highly defective influenza A virus mutant from its temperature-sensitive phenotype by extragenic suppression and other types of mutation. *Ann. N.Y. Acad. Sci.* **354:** 172.

Palese, P. 1977. The genes of influenza virus. *Cell* **10:** 1.

Rott, R. 1979. Molecular basis of infectivity and pathogenicity of myxovirus. *Arch. Virol.* **59:** 285.

―――. 1982. Determinants of influenza virus pathogenicity. *Hoppe-Seyler's Z. Physiol. Chem.* **363:** 1273.

Rott, R. and C. Scholtissek 1982. The molecular basis of biological properties of influenza viruses. In *Basic and applied influenza research* (ed. A.S. Beare), p. 189. CRC Press, Boca Raton, Florida.

Rott, R., M. Orlich, and C. Scholtissek. 1976. Attenuation of pathogenicity of fowl plague virus by recombination with other influenza viruses nonpathogenic for fowl: Nonexclusive dependence of pathogenicity on hemagglutinin and neuraminidase of the virus. *J. Virol.* **19:** 54.

―――. 1979. Correlation of pathogenicity and gene constellation of influenza viruses. III. Nonpathogenic recombinants derived from highly pathogenic parent strains. *J. Gen. Virol.* **44:** 471.

―――. 1981. Intrinsic interference between swine influenza and fowl plague virus. *Arch. Virol.* **69:** 25.

―――. 1982. Differences in multiplication at elevated temperature of influenza virus recombinants pathogenic and nonpathogenic for chicken. *Virology* **120:** 215.

―――. 1983. Pathogenicity reactivation of nonpathogenic influenza virus recombinants under von Magnus conditions. *Virology* **126:** 459.

Rott, R., C. Scholtissek, H.-D. Klenk, and M. Orlich. 1978. Structure and pathogenicity of influenza viruses. In *Negative strand viruses and the host cell* (ed. B.W.J. Mahy and R.D. Barry), p. 653. Academic Press, New York.

Scholtissek, C. 1978. The genome of the influenza virus. *Curr. Top. Microbiol. Immunol.* **80:** 139.

Scholtissek, C. and S. Spring. 1982. Extragenic suppression of temperature-sensitive mutations in RNA segment 8 by replacement of different RNA segments with those of other influenza A virus prototype strains. *Virology* **118:** 28.

Scholtissek, C., I. Koennecke, and R. Rott. 1978. Host range recombinants of fowl plague (influenza A) virus. *Virology* **91:** 79.

Scholtissek, C., R. Rott, M. Orlich, E. Harms, and W. Rohde. 1977. Correlation of pathogenicity and gene constellation of an influenza A virus (fowl plague). I. Exchange of a single gene. *Virology* **81:** 74.

Scholtissek, C., A. Vallbracht, B. Flehmig, and R. Rott. 1979. Correlation of pathogenicity and gene constellation of influenza A viruses. II. Highly neurovirulent recombinants derived from non-neurovirulent or weakly neurovirulent parent virus strains. *Virology* **95:** 492.

Tolpin, M.D., J.G. Massicot, M.G. Mullinix, H.W. Kim, R.H. Parrott, R.M. Chanock, and B.R. Murphy. 1981. Genetic factors associated with loss of the temperature-sensitive phenotype of the influenza A/Alaska/77-ts-1 A2 recombinant during growth *in vivo*. *Virology* **112:** 505.

Vallbracht, A., B. Flehmig, and H.-J. Gerth. 1979. Influenza virus: Appearance of high mouse-neurovirulent recombinants. *Intervirology* **11:** 16.

Vallbracht, A., C. Scholtissek, B. Flehmig, and H.-J. Gerth. 1980. Recombination of influenza A strains with fowl plague virus can change pneumotropism for mice to a generalized infection with involvement of the central nervous system. *Virology* **107:** 452.

Evolution of the Oral Polio Vaccine Strains in Humans Occurs by Both Mutation and Intramolecular Recombination

Olen M. Kew and Baldev K. Nottay
Division of Viral Diseases
Centers for Disease Control
Atlanta, Georgia 30333

Polioviruses are capable of rapid evolution upon replication in humans. This process is characteristic of both wild strains during epidemic transmission and the live-virus vaccines during growth in vaccinees (Kew et al. 1981). For the vaccine strains, the rapid evolution is manifested by changes in genetic and antigenic characters and by occasional increases in neurovirulence, which, in very rare instances, result in cases of paralytic disease among vaccinees or their contacts. In previous studies, we examined vaccine-derived case isolates by oligonucleotide fingerprinting of virion RNA and SDS-polyacrylamide gel electrophoresis (SDS-PAGE) of the viral intracellular proteins. Different case isolates appeared to have evolved along independent pathways of variation, involving changes in both capsid and noncapsid proteins. For many case isolates, the extent of genomic change suggested that multiple rounds of mutation and selection had occurred. However, it was also found that neurovirulence could potentially be restored to the vaccine strain by a small number of mutational steps (Kew et al. 1981).

To follow the dynamics of polio vaccine variation in humans, as a model for the changes occurring in paralytic cases, isolates from normal, presumably typical, immunizations were examined. In a companion study, some highly modified vaccine-associated case isolates were found to be not only multisite mutants, but also intramolecular recombinants of the vaccine strains.

Periodic Selection of Sabin-1-derived Mutational Variants in Normal Vaccinees

Nakano et al. (1963) have described serologic studies of isolates collected serially during 2–28 days after immunization of healthy infants with monovalent oral

357

polio vaccine type 1 (MOPV1). Periodic selection for new antigenic variants of Sabin 1 was observed in four (infants 1–4) of the eight infants studied. In these children, antigenic drift of the vaccine typically became evident at 8–10 days postvaccination, and new predominating variants arose over short (2–7 days) intervals. These early serologic findings have recently been confirmed by analyses using neutralizing monoclonal antibodies (Humphrey et al. 1982; Crainic et al. 1983) and extended by biochemical studies (Table 1). Oligonucleotide fingerprint analyses of all isolates from infants 1 and 3 indicated that amplification of new genotypic variants occurred as early as 6 days postvaccination and that these were replaced by other variants at later times. The only altered oligonucleotides that have been mapped (Kitamura et al. 1981) derived from the region encoding polypeptide X. The function of this noncapsid protein is unknown, and the possible significance of these findings is unclear. SDS-PAGE of the viral proteins of the same isolates showed successive alterations in the mobilities of VP1 beginning at day 10.

The sequences of nucleotides 1–375 of the VP1 region were determined for Mahoney, Sabin 1, and eight isolates from infant vaccinees 1, 2, and 3 (Fig. 1). This region was selected for analysis because it encompassed a cluster of missense mutations distinguishing Sabin 1 from its antigenically distinct (Nakano et al. 1963; Humphrey et al. 1982; Crainic et al. 1983) neurovirulent parent, Mahoney (Nomoto et al. 1982), and a set of sequences near the 5′ end of the VP1 region, which is poorly conserved across the three poliovirus serotypes (A. Nomoto, pers. comm.). Sequence changes among the vaccine isolates were observed in only two positions. A consistent change from threonine to alanine at

Table 1
Properties of Sabin-1-derived Isolates from Healthy Infants Fed MOPV1

Source of isolate	Days postvaccine	Characteristic neutralization antigens[a]			Altered viral proteins[b]	Amino acid substitutions (and positions) in residues 1–125 of VP1[c]
		Sab 1	Mah$_a$	Mah$_b$		
Infant 1	4	+	−	−	none	none
	10	−	−	−	VP1	none
	28	−	+	+	VP1	Thr→Ala (106)
Infant 2	10	−	−	−	n.d.	Thr→Ala (106)
Infant 3	2	+	−	−	none	none
	8	−	±	−	none	none
	21	−	+	−	VP1	Thr→Ala (106); Lys→Glu (99)
	28	n.d.	n.d.	n.d.	VP1	Thr→Ala (106); Lys→Glu (99)

[a]Summarized from Crainic et al. (1983). n.d. indicates not done. (+) Virus neutralized by specific monoclonal antibodies; (−) virus not neutralized by specific monoclonal antibodies; (±) virus neutralized by high levels of monoclonal antibody.

[b]Detected as variations in mobility upon electrophoresis of radiolabeled infected cell lysates on SDS-polyacrylamide gels.

[c]Nucleic acid sequences were determined by extension of synthetic (Genentech, Inc., given to us by J. Obijeski) or restriction fragment primers, hybridized to virion RNA, with AMV reverse transcriptase in the presence of dideoxynucleoside triphosphates. Amino acid sequences were deduced from the genomic RNA sequences by comparison with the results of Kitamura et al. (1981).

VP1 codon 106 was seen in the late antigenically drifted isolates from all three infants (Fig. 1). Apparently, restoration of the Mahoney residue at position 106 confers a selective advantage to continued replication in the human intestine. A second mutation, encoding the substitution of glutamic acid for lysine, in VP1 codon 99 of two late isolates from infant 3, was also detected.

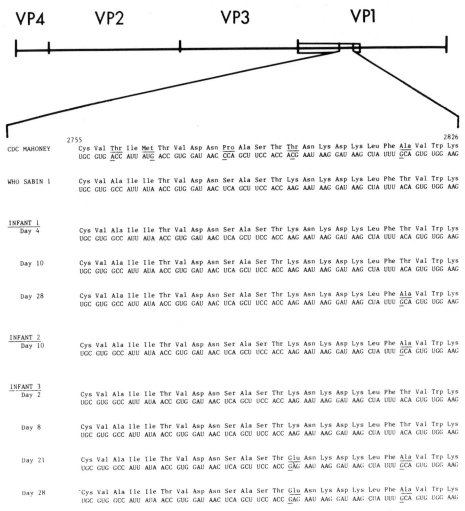

Figure 1

Sequences of nucleotide residues 2755–2826 (corresponding to VP1 amino acid residues 86–109) of Mahoney (CDC strain), its attenuated derivative, Sabin 1 (LSc 2ab; WHO master vaccine seed), and eight isolates from healthy infants fed MOPV1 (Table 1). The enclosed region, corresponding to the first 375 nucleotides encoding VP1, was sequenced as described in Table 1. The only sequence differences detected in the vaccine isolates relative to those of the Sabin-1 reference strain were found in the expanded region. Nucleotide and deduced amino acid residues that differed from Sabin 1 are underlined.

We did not find a strict correlation between antigenicity and observed sequence changes in nucleotide residues 1–375 (Table 1). However, because isolates that had identical nucleotide sequences over this interval had distinguishable VP1 mobilities, we are seeking additional mutations in other regions of VP1.

The kinetics of antigenic variation, and the localization of the observed sequence changes to a region of VP1 found to contain epitopes important to neutralization of type 1 (Emini et al. 1983; van der Werf et al. 1983) and type 3 (Evans et al. 1983) polioviruses, suggest that antibody pressure is a major selective factor for change. However, other factors may also be involved, as the polio vaccines also evolve rapidly in immunodeficient persons (Yoneyama et al. 1982; O.M. Kew and B.K. Nottay, unpubl.).

Natural Intramolecular Recombinants of the Oral Polio Vaccines

Laboratory recombinants of polioviruses have been known for two decades (Cooper 1977), and biochemical evidence for intertypic recombination between defined mutants has been described for polioviruses (Tolskaya et al. 1983) and for foot-and-mouth disease viruses (King et al. 1982). However, no conclusive evidence for natural genetic recombinants among polioviruses has yet been reported.

The general use of trivalent oral polio vaccine (TOPV) establishes conditions permissive for mixed infection and possible intertypic recombination among the vaccine strains. Several case isolates involving TOPV have oligonucleotide fingerprint patterns expected for intertypic recombinants. Two of these recombinants have been characterized in more detail.

Fingerprint analysis of one (serotype 3) isolate revealed that the Sabin-3 capsid region oligonucleotides were present, but that the noncapsid oligonucleotides distal to the middle of the X region were derived from Sabin 2. The crossover junction in the second isolate, a Sabin 2/Sabin 1 recombinant, occurred near the 3' end of the X region (Fig. 2). Sequence analysis localized the crossover site to within an 18-base region that is identical between Sabin 1 and Sabin 2. The crossover event did not alter the number of codons. Three mutations to synonymous codons were also detected in the 546 bases analyzed.

The nucleotide sequences in the vicinity of the crossover region do not contain prototype splice-site sequences (Breathnach and Chambon 1981) signaling the processing of cellular RNAs. A preliminary conclusion from this observation is that recombination in polioviruses may not involve the splicing enzymes but may arise instead by template switching of the viral RNA polymerase over regions of extended sequence homology.

We believe that the recombination events occurred in humans, rather than during the isolation process, because standard methods of poliovirus isolation from clinical specimens generally select against mixed infections. Furthermore, because the recombinants described here were obtained from contacts of TOPV vaccinees, the possibility exists that intertypic recombinants may not only be amplified in humans, but also be transmitted at low levels to others.

DISCUSSION

The studies with the infant vaccinees illustrate the genetic mutability of live polio vaccines during normal immunizations. Although these isolates showed only a

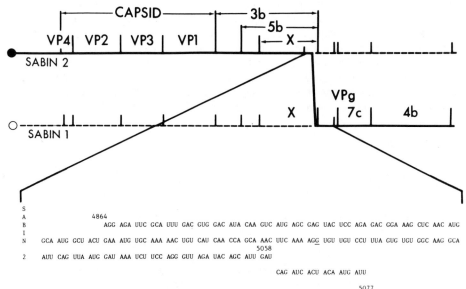

Figure 2
Nucleotide sequence of the region of genetic crossover of a Sabin 2/Sabin 1 intramolecular recombinant, isolated from a vaccine-contact case of paralytic poliomyelitis. Parental origins of isolate 151 sequences were identified by sequence analysis of the same regions of Sabin 1 and 2 and by comparison with the genomic sequences for these vaccine strains determined by Nomoto et al. (1982; A. Nomoto, pers. comm.). The sequences indicated as being derived from Sabin 2 (4864–5058) differed from the corresponding Sabin-1 sequences at 31 positions; those designated as Sabin 1 (5077–5409) differed from Sabin 2 at 55 positions. The recombination event(s) occurred between nucleotide residues 5058 and 5077. The precise location of the crossover site(s) is indeterminable because the 18-base sequence in positions 5059–5076 is strictly conserved between the parental strains. Underlined residues indicate transition mutations to synonymous codons in isolate 151. Genomic RNA of 151 was sequenced by the reverse transcriptase–dideoxy method for extending synthetic (Genentech, Inc.) and restriction fragment (from Mahoney DNA clone pVR104; Racaniello and Baltimore 1981, given to us by V. Racaniello) primers.

slight increase in neurovirulence (B. Elisberg, pers. comm.), we are currently examining other strains that differ in neurovirulence to find sequence correlations with this trait. The antigenic instability of the Sabin-1 vaccine strain during natural replication highlights the importance of using immunogens with broad antigenic specificities in any future candidate polio vaccines.

The significance of recombination in the polio vaccine to human disease is unclear. Epidemiologic studies have not shown an increase in vaccine-associated poliomyelitis by the replacement of MOPV with TOPV (L. Schonberger, pers. comm.). Moreover, most of our case isolates do not appear to be intertypic recombinants. The demonstration that intertypic recombination of vaccine strains occurs in the natural host clearly suggests that recombination among variants of the same strain also occurs. Thus, recombination appears to provide a second mechanism for the rapid evolution of vaccine and wild poliovirus strains. If the chief determinants for attenuation are located in different regions of the genome for each of the three polio vaccine serotypes, it may be desirable to construct live polio vaccine strains having common noncapsid sequences to minimize the chances for phenotypic reversion resulting from intertypic recombination.

REFERENCES

Breathnach, A. and P. Chambon. 1981. Organization and expression of eukaryotic split genes coding for proteins. *Annu. Rev. Biochem.* **50:** 349.

Cooper, P.D. 1977. Genetics of picornaviruses. In *Comprehensive virology* (ed. H. Fraenkel-Conrat and R.R. Wagner), vol. 9, p. 133.

Crainic, R., P. Couillin, B. Blondel, N. Cabau, A. Boue, and F. Horodniceanu. 1983. Natural variation of poliovirus epitopes. *Infect. Immun.* **41:** 1217.

Emini, E.A., B.A. Jameson, and E. Wimmer. 1983. Priming for the induction of anti-polio-virus neutralizing antibodies by synthetic peptides. *Nature* **304:** 699.

Evans, D.M.A., P.D. Minor, G.S. Schild, and J.W. Almond. 1983. Critical role of an eight-amino acid sequence of VP1 in neutralization of poliovirus type 3. *Nature* **304:** 459.

Humphrey, D.D., O.M. Kew, and P.M. Feorino. 1982. Monoclonal antibodies of four different specificities for neutralization of type 1 polioviruses. *Infect. Immun.* **36:** 841.

Kew, O.M., B.K. Nottay, M.H. Hatch, J.H. Nakano, and J.F. Obijeski. 1981. Multiple genetic changes can occur in the oral poliovaccines upon replication in humans. *J. Gen. Virol.* **56:** 337.

King, A.M.Q., D. McCahon, W.R. Slade, and J.W.I. Newman. 1982. Recombination in RNA. *Cell* **29:** 921.

Kitamura, N., B.L. Semler, P.G. Rothberg, G.R. Larsen, C.J. Adler, A.J. Dorner, E.A. Emini, R. Hanecak, J.J. Lee, S. van der Werf, C.W. Anderson, and E. Wimmer. 1981. Primary structure, gene organization and polypeptide expression of poliovirus RNA. *Nature* **291:** 547.

Nakano, J.H., H.M. Gelfand, and J.T. Cole. 1963. The use of a modified Wecker technique for the serodifferentiation of type 1 polioviruses related and unrelated to Sabin's vaccine strain. II. Antigenic segregation of isolates from specimens collected in field studies. *Am. J. Hyg.* **78:** 215.

Nomoto, A., T. Omata, H. Toyoda, S. Kuge, H. Horie, Y. Kataoka, Y. Genba, Y. Nakano, and N. Imura. 1982. Complete nucleotide sequence of the attenuated poliovirus Sabin 1 strain genome. *Proc. Natl. Acad. Sci.* **79:** 5793.

Racaniello, V.R. and D. Baltimore. 1981. Cloned poliovirus complementary DNA is infectious in mammalian cells. *Science* **214:** 916.

Tolskaya, E.A., L.A. Romanova, M.S. Kolesnikova, and V.I. Agol. 1983. Intertypic recombination in poliovirus: Genetic and biochemical studies. *Virology* **124:** 121.

van der Werf, S., C. Wychowski, P. Bruneau, B. Blondel, R. Crainic, F. Horodniceanu, and M. Girard. 1983. Location of a poliovirus type 1 neutralization epitope in viral capsid polypeptide VP1. *Proc. Natl. Acad. Sci.* **80:** 5080.

Yoneyama, T., H. Hagiwara, M. Hara, and H. Shimojo. 1982. Alteration in oligonucleotide fingerprint patterns of the viral genome of poliovirus type 2 isolated from paralytic patients. *Infect. Immun.* **37:** 46.

ISCOM, a Cagelike Immunostimulating Complex of Membrane Proteins

Bror Morein
Institute of Veterinary Microbiology
Department of Virology, The Swedish
University of Agricultural Science
Uppsala, Sweden

Bo Sundquist
National Veterinary Institute
Uppsala, Sweden

Stefan Höglund
Institute of Biochemistry
Uppsala University, Sweden

Kristian Dalsgaard
State Veterinary Institute for Virus Research
Lindholm, Kalvehave, Denmark

Albert Osterhaus
National Institutes of Health
Bilthoven, Holland

Ideally, a vaccine should only contain the structures important for induction of protective immunity, and this has led to the development of the subcutaneous subunit vaccines. Most of these studies have been done with influenza viruses. However, the subunit vaccines have often turned out to be inferior to whole-virus vaccines. No consistent explanations have been given concerning the low efficacy of many of the subunit vaccines. One likely reason is that, in most cases, the experimental or commercial vaccines prepared have not been defined with respect to their composition or to the physical form in which the antigenic proteins are present. Previous work has shown that monomeric forms of viral envelope proteins are weakly immunogenic, whereas multimeric forms are strongly immunogenic (Morein et al. 1978, 1983).

Preparation and Structure of the Immunostimulating Complex

A new type of *immunostimulating complex* (ISCOM) has been constructed that is highly immunogenic. The first studies with this complex were done with parain-

363

fluenza-3 virus (Morein et al. 1984). The virus was solubilized with a nonionic detergent (Triton X-100) and centrifuged through a layer of sucrose containing Triton X-100 into a layer of a 20–50% sucrose gradient containing a glycoside extracted from a South American tree, Quillaja Saponaria Molina (Dalsgaard 1978). The sugar and surplus glycoside were removed by dialysis, and the preparation was then concentrated by lyophilization. The ISCOM was formed only if the concentration of glycoside was above the critical micellar concentration in the sucrose gradient, i.e., 0.03%.

We hypothesize that the glycoside micelles capture the monomer forms of membrane proteins when they migrate into the gradient containing the glycoside. ISCOMs have been prepared from a variety of viruses, e.g., myxo-, paramyxo-, herpes-, rhabdo-, and retroviruses.

The ISCOM was characterized (1) by electron microscopy as having a cagelike structure of about 35 nm in diameter built up by ringlike subunits of 12 nm (see Fig. 1), (2) by its sedimentation coefficient of 19S in a sucrose gradient compared with 30S of micelles containing the same proteins, and (3) by its protein profile in an SDS-polyacrylamide gel in which only the envelope proteins hemagglutinin-neuraminidase and fusion were found.

Immunization Experiments

In immunization experiments in mice, which were immunized twice with ISCOMs containing the envelope protein hemagglutinin and neuraminidase from influenza virus (Fig. 2), the following conclusions could be drawn. First, up to 50 times more influenza virus envelope proteins could be included in the micelles than in the ISCOMs and still the ISCOMs induced higher antibody response. Second, one immunization with 5 μg of ISCOMs induced as high a level of antibody response as two immunizations with 5 μg of micelles. The ISCOMs also induced about ten times higher hemagglutination-inhibiting (HI) antibody titers than the micelles. Similar results were obtained in immunization experiments with ISCOMs in guinea pigs, i.e., 10 μg induced about ten times higher HI antibody titers than commercial horse influenza vaccines, and 1 μg of ISCOMs induced as high an HI antibody titer or higher than the commercial vaccines tested.

ISCOMs enriched in the fusion protein from measles virus induced after one immunization with 5 μg about a tenfold higher HI antibody titer in serum of rats than a β-propiolactone-killed virus containing a similar amount of envelope proteins. The ISCOMs also induced high hemolysis-inhibition titers, whereas the killed virus did not (Fig. 3). It should be mentioned that ISCOMs were prepared from β-propiolactone-killed virus. These results are of interest regarding the development of killed paramyxovirus vaccines, since there is a general opinion that paramyxovirus vaccines should induce an immune response to the fusion protein in order to elicit full protection. So far, killed experimental or commercial vaccines have not done so (for references, see Merz et al. 1980; Choppin et al. 1981). Micelles containing the fusion protein from parainfluenza-3 virus also seem to induce antibody to the fusion protein (Morein et al. 1983). It has been suggested that the inactivation process of the virus denatures the fusion protein, and this results in a loss of its antigenicity. Our studies suggest that in the complete virion, the fusion protein is hidden, rather than denatured, by the hemagglutinin-neuraminidase protein, as indicated by the work of Armstrong et al. (1982).

Why is an ISCOM more immunogenic than a micelle? The morphology of the ISCOM is different from that of a protein micelle and the envelope proteins are openly exposed. The glycoside has an adjuvant activity (Dalsgaard 1978; Egerton et al. 1978), and in mice, 10 μg of the glycoside is needed to exert adjuvant activity. In the ISCOM preparations used, the amount of the glycoside ranged from 0.05 μg to 1 μg, depending on the dose used. It is not known whether the linkage of the glycoside to the antigens makes it active as adjuvant at lower

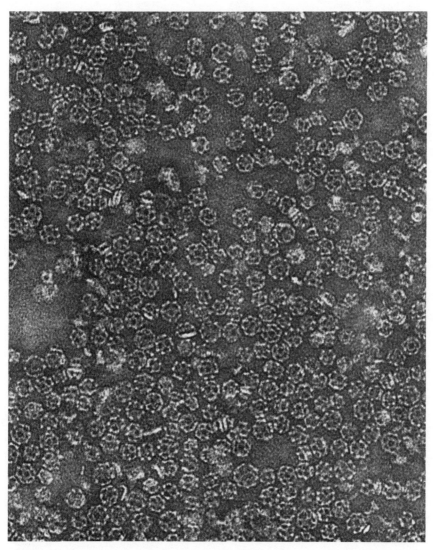

Figure 1
Electron micrograph of ISCOMs of influenza virus (PR8 strain) at high concentration. The specimen was negatively stained by 2% neutralized ammonium molybdate. Most projections appear round with ringlike subunits. Magnification, 140,000 ×.

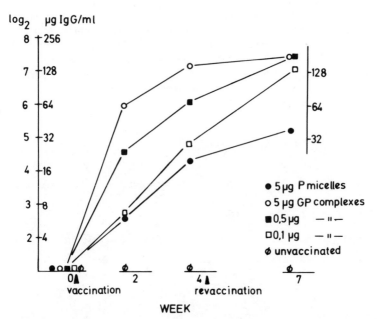

Figure 2
Antibody response in serum of BALB/c mice following two immunizations with ISCOMs containing the envelope protein of horse influenza virus H_3N_8.

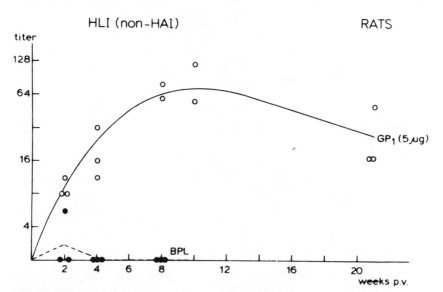

Figure 3
Antibody response in serum of rats following one immunization with 5 μg of ISCOMs containing the envelope proteins of measles virus. Approximately the same amounts of fusion and hemagglutinin proteins were included in the complex.

concentrations, as shown by Arnon et al. (1980), where MDP had adjuvant activity in much lower concentrations when covalently linked to a synthetic antigen. The ISCOMs give practically no side effects; they can be defined in structure by electron microscopy and by their sedimentation coefficient. They are highly immunogenic, making the proteins accessible for the immune system, and may therefore be an interesting structure for vaccines.

ACKNOWLEDGMENT

This work was supported by grants from the Swedish Board for Technical Development (79-6389) and the Swedish Medical Research Council (B84-16X-04920-09).

REFERENCES

Armstrong, M.A., K.B. Frazer, E. Dermott, and P.V. Shirodaria. 1982. Immunoelectron microscopic studies on haemagglutinin and haemolysin of measles virus in infected HEp2 cells. *J. Gen. Virol.* **59:** 187.

Arnon, R., M. Sela, M. Parant, and L. Chedid. 1980. Antiviral response elicited by a completely synthetic antigen with built-in adjuvanticity. *Proc. Natl. Acad. Sci.* **77:** 6769.

Choppin, R.W., C.D. Richardson, D.C. Merz, and A. Scheid. 1981. In adhesion and microorganism pathogenicity. *Ciba Found. Symp.* **80:** 252.

Dalsgaard, K. 1978. A study of the isolation and characterization of the saponin Quil A. Evaluation of its adjuvant activity with special reference to the application in the vaccination of cattle against foot and mouth disease. *Acta. Vet. Scand. Suppl.* **69:** 1.

Egerton, J.R., E.A. Laing, and C.M. Thorley. 1978. Effect of Quil A saponin derivate on the response of sheep to alum precipitated *Bacteroides nodosus* vaccines. *Vet. Sci. Commun.* **2:** 247.

Merz, D.C., A. Scheid, and P.W. Choppin. 1980. Importance of antibodies to the fusion glycoprotein of paramyxoviruses in the prevention of spread of infection. *J. Exp. Med.* **151:** 275.

Morein, B., M. Sharp, B. Sundquist, and K. Simons. 1983. Protein subunit vaccines of parainfluenza type 3 virus: Immunogenic effect in lambs and mice. *J. Gen. Virol.* **64:** 1557.

Morein, B., B. Sundquist, S. Höglund, K. Dalsgaard, and A. Osterhaus. 1984. Iscom, a novel structure for antigenic presentation of membrane proteins from enveloped viruses. *Nature* (in press).

Morein, B., A. Helenius, K. Simons, R. Pettersson, L. Kääriäinen, and V. Schirrmacher. 1978. Effective subunit vaccines against an enveloped virus. *Nature* **276:** 715.

Use of Palmitic Acid as a Carrier for Chemically Synthesized Vaccines

Thomas P. Hopp
Immunex Corporation
Seattle, Washington 98101

Chemically synthesized peptide immunogens are being used in an increasing number of laboratories to raise antisera or hybridoma antibodies against a variety of proteins, and they are currently under investigation as potential vaccines for prevention of viral and other diseases. One of the major technical obstacles to successful immunization with synthetic peptides is the necessity to couple them to proteins or other macromolecules in order to elicit a useful antibody response. This usually results in acceptable antipeptide responses, but, in most cases, a strong response is also obtained against the carrier. Such anticarrier responses may make it difficult to boost the desired antipeptide titers and could lead to sensitization against the carrier, with the potential for anaphylactic responses. Furthermore, coupling to protein or polypeptide carriers must be carried out using coupling reagents that are themselves haptenic, and which usually lead to products of variable composition that are hard to characterize and reproduce. Dipalmityl lysine carrier has been developed in my laboratory as a readily produced peptide carrier moiety capable of improving antipeptide titers, compared with those obtained with free peptides or keyhole limpet hemocyanin conjugates (Hopp 1984). In this paper, I present evidence that immunizations with different peptides conjugated to the dipalmityl lysyl moiety generate little or no cross-reacting antibody, suggesting that the responses are relatively free of antibody specific for the common carrier portion of the conjugates.

Peptide Synthesis

Peptide immunogens corresponding to three sites on the hepatitis-B virus surface antigen were synthesized by the Merrifield procedure (Barany and Merrifield

369

1980). They corresponded to residues 138–149 (HP1), 26–37 (HP2), and 114–125 (HP3), chosen because they were predicted as antigenically relevant regions by their hydrophilicity (Hopp and Woods 1981). The carrier portion was attached as described previously (Hopp 1984). As shown in Figure 1 (for HP1), the synthesis was continued through a spacer consisting of two glycyl residues on the amino-terminal end of the peptide, followed by a lysyl residue that was subsequently derivatized at both the a- and ε-amino groups with palmitic acid. All couplings were made using the symmetrical anhydride method typically used in the Merrifield synthesis, including the palmitic acid couplings.

Immunizations

Because it is of interest to produce a significant titer with a minimum of immunizations, especially for vaccine purposes, the immunization schedule was deliberately kept simple. Two injections were given to each rabbit, with 3 weeks intervening. Doses were 50 μg of conjugate for the first immunization and 200 μg for the second in 1 ml of phosphate-buffered saline (PBS)/Freund's complete adjuvant. Four rabbits were immunized with each conjugate.

Assays

Antipeptide titers were measured by an ELISA procedure. Plates were coated with peptides at a concentration of 0.1 mg/ml in 0.05 M NaHCO$_3$ (pH 9.6), 200 μl per well, and then blocked with 1% bovine serum albumin in PBS. After incubation with antiserum (diluted, 1:33), bound antipeptide antibody was detected by incubation with horseradish-peroxidase-conjugated swine anti-rabbit immunoglobulin (Dalko) and o-phenylenediamine. Color was measured at 492 nm, either manually or with an automatic plate reader.

RESULTS

Immunizations

Each of the peptide conjugates stimulated strong antipeptide responses in all animals. Antibody was detectable at 21 days and continued to increase to maxi-

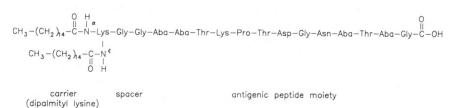

Figure 1
Structure of dipalmityl lysyl peptide conjugate HP1. The cysteine residues occurring in the natural HBsAg sequence have been replaced by L-a-aminobutyric acid (Aba) residues. Two glycyl residues act as a spacer between the antigenic peptide moiety and the hydrophobic dipalmityl lysyl carrier moiety. Peptides HP2 and HP3 were synthesized in analogous fashion, with the dipalmityl-Lys-Gly-Gly sequence attached to their amino termini.

mum at day 135. Anti-HP1 titers, which were tested for a longer period, declined slightly after day 135. In all cases, the maximum titers measured at day 135 were in excess of 1/10,000 (maximum dilution greater than twice background).

No Detectable Anticarrier Antibody

Figure 2 shows the results obtained when antisera raised against the three hepatitis peptides were tested for cross-reactivity in an ELISA assay. In each case, the antiserum reacts strongly with the immunizing conjugate, but not with the other two conjugates. This result strongly implies that no antibody against the common dipalmityl lysyl moiety has been produced in any of the immunizations. This presumably results because the dipalmityl lysyl moiety is internalized in the aggregate or micelle by hydrophobic interactions and is therefore not exposed to the immune system.

DISCUSSION

Dipalmityl lysyl peptides are readily produced by the Merrifield procedure and can be prepared rapidly and in high yield. They eliminate the problems of carrier conjugation variability that are encountered with protein and polypeptide carriers

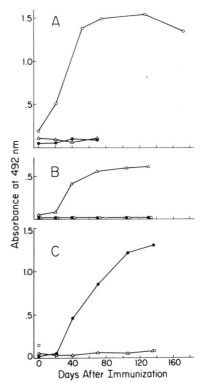

Figure 2
Peptide antigen-antibody reactions measured by ELISA. Plates were coated with HP1 (*A*), HP2 (*B*), and HP3 (*C*). Antisera were anti-HP1 (○), anti-HP2 (△), and anti-HP3 (●). Points represent the average result for four rabbits.

and yield high-titer antibody responses after a simple immunization procedure. Their most striking difference, when compared with classical macromolecular carriers, is the absence of a detectable antibody response against any part of the carrier moiety. These findings make it clear that conjugation to fatty acids is a useful alternative for the enhancement of immune responses to peptide immunogens.

ACKNOWLEDGMENT

I wish to thank Heidi Rubino for excellent technical assistance.

REFERENCES

Barany, G. and R.B. Merrifield. 1980. Solid-phase peptide synthesis. In *The peptides* (ed. E. Gross and J. Meienhofer), vol. 2, p. 1. Academic Press, New York.

Hopp, T.P. 1984. Immunogenicity of a synthetic HBsAg peptide: Enhancement by conjugation to a fatty acid carrier. *Mol. Immunol.* 21: (in press).

Hopp, T.P. and K.R. Woods. 1981. Prediction of protein antigenic determinants from amino acid sequences. *Proc. Natl. Acad. Sci.* 78: 3824.

Rabies Immunosomes: Candidate for an RNA-free Vaccine

Lise Thibodeau
Institut Armand Frappier
Université du Québec
Laval, P.Q., Canada H7V 1B7

Pierre Perrin and Pierre Sureau
Institute Pasteur, Paris, France

Most current vaccines are made of inactivated or attenuated viruses. Although very efficient, they may contain substances that present potential risks, such as nucleic acids and other reactogenic contaminants. An ideal vaccine should contain only the relevant antigenic determinants. However, if subunit vaccines have the advantage of being virtually devoid of side effects, they are generally much less immunogenic than whole virus. We have previously shown that influenza hemagglutinin and rabies G glycoprotein, in the form of rosette aggregates, interact poorly with the cells of the immune system (Thibodeau et al. 1981; P. Perrin et al., in prep.). In most enveloped viruses, the surface glycoproteins are the major antigens; these molecules are membrane-associated and form spikelike projections on the surfaces of mature virions. Taking advantage of this particular structure, we have developed a methodology that enables the insertion of purified influenza hemagglutinin and neuraminidase into the bilayer of preformed liposomes. With this technique, it was possible to recreate a structure (immunosomes) in which the molecules have an orientation similar to that found in the native virus, as judged from the restoration of their immunological properties (Thibodeau et al. 1981).

In this paper, we describe the preparation of immunosomes using purified G protein. A preliminary study of their immunological properties, namely, their potential to elicit antibody production and their capability to protect animals upon challenge with live viruses, is also presented.

373

Rabies Immunosomes

Rabies virus belongs to the family Rhabdoviridae; its genome is made of a single negative-strand RNA that encodes four major polypeptides; G, M_1, M_2, and N. The glycoprotein (G) is the only viral antigen that induces the production of neutralizing antibodies. The G protein is anchored in the viral membrane by its hydrophobic sequence and can be easily extracted with mild detergents.

The glycoprotein was extracted from inactivated purified virus with 2% octyl-β-D-glucopyranoside (OGP) in the presence of 0.3 M NaCl and further purified by ultracentrifugation on a linear sucrose gradient. The immunosomes were prepared as described previously for influenza (Thibodeau et al. 1981). Briefly, the liposomes (phosphatidylcholine, cholesterol, and lysolecithin; molar ratio 16:2:1) were formed by injecting the lipids (solubilized in OGP) in cold phosphate saline buffer and further purified on a small Sephadex G-75 column. The anchorage of the G protein onto the liposome membrane was achieved during a dialysis against a decreasing gradient of OGP. Electron microscopic analysis of immunosomes showed structures of 50–70 nm, in which the G protein, anchored on the liposome membrane, forms a fringe around the particle (Fig. 1).

Immunological Properties of Immunosomes

Rabies immunosomes were compared with purified G protein for their ability to induce serum antibody production as well as protection in mice. For antibody production, each group of five mice were injected with a single dose of an equal amount of antigen either in the form of purified G protein or as immunosomes. Antibody titers were measured by an enzyme immunoassay (EIA) in plates sensitized with inactivated rabies virus. Neutralization titers were measured by the rabies fluorescent focus inhibition technique (Zalan et al. 1979). IgG was evaluated by EIA with a reference mouse serum and expressed in equivalent units (EU). IgM was measured by EIA using a horseradish-peroxidase-conjugated anti-mouse IgM.

Figure 2A shows that anti-rabies IgM antibodies were first detected 3 days postinjection with both immunogens. The immunosomes produced a peak titer at 7 days and an overall higher response than for the purified G protein alone. Specific IgG antibodies induced by the immunosomes were detected 7 days earlier (day 7 postinjection) than those induced by the purified G protein and were also present in higher titers (Fig. 2B). Similarly, neutralizing antibodies appeared 7 days earlier in the sera of mice inoculated with the immunosomes, and titers, expressed in international units (IU), were approximately three times higher than those found in mice immunized with the purified G protein (Fig. 2C).

The protection induced in mice by the different rabies preparations was tested by a modified National Institutes of Health protocol in which a single vaccine dose, in the form of purified G protein or immunosomes, was injected into animals, followed by a challenge with live virus 14 days later. The protective power is expressed in IU after comparison with an international reference vaccine. Table 1 shows that a glycoprotein solution of 1 mg/ml has a protective power of 6 IU, whereas when the same amount of glycoprotein is anchored onto liposomes, a value of 73 IU is obtained. However, the protective power of the immunosomes is still three times lower than that obtained with inactivated whole virus.

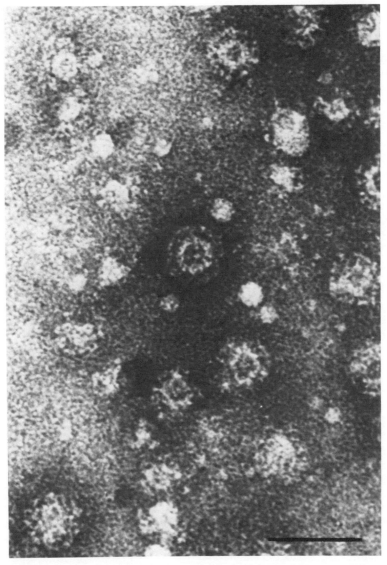

Figure 1
Electron micrograph of rabies immunosomes negatively stained with 3% phosphotungstic acid. Bar, 100 nm.

CONCLUSION

These results clearly indicate that the structural feature of the antigen is of great importance for eliciting an adequate immune response. In previous studies, Atanasiu et al. (1981) showed that spontaneous association of G protein with viral lipids or a reconstitution of the G protein with exogenous lipids (lecithin) was not

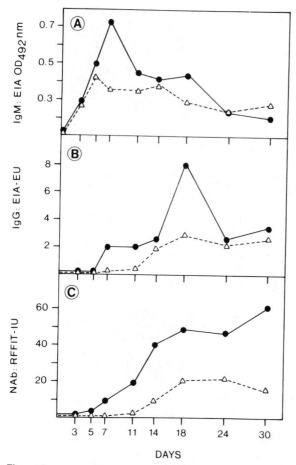

Figure 2

Antibody production following a single injection of 2 μg of purified G protein (△) or immunosomes (●). At different times postimmunization, mice were bled and sera were assayed for circulating antibodies. (*A*) Anti-rabies IgM (EIA OD_{492nm}); (*B*) anti-rabies IgG measured by EIA and expressed in equivalent units (EU); (*C*) neutralizing antibody titer (NAb) measured by the fluorescent focus inhibition technique (RFFIT) and expressed in international units (IU).

more efficient than the purified glycoprotein alone in protecting animals upon challenge. It thus appears that the anchorage of the G protein on preformed liposomes not only avoids entrapment of the antigen in the aqueous compartment, but also allows the molecules to fold into a structure that mimics its natural state. The protective power of the immunosomes may also come from the fact that they are large particles suitable for effective interaction with the cells of the immune system.

Because it is structurally and immunologically similar to the viral particle, the

Table 1
Protective Power of the G Glycoprotein before and after Anchorage on Liposomes

Samples	Protein ($\mu g/ml$)	ED_{50} dilution	$\mu g/ED_{50}$[a]	Protective power IU	Protective power IU/mg[b]
G before anchorage on liposome	760	1/1063	0.715	5.07	6.0
Immunosomes	70	1/1078	0.065	5.14	73
Virus used to prepare G protein	750	1/44480	0.018	171	228

[a] $\mu g/ml$ for 1 ED_{50}.
[b] IU for 1 mg/ml solution.

immunosome could be considered a good candidate for a subunit vaccine. Further studies are under way to increase the protective power of the immunosome in preventive vaccination so that it is as close as possible to that of whole virion.

ACKNOWLEDGMENTS

The excellent technical assistance of Pierre Versmisse is gratefully acknowledged. This work was supported in part by le Ministère de la Science et de la Technologie of Québec.

REFERENCES

Atanasiu, P., P. Perrin, G. Gerfaux, and P. Sureau. 1981. Rabies glycoprotein affinity for lipids. II. Analysis of immunogenic and protective properties of spontaneous and induced associations. *Microbiologica* 4: 383.

Thibodeau, L., P. Naud, and A. Boudreault. 1981. An influenza immunosome: Its structure and antigenic properties. A model for a new type of vaccine. *ICN-UCLA Symp. Mol. Cell. Biol.* 21: 587.

Zalan, E., S. Wilson, and D. Pukitis. 1979. A microtest for the quantitation of rabies virus neutralizing antibodies. *Biol. Stand.* 7: 213.

Use of MHC Molecules to Augment Immunogenicity: Widely Applicable MHC1 Purification Technology and More Evidence for Superior Carrier Function

Arnold R. Sanderson
MRC Immunology Team, Medical School
Guy's Hospital, London SE1 9RT, England

Probably the most dramatic and easily observable *primary* immune response, in the absence of any adjuvant, is a full-thickness skin graft between two genetically dissimilar members of the same species. If the model comprises two mice from congenic strains differing only at the major histocompatibility complex (MHC) (H2) region, the 100 mg of tissue involved probably contains only a few nanograms of MHC substances as the antigenic stimulus. Nevertheless, the response is most impressive and is accompanied by massive infiltration of the grafted tissue by T lymphocytes.

One commonly accepted explanation (Simonsen 1968) is that the graft MHC molecules engage the attention of a large proportion of the host's T cells. Estimates vary from 1% to 10%, compared with 10^{-3} to 10^{-4} times fewer T cells in primary immune responses to any other antigen. It can therefore be argued that allo-MHC molecules are superimmunodominant (the so-called *strong* transplantation antigens of a decade ago). It is also to be expected that the subsequent anamnestic component of such a strong primary stimulus would be weak, compared with secondary responses to other antigens, where memory gives a profound reaction in previously sensitized animals.

It is now part of immunological dogma that all antigens (except allo-MHC molecules) are processed by being associated with self-MHC molecules throughout all stages of an immune response, from initial recognition to the final effector mechanism (Zinkernagel and Doherty 1979). Furthermore, tolerance, even to a few MHC alloantigens, other than by clonal (i.e., fetal) deletion, is difficult to achieve and easily broken. Tolerance in any given individual to all MHC alloantigens of the species is probably impossible.

All MHC molecules so far examined (in mammals, birds, and fish) are similarly organized at the genetic level. One chromosomal region in the genome determines a number of polymorphic peptides that occur on membranes of all normal nucleated cells of that species. They form two types of molecules on the membrane, called class I and class II. Class II molecules comprise two highly polymorphic peptide chains that have constant and variable regions, and both chains are anchored in, and probably through, the cell membrane. Class I molecules comprise one polymorphic chain having properties similar to those described for class II and a nonpolymorphic smaller peptide determined by a different chromosome that is not an integral membrane component. Interchain bonds are strong but not covalent. The smaller (12 kD) nonpolymorphic chain of class I molecules is unique in at least two respects: It is not glycosylated, and it can be prepared in reasonable quantity from the urine of animals with tubular renal disease. The other polypeptide chains (29 kD and 34 kD for class II molecules and 45 kD for class I molecules) occur naturally as glycoproteins.

It is my hypothesis that augmented primary immunogenicity will be conferred on any foreign epitope that is deliberately linked (i.e., before administration to an animal) to a mixture of MHC molecules of the species in question. In using a mixture of MHC molecules covalently linked to an antigen, it should be appreciated that the host will regard some of these as self-MHC and others as allo-MHC. It has been proposed that the combination will represent an obligatory and dominant set of signals; some will mimic an animal's normal immune physiology and others will reflect the signals that only occur naturally in pregnancy, but together they will present the most powerful of immune stimuli.

Current understanding of immune physiology might suggest that MHC2 molecules would prove even more efficacious in promoting immune stimuli. However, the first evidence was obtained (Sanderson 1977) using the class I molecule, and as shown below, the B2-microglobulin (B2M) component is particularly useful for obtaining data. Furthermore, although it is entirely possible that strategies using MHC2 molecules alone, or a mixture of MHC1 and MHC2 molecules deliberately associated with antigen, may prove even more efficient, there is as yet no evidence to suggest that immune pathways are absolutely exclusive in dependence on one or another MHC moiety; rather, one may be more fundamentally involved in some stages of immune processing than the other. Furthermore, the known amino acid sequence homology between these molecules may result from gene duplication during evolution, suggesting that some overlap of function is plausible.

If the results obtained are to be translated into useful clinical or veterinary application, then it will be necessary to purify MHC molecules in quantity from natural or genetically engineered sources. This paper additionally outlines how this may be done very simply and with wide applicability.

RESULTS AND DISCUSSIONS

Purification of MHC Molecules on Insolubilized Xenospecific B2M

It has been known for some time that human B2M can be inserted into the MHC1 molecules of nonhuman species. In so doing the native B2M is displaced, although the specific allogenic integrity is precisely preserved. Under appropriate conditions, it has also been shown that "altered" (derivatized) human B2M can also be inserted into HLA molecules and that the native B2M is displaced. Careful measurement of the equilibrium constant of this reaction revealed the surprising finding that the MHC1 allospecific glycoprotein chain showed preferential association with derivatized B2M (Ward and Sanderson 1983). This suggested that nonhuman allospecific MHC1 chains could therefore be purified particularly efficiently on columns of human B2M, because the amino acid differences in B2M between the species concerned would be regarded as several positions of alteration or derivatization. This proved to be the case and has been used to purify MHC1 molecules from mice (Sanderson et al. 1983); a related technique has been successful in fish and birds (Schmidt and Sanderson 1983). Further experiments are in progress to validate other models, such as the purification of HLA antigen on columns of nonhuman B2M, e.g., bovine B2M.

Augmented Immunogenicity Extended to Epitopes
Covalently Bound to MHC1 Molecules

There is good evidence to suggest that man and nonhuman primates are very similar with respect to their MHC genes. Many primate diseases are pathogenic in man, and allospecific sera raised in one species of primate recognize alloantigens in another species of primate. It is therefore not unreasonable to suggest that primates will regard HLA molecules as if they were allo-MHC molecules. The same is true of the B2M component of MHC1 molecules. B2M amino acid sequences are very strongly preserved throughout mammalian species, and there is evidence that certain monkeys may only recognize two epitope sites on human B2M.

To demonstrate augmented immunogenicity the following model was chosen. Free human B2M was dinitrophenylated so that an average of about 1.0 dinitrophenyl residue (DNP) was incorporated per molecule of B2M. This derivatized B2M was then incorporated into HLA antigen by incubation with the native papain-solubilized molecule. Using tritiated DNP ($[^3H]DNP$) as a marker, it was possible to re-isolate HLA molecules in which B2M(DNP) was now associated with the MHC1 allospecific glycoprotein chain. The use of trace label also facilitated calculation of the extent of incorporation of epitope(DNP) into the HLA molecule. Primates were then immunized with B2M(DNP), HLA-B2M(DNP), and ovalbumin(DNP). Ovalbumin has the same molecular weight as papain-solubilized HLA-B2M and was dinitrophenylated to a similar extent. Identical doses of antigen (about 3 μg in oil, but without Freund's adjuvant) were administered, and serial bleeds were taken before and after each administration. The results are shown in Tables 1 and 2.

Table 1 confirms previous results (Sanderson 1977) in that substantially augmented immunogenicity to human B2M in primates is observed when it is administered as part of the HLA molecule. From these and similar results with many animals, it is possible to calculate approximately that antibodies are detected after a single immunization without adjuvant and rise to titers of about one to two orders of magnitude greater in animals immunized with 10^{-2} times the quantity

Table 1
Immunization of Primates with Ovalbumin(DNP), Human B2M(DNP), and
HLA-B2M(DNP): Anti-B2M Titers

Antigen	Inoculum (days after)[a]				
	Pre(1)	1(24)	2(14)	3(7)	4(7)
Ovalbumin(DNP)	0	0	0	0	0
Human B2M(DNP)	0	0	0	0	3[b]
HLA-B2M(DNP)	0	7	125	200	330

Farr assay with ^{125}I-labeled B2M.
[a]3 μg protein intramuscularly (incomplete Freund's adjuvant).
[b]100 μg B2M(DNP).

of B2M as part of the HLA molecule than when free B2M peptide alone is used
as antigen.

It was not particularly easy to demonstrate anti-DNP antibodies using these
immunizing antigens in Farr precipitin radioimmunoassays, because dinitrophenylation at a low level frequently results in considerable reorientation of polypeptide so that the DNP moiety is buried in hydrophobic regions of the molecule.
Extensive dinitrophenylation of B2M resulted in precipitation of the molecule from
solution. However, iodination of GAT(DNP) resulted in a molecule suitable for
Farr radioimmunoassays, and a second assay is also shown using a methodology derived from Jerne plaque assays for anti-DNP-producing B cells. In each
case it is clear that substantially augmented immunogenicity is imparted to DNP
epitopes covalently linked to the B2M component of HLA molecules, compared

Table 2
Immunization of Primates with Ovalbumin(DNP), Human B2M(DNP), and
HLA-B2M(DNP): Anti-DNP Titers

(a) *Farr assay,* [125]*I-labeled GAT(DNP)*

Antigen	Inoculum (days after)				
	Pre(1)	1(24)	2(14)	3(7)	4(7)
Ovalbumin(DNP)	0	0	0	45	30
Human B2M(DNP)	0	19	100	220	110
HLA-B2M(DNP)	0	11	300	180	140

(b) *50% ^{51}Cr-lytic assay*[a]

Antigen	Inoculum (days after)				
	Pre(1)	1(25)	2	3(7)	4(7)
Ovalbumin(DNP)	100[b]	147	n.d.	129	119
Human B2M(DNP)	100	123	n.d.	384	323
HLA-B2M(DNP)	100	200	n.d.	700	800

[a][51]Cr-labeled sheep red blood cell (RBC) coated with DNP-(Fab) fragment of rabbit anti-
sheep RBC; Guinea pig complement. n.d. indicates not done.
[b]Normal primate sera contained anti-sheep hemolysins. Values are normalized to the
preimmune titer taken as 100 after three absorptions with packed sheep RBC.

with the immune response to the same epitope linked at the same density and presented on the same dose of ovalbumin as a carrier protein.

It is interesting to note that DNP associated with human B2M alone also enjoyed augmented immunogenicity. Perhaps this is because the DNP moiety was sufficiently small that it did not prevent the human B2M exchanging into primate self-MHC1 molecules either on lymphocyte or other cell surfaces or in solution and enjoying special treatment as a consequence. However, it seems unlikely that this strategy could be deliberately exploited, except for very small epitopes, because deliberate binding to larger antigens would presumably sufficiently alter the B2M shape or obscure the molecule entirely so that the crucial association with MHC1 would not be possible. In this case the simplest procedure would be to link the whole MHC1 molecule deliberately to the antigen in question. This is presently being examined.

CONCLUSIONS

MHC1 molecules can be rapidly and simply purified on columns of xenospecific B2M. This principle may be extendable to other strongly associated, but noncovalently linked, heterodimers.

MHC1 molecules provide augmented immunogenicity when covalently associated with antigenic epitopes. The augmentation is superior to that provided by other molecules of similar size and is promising as a general adjuvant strategy.

ACKNOWLEDGMENT

I am grateful to Philip Ward, Peter J. Robinson, Keith Wood, Tim Hilditch, and Barbara Springett for help in various aspects of this work.

REFERENCES

Sanderson, A.R. 1977. HLA "help" for human B2-microglobulin across species barriers. *Nature* **269:** 414.

Sanderson, A.R., P. Robinson, and P.J. Ward. 1983. Interchange of allospecific MHC class I peptide chains with xenospecific B2-microglobulin and its implications for genetic restriction. In *Peptides of the biological fluids* (ed. R. Peters). Pergamon Press, London (In press.)

Schmidt, W. and A.R. Sanderson. 1983. Reversible association with B2-microglobulin as a tool for phylogenetic studies of major histocompatibility antigens. *Transplant. Proc.* (in press).

Simonsen, M. 1968. The clonal selection hypothesis evaluated by grafted cells reacting against their hosts. *Cold Spring Harbor Symp. Quant. Biol.* **32:** 517.

Ward, P.J. and A.R. Sanderson. 1983. The interchange of derivatives of human B2-microglobulin in HLA antigens. *Immunology* **48:** 87.

Zinkernagel, R.M. and P.C. Doherty. 1979. MHC-restricted cytotoxic T cells: Studies on the biological role of polymorphic major histocompatibility antigens determining T cell restricted specificity, function, and responsiveness. *Adv. Immunol.* **27:** 52.

Development of Hepatitis-B Polypeptide Micelle Vaccines

Colin R. Howard, Paul R. Young,
Kwesi N. Tsiquaye, and Arie J. Zuckerman
WHO Collaborating Centre for Reference
and Research on Viral Hepatitis
Department of Medical Microbiology
London School of Hygiene and Tropical Medicine
London WC1E 7HT, England

The historical perspective of hepatitis B is unique in virology in that development and application of genome sequencing are preceding the isolation and study of the intracellular replication cycle, owing to the failure by numerous investigators to propagate hepatitis-B virus (HBV) in vitro. This drawback has prevented the development of conventional vaccines from virus grown in cell culture. Attention has therefore been directed to the use of alternative sources of viral antigen for active immunization, including the use of hepatitis-B surface antigen (HBsAg), the noninfectious surplus protein coat of the virus, purified from the plasma of asymptomatic human carriers and subsequently subjected to an inactivation procedure. Since HBsAg leads to the production of neutralizing or protective surface antibody, as shown by serological surveys and experimental transmission studies to human volunteers and chimpanzees susceptible to hepatitis-B infection, purified 22-nm spherical surface-antigen particles have been developed as vaccines. It is generally accepted that the preparation of the 22-nm particles, when pure, is free of nucleic acid and therefore noninfectious, but the fact that the starting material is human plasma obtained from persons infected with HBV means that extreme caution must be exercised to ensure that the preparations of antigen are free of all harmful contaminating material, including host components.

The advantages of a polypeptide vaccine derived from any source include precise biochemical characterization, exclusion of genetic material of viral origin, and exclusion of host or donor-derived substances. The disadvantages of polypeptide vaccines include low yield when strong ionic detergents are used for separation, although the yield has been substantially improved by the use of nonionic detergents.

385

The two major polypeptides of purified HBsAg, with molecular weights of 25,000 (p25) and 30,000 (gp30), contain both the group-specific *a* determinant and the subtype-specific determinants as shown by precipitation by antiserum to the native surface antigen and by antisera prepared against the separated polypeptides, thereby indicating a high degree of serological relationship among these three components. Both polypeptides may exist as a 49,000-molecular-weight complex under nonreducing conditions and have identical amino acid sequences at both amino and carboxyl termini, indicating that the larger polypeptide represents a glycosylated form of the smaller nonglycosylated polypeptide.

Preparation of Hepatitis-B Micelles

The purification of viral coat subunits in large quantities presents considerable problems, particularly with viruses possessing a lipoprotein envelope in which the immunogenic components are integral membrane proteins, highly hydrophobic, and insoluble in aqueous media. Nucleotide sequence analysis of the HBV genome has shown that the surface-antigen gene product contains an internal sequence of 19 hydrophobic amino acids (Valenzuela et al. 1980), representing the site of polypeptide intercalation into the lipid bilayer of the 22-nm HBsAg particles. Solubilization of both p25 and gp30 polypeptides is readily accomplished by disruption of the lipid bilayer with the nonionic detergent Triton X-100 (Skelly et al. 1979). The biological and antigenic properties of viral proteins are preserved by this method, in contrast to the use of strongly ionic detergents such as SDS. Both virus-specific polypeptides can be extracted as a 3.9S complex from intact 22-nm HBsAg particles by Triton X-100 solubilization and affinity chromatography on concanavalin A–Sepharose, with full retention of antigenic activity. The binding efficiency for the plant lectin is close to 100% and recovery following elution with methyl-D-mannoside is greater than 90% (Young et al. 1982).

Polypeptides maintained as monomers in the presence of detergent are not a suitable form of vaccine and remain weakly immunogenic. Detergent removal is thus critical for the reassociation of polypeptides into a suitable immunogenic form and may be accomplished by sedimentation of solubilized gp30-p25 polypeptide complexes into a detergent-free sucrose gradient under defined conditions, resulting in the formation of polypeptide micelles (Skelly et al. 1981). The protein micelle structure remains water-soluble due to the presence on its outer surface of hydrophilic regions of the polypeptides, which reassociate by way of their hydrophobic portions.

Physicochemical Properties

The buoyant density of hepatitis-B micelles in sucrose was found to be 1.24 g/cm^3 and 1.22 g/cm^3 for material prepared from 22-nm HBsAg particles of human and chimpanzee origin, respectively, representing an increase from 1.16 g/cm^3, consistent with the removal of most of the lipid by the solubilization procedure. Examination of micelle preparations by electron microscopy revealed spheroidal particles of variable diameter in the range of 140–250 nm (Fig. 1). Measurement of over 200 particles of each preparation indicates that the human micelles are slightly larger, with a mean diameter of 200 nm, compared with 180 nm for the micelles prepared from chimpanzee HBsAg material (Fig. 1) (Young

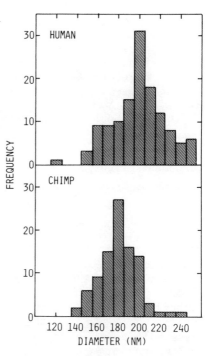

Figure 1
Comparative size distribution of micelles prepared from HBsAg of chimpanzee and human origin.

et al. 1982). Morphologically, however, both preparations are identical, the surface of the particles being composed of discrete globular and stranded units (Fig. 2a).

The SDS-polyacrylamide gel electrophoresis (SDS-PAGE) profiles of hepatitis-B micelles prepared from either human or chimpanzee serum show that the two component polypeptides were present in the same stoichiometric ratio as in the original intact HBsAg particles, indicating that neither polypeptide was preferentially packaged (Fig. 2). This can also be inferred from the evident linkage between the two proteins, which is demonstrated by the retention of the nonglycosylated 25,000-molecular-weight component to concanavalin A–Sepharose. When samples of HBsAg were solubilized prior to SDS-PAGE in the absence of 2-mercaptoethanol, it was found that approximately 2% of the total complement of gp30 and p25 existed as a dimer with a molecular weight of 50,000 in the intact 22-nm particle (Fig. 3). Approximately 5% was present as individual polypeptides, but more than 90% of these two proteins found in the intact 22-nm particles remained at the top of the gel. These observations suggest that the gp30-p25 complex exists in its native form as an extensive, disulfide-linked oligomer.

This is further supported by electron microscopy which shows that detergent solubilization of HBsAg particles with either Triton X-100 or SDS results in large protein aggregates and occasional spherical particles with a "hazy" surface and a diameter only marginally less than that of the intact 22-nm HBsAg particle (Young et al. 1982). Such large aggregates of hepatitis-B-specific proteins are also found in the eluate from concanavalin A–Sepharose columns and may ex-

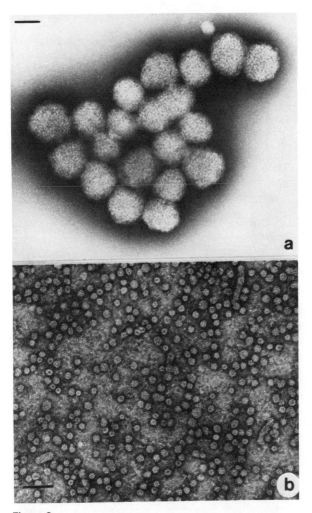

Figure 2
Electron microscopy of hepatitis-B micelles (*a*) and intact 22-nm HBsAg particles (*b*) negatively stained with 1% uranyl acetate (pH 4.4).

plain the formation of the large micelle forms. The final yield of the two polypeptides in micelle form was estimated at 60–70% of the amount originally present in the intact 22-nm particles. The good recovery of total protein confirms the suitability of the method for large-scale production of hepatitis polypeptide vaccine.

Immunogenicity Studies

Immune electron microscopy has shown that the micelles formed complexes and coaggregated with intact 22-nm particles in the presence of anti-HBs (Al-

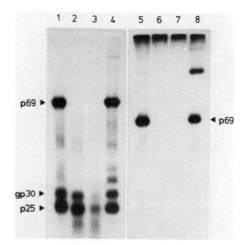

Figure 3
SDS-PAGE of HBsAg and micelle preparations of human (*1,2,5,6*) and chimpanzee (*3,4,7,8*) origin run in either the presence (*1–4*) or absence (*5–8*) of 2-mercaptoethanol.

meida et al. 1981). To obtain a more precise definition of the antigenic reactivity and specificity of hepatitis-B micelle preparations, Skelly et al. (1981) compared the latter with intact HBsAg particles in a competitive radioimmunoprecipitation test. It is estimated that the competitive ability of the micelles was about 40% that of the intact protein, although differences in surface area and in surface distribution of antigenic sites may account for the somewhat lower recovery of serologic activity compared with the final yield of HBsAg-specific protein.

The immunogenicity of the micelles has been compared with that of intact 22-nm particles in a mouse potency test (Skelly et al. 1981). In early studies, it was found that the use of SWR/J mice (H-2^q) produced particularly high levels of antibody (Howard et al. 1982). Consistently higher levels of anti-HBs were induced in animals receiving micelles, possibly also with a higher affinity as indicated by the steeper slope of the dilution curve, compared with that obtained with sera from mice receiving intact particles. Several factors may singly or in combination account for the greater immunogenicity of the micelles, including their large size, altered distribution sites, and the absence of host-derived serum proteins such as albumin. The HBsAg virus-specific polypeptides as gp30-p25 complexes, isolated in high yield from intact 22-nm particles, can therefore be reassociated into a highly immunogenic micellular form, as has been similarly described for other viral envelope proteins.

Hepatitis B may be successfully transmitted to chimpanzees, and although the infection is generally mild, the biochemical, histological, and serological responses in these primates are very similar to those in humans. It has been shown that the 3.9S complex prepared by Triton X-100 solubilization of HBsAg particles is only mildly immunogenic in chimpanzees when administered in aqueous form (Tabor et al. 1982). Although, in this study, no attempt has been made to produce larger, organized morphological forms of the gp30-p25 complexes, the components were effective in conferring protection to susceptible chimpanzees challenged with infectious virus. In a further experiment, the protective efficacy of hepatitis-B micelles was examined using three chimpanzees with no serological evidence of previous exposure to hepatitis B. One animal received the original

22-nm HBsAg particle preparation, itself of chimpanzee origin. The remaining animals received the polypeptide micelle vaccine. The anti-HBs response is shown in Figure 4. Consistently higher levels of antibody were induced in both animals receiving the hepatitis-B micelle preparation. At 6 months, all three animals were challenged with 10^3 chimpanzee-infectious doses of live virus. There was no serological or biochemical evidence of hepatitis B in any of the three animals, thereby confirming the protective efficacy of the micelle preparation.

CONCLUSION

The chemical purity, specific serological activity, and immunogenicity of the micelles, taken together with ease of preparation on a large scale, strongly favor their development as an alternative "second-generation" hepatitis-B vaccine. Consistently higher levels of anti-HBs were induced in animals receiving micelles, possibly also with a higher affinity. These findings have been confirmed by Sanchez et al. (1983), who demonstrated up to 125-fold increases in the level of anti-HBs in mice immunized with hepatitis-B micelles. Several factors may, singly or in combination, account for the greater immunogenicity of the micelles, including their large size and altered distribution of antigenic sites. Alternatively, the absence in them of host-derived serum proteins, such as albumin and associated lipoproteins, may mask a proportion of relevant epitopes and/or depress the immune response to virus-specific antigens.

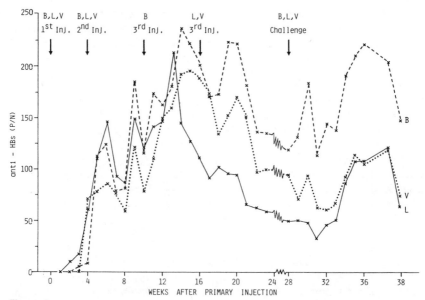

Figure 4
Anti-HBs responses in chimpanzees inoculated with either hepatitis-B micelles (B,L) or intact 22-nm HBsAg (V) particles of chimpanzee origin. Antibody levels are expressed as ratios with respect to a series of negative control values.

The preparation of hepatitis-B micelles may also be suitable for vaccines prepared using HBsAg polypeptides produced by the expression of cloned gene sequences in *Escherichia coli* or other hosts. Synthetic peptides have also recently been shown to aggregate in micelle form (Sanchez et al. 1982), confirming the validity of this approach for the manufacture of safe, effective hepatitis-B vaccines from alternative sources.

ACKNOWLEDGMENTS

The hepatitis-B vaccine development program at the London School of Hygiene and Tropical Medicine is generously supported by the British Technology Group and the Department of Health and Social Security. We are most grateful to Drs. I.M. Murray-Lyon and M. Anderson of Charing Cross Hospital, London, for the supply of human plasma.

REFERENCES

Almeida, J.D., J. Skelly, C.R. Howard, and A.J. Zuckerman. 1981. The use of markers in immune electron microscopy. *J. Virol. Methods* **2:** 169.

Howard, C.R., J. Skelly, E. Tabor, R.J. Gerety, J. Kremastinou, and A.J. Zuckerman. 1982. The development and properties of alternative hepatitis B polypeptide vaccines. In *Viral hepatitis* (ed. H. Alter et al.), p. 411. The Franklin Institute Press, Philadelphia, Pennsylvania.

Sanchez, Y., I. Ionescu-Matiu, J.L. Melnick, and G.R. Dreesman. 1983. Comparative studies of the immunogenic activity of hepatitis B surface antigen (HBsAg) and HBsAg polypeptides. *J. Med. Virol.* **11:** 115.

Sanchez, Y., I. Ionescu-Matiu, J.T. Sparrow, J.L. Melnick, and G.R. Dreesman. 1982. Immunogenicity of conjugates and micelles of synthetic hepatitis B surface antigen peptides. *Intervirology* **18:** 209.

Skelly, J., C.R. Howard, and A.J. Zuckerman. 1979. Analysis of hepatitis B surface antigen components solubilized with Triton X-100. *J. Gen. Virol.* **44:** 679.

———. 1981. Hepatitis B polypeptide vaccine preparation in micelle form. *Nature* **290:** 51.

Tabor, E., C.R. Howard, J. Skelly, A. Goudeau, A.J. Zuckerman, and R.J. Gerety. 1982. Immunogenicity in chimpanzees of experimental hepatitis B vaccines prepared from intact hepatitis B virions. *J. Med. Virol.* **10:** 65.

Valenzuela, P., M. Quiroga, J. Zaldivar, P. Gray, and W.J. Rutter. 1980. The nucleotide sequence of the hepatitis B viral genome and the identification of the major viral genes. In *Animal virus genetics* (ed. B.N. Fields et al.), p. 57. Academic Press, New York.

Young, P., M. Vaudin, J. Dixon, and A.J. Zuckerman. 1982. Preparation of hepatitis B polypeptide micelles from human carrier plasma. *J. Virol. Methods* **4:** 177.

Characterization of a Hapten-carrier Conjugate Vaccine: H. influenzae–Diphtheria Conjugate Vaccine

Lance K. Gordon
Connaught Research Institute
Willowdale, Ontario M2R 3T4, Canada

Haemophilus influenzae type b (H-flu-b) is the major cause of bacterial meningitis in children under the age of 5 years (Fraser et al. 1974). This organism is protected from phagocytosis, and to a lesser extent from antibody to outer membrane proteins, by a polysaccharide capsule that is a repeating polymer of ribose, ribitol, and phosphate (PRP). A purified capsular polysaccharide vaccine has been shown to provide effective prophylaxis against *H. influenzae* disease in children over 18 months of age (Makela et al. 1977). However, the peak incidence of disease is at 6–9 months, an age at which PRP is not immunogenic.

PRP is a T-independent antigen in older children and adults in which it is immunogenic. Although it induces a good primary antibody response in adults, the polysaccharide vaccine does not elicit either booster responses or sequential increases in the proportion of IgG to IgM antibody.

The vaccine described here (H-flu-VAX™) is a covalent conjugate of H-flu-b polysaccharide (PRP) and diphtheria toxoid (D). The biological criteria for this vaccine included safety, immunogenicity, and T-dependent characteristics, e.g., booster responses, an immunoglobulin class switch, and carrier priming. The physical criteria set for this vaccine included the use of a clinically acceptable carrier protein, synthesis of a stable covalent link between the two components, purity, and the ability to define the conjugate chemically and to control the preparation of the vaccine.

393

Vaccine

The diphtheria toxoid component is routinely used in the licensed adult tetanus-diphtheria (Td) vaccine and pediatric diphtheria-tetanus-pertussis (DTP) vaccine manufactured at Connaught Laboratories. Capsular polysaccharide was isolated from H-flu-b bacteria (strain Eagan) grown in fermenter cultures. Methods used for the isolation and purification were similar to those used to produce licensed meningococcal polysaccharide vaccines.

The conjugate vaccine was prepared according to the methods developed at Connaught Laboratories, Inc. (Swiftwater, Pennsylvania). Adipic dihydrazide (ADH) and cyanogen bromide (CNBr) were used in the conjugation process, as previously suggested by Schneerson et al. (1980). Purified diphtheria toxoid was derivatized with ADH. One of the hydrazide residues was consumed by attachment to the protein, and the unreacted ADH was removed by dialysis. PRP was activated with CNBr and reacted with ADH-derivatized diphtheria toxoid (D-AH). The product, PRP-diphtheria toxoid conjugate (PRP-D™), was purified by Sephacryl S-300 chromatography, removing unconjugated D-AH and any additional low-molecular-weight ($< 140,000$) material. The purified conjugate was stored at $4°C$.

RESULTS

H-flu-VAX (PRP-D) is a clear colorless liquid at final dose concentration. The vaccine is formulated to contain 10 μg ribose per 0.5-ml dose. In conjugates containing equal weights of PRP and diphtheria toxoid, the calculated molecular composition is nine diphtheria toxoid molecules covalently linked to each polysaccharide molecule. The calculated average molecular weight for a conjugate with the formula PRP_1-D_9 is 2.1×10^6.

Stability of the covalent bond between PRP and diphtheria toxoid was studied using SDS-polyacrylamide gel electrophoresis. PRP-D showed a single band at the origin of the gel (m.w. $\geq 330,000$), whereas a sample of free diphtheria protein bands at approximately halfway into the rod gel. In stability studies, PRP-D could not be split into its components by incubation at $100°C$ for 30 minutes or at $56°C$ for 18 hours.

The PRP-D vaccine has been shown to present the polysaccharide as a T-dependent antigen (Fig. 1). Animals immunized with PRP alone, or mixed with diphtheria toxoid, do not respond to the polysaccharide. When immunized with PRP-D, they respond with sequential increases in the level of anti-PRP antibody (booster responses) and in the ratio of IgG antibody to IgM antibody (immunoglobulin class switch). Preimmunization with diphtheria toxoid enhances the antibody response, whereas tetanus toxoid had no effect (antigen-specific carrier priming).

Clinical trials have shown PRP-D to be safe and significantly more immunogenic than PRP alone. In adults, a single dose of PRP-D induced 2.8 to 3.9 times as much anti-PRP immunoglobulin as a PRP vaccine ($P < 0.01$) (Boies et al. 1983). Current studies in 1 year olds, conducted by Dr. M. Lepow (Albany Medical Center), show one dose of PRP-D induces over 1 μg of anti-PRP immunoglobulin in more than 90% of the children, whereas PRP induces a response in approxi-

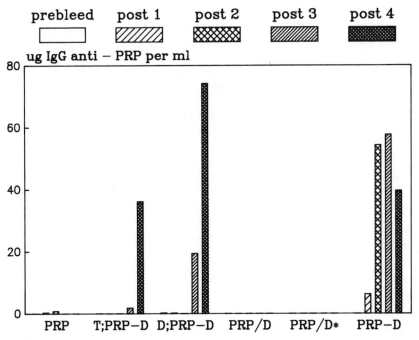

Figure 1
Immunogenicity testing of H-flu-VAX. Groups of three rabbits each were immunized with either 20 μg of PRP, 20 μg of diphtheria toxoid, mixtures of the two, or the conjugate vaccine containing an equal amount of PRP and D. The graph represents the geometric mean level of IgG anti-PRP, 10 days after each injection, measured by a class-specific solid-phase radioimmunoassay. Group 1 received four injections of PRP. Group 2 received two injections of tetanus toxoid, followed by two injections of PRP-D. Group 3 received two injections of diphtheria toxoid, followed by two injections of PRP-D. Group 4 received four injections of PRP mixed with conventional diphtheria toxoid. Group 5 received four injections of PRP mixed with AH-derivatized diphtheria toxoid (not conjugated). Group 6 received four injections of the PRP-D covalent conjugate.

mately 20% of the subjects. PRP-D also induced more than a threefold increase in diphtheria antitoxin. Clinical trials are in progress in children 2 and 3 months of age. This approach to vaccine development is being used for other polysaccharides, as well as proteins and small peptides.

ACKNOWLEDGMENT

The author wishes to acknowledge the contributions of the staff from all departments at Connaught Laboratories, Inc., and the clinical investigators associated with the vaccine project.

REFERENCES

Boies, E.G., D.M. Granoff, R.S. Munson, J. Samuelson, and L.K. Gordon. 1983. Enhanced immunogenicity of PRP-D, a new synthetic conjugate vaccine which induces biologically active anti-PRP. *Intersci. Conf. Antimicrob. Agents Chemother. Proc.* p. 259.

Fraser, D.W., C.C. Giel, and R.A. Felman. 1974. Bacterial meningitis in Bernalillo County, New Mexico: A comparison with three other American populations. *Am. J. Epidemiol.* **100:** 29.

Makela, P.H., H. Peltola, H. Kayhty, H. Jousimies, O. Pettay, E. Rouslahti, A. Sivonen, and O.V. Renkonen. 1977. Polysaccharide vaccines of group A *Neisseria meningitidis* and *Haemophilus influenzae* type b: A new field trial in Finland. *J. Infect. Dis.* **136:** S43.

Schneerson, R., O. Barrera, A. Sutton, and J.B. Robbins. 1980. Preparation, characterization and immunogenicity of *Haemophilus influenzae* type b polysaccharide-protein conjugates. *J. Exp. Med.* **152:** 361.

Of Antigens, Adjuvants, and Carriers in Synthetic Vaccines

Françoise Audibert and Louis Chedid
GR 31 du CNRS, Immunothérapie Expérimentale
Institut Pasteur, 75724 Paris, Cedex 15, France

Very recently, several promising results have been obtained with new synthetic bacterial, viral, and hormonal vaccines (Sutcliffe et al. 1983). In all these studies it was clear that besides the selection of the appropriate antigenic structures, the choice of the adjuvant and the carrier was also of utmost importance. Since synthetic antigens of the future are likely to be weak immunogens, they will require the addition of appropriate adjuvants. In several models of classical vaccines and also of synthetic vaccines, Freund's complete adjuvant (FCA) can be replaced by MDP (NAcMur-L-Ala-D-isoGln), which is a copy of the bacterial cell wall (Ellouz et al. 1974). (An analog of MDP, NAcMuramyl-L-Ala-D-Gln-*a*-*n*-butyl-ester, called murabutide [Chedid et al. 1982] is currently undergoing clinical trials.)

Several investigators have advocated the use of tetanus toxoid, which is a strong carrier and has the additional advantage of being widely used in humans. It must be strongly stressed, however, that the utilization of such carriers raises many problems that are far from being solved. These limitations can be summarized as follows.

1. *Dosage.* Tetanus toxoid, for example, is usually administered in amounts of 5 μg (50 μg is considered a maximum) on which one cannot couple more than approximately 1 μg of the peptide.
2. *Sensitization.* The carrier can sensitize with at least the risk of rapid clearance of the haptenic determinants and even greater hazards.
3. *Specific epitopic suppression.* Epitopic suppression using DNP as a hapten conjugated to serum albumin or to immunoglobulins was described by Her-

397

zenberg and Tokuhisa in 1982. They found that immunizing carrier-primed mice with a "new" epitope (absent in the priming) coupled to the priming carrier induces an epitope-specific system to suppress antibody production. Antibody responses to the newly introduced epitope are selectively suppressed, and anticarrier responses proceed normally.

We have confirmed such results by using a diphtheria synthetic octodecapeptide (SODP) conjugated to tetanus toxoid (TT). As shown in Table 1, BALB/c mice, pretreated with TT (10 μg and 100 μg), received 1 and 2 months later the same carrier coupled to SODP. Controls were immunized under the same conditions with the conjugate, but without receiving a previous injection of TT. Primary and secondary responses of mice pretreated with TT were suppressed. Since, in most countries, there are very few adults who have not been exposed to tetanus, such experimental results must be given very serious consideration. It must be noted that in certain cases the use of appropriate adjuvants can overcome such a suppression (data not shown).

We describe below three models of synthetic vaccines that have allowed us to sidestep the above-mentioned difficulties by using a synthetic carrier or by administering the synthetic antigen coupled to a synthetic adjuvant, or even alone after polymerization.

Protection against Diphtheria Toxin

Following the demonstration that a synthetic fragment of diphtheria toxin (SODP) could elicit protective antibodies (Audibert et al. 1981), we showed that a totally artificial immunogen containing SODP coupled to MDP-A--L (MDP conjugated to a synthetic carrier, multi-poly-DL-Ala–poly-L-Lys) produced an active antitoxic immunization (Audibert et al. 1982). Interestingly, separate studies showed that no sensitization to MDP-A--L could be detected in guinea pigs receiving the conjugate in saline.

Table 1
Hapten-specific Suppression Induced by Pretreatment with the Carrier

Pretreatment (day 1)	Immunization (days 30 and 60)	Responses to SODP (OD 492 nm)	
		primary	secondary
None	SODP-TT[a]	1.5	1.6
TT (10 μg)	SODP-TT	0.8	0.2
TT (100 μg)	SODP-TT	0.3	0.5

Mice (BALB/c) were divided into three groups of eight mice each. On day 0, two groups received subcutaneously TT in 0.2 ml of phosphate-buffered saline. On days 30 and 60, the three groups received 100 μg of SODP-TT. Responses to SODP were measured by ELISA on sera diluted 1:1000.

[a]SODP covalently linked to tetanus toxoid (15–20 μg of peptide in 100 μg of conjugate).

Immunological Castration

A very promising model of a synthetic vaccine that avoids the use of carrier was found by conjugating the decapeptide LH-RH (luteinizing hormone-releasing hormone) to MDP or MDP-Lys. Such a conjugate administered in saline to mice elicited immunological castration and anti-LH-RH antibodies (Carelli et al. 1982). Surprisingly, the effect was stronger than when LH-RH was injected coupled to immunoglobulins and emulsified in FCA.

Antistreptococcal Vaccine

It was recently shown that for secondary immunization, polymerized synthetic antigens can evoke strong responses. A synthetic fragment (35 amino acids long, called S-CB7 for synthetic cyanogen bromide fragment no. 7) had been previously reported to be capable of evoking antistreptococcal S-CB7 antibodies (Beachey et al. 1981). More recently, we have shown that a strong protective epitope-specific response can be obtained by injecting the polymerized S-CB7 without carrier or adjuvant into mice previously primed with the natural M24 protein. These results are reported in Table 2. It can be seen that the administration of protein M24 alone induces low antibody titers. Conversely, when polymerized S-CB7 was given as a booster, high levels of antibodies were obtained that recognized both S-CB7 and protein M24. There was evidence (data not shown) that these antibodies are protective.

CONCLUSIONS

It is reasonable to predict that whatever their mode of preparation, artificial specific determinants are likely to be poor immunogens and will need the help of a carrier (in most cases) and of immunoadjuvants. It seems unfair to consider adjuvants as simple delivery systems, since they represent the active nonspecific stimulating component of the immune response.

Table 2
Antistreptococcal Peptide S-CB7 and Antiprotein M24 Responses of Mice Primed with Protein M24 and Boosted by Polymerized Synthetic S-CB7

		Day 225	
Response to	*Day 100*	*nonboosted*	*boosted*
Peptide S-CB7	380–<100	300–<100	45,000–4,500
	(<135)	(<200)	(24,400)
Protein M24	780–<100	400–<100	37,000–3,100
	(<225)	(<200)	(19,900)

Swiss mice (eight per group) were immunized with 10 μg of protein M24 given in saline on days 1 and 60. On days 115 and 225, four mice were injected with 50 μg of monomeric S-CB7 and of polymerized S-CB7, and four mice received no further treatment. Antipeptide and antiprotein responses were measured by ELISA. Results are given as the maximal dilution giving an absorbance twice as high as a normal serum diluted 100 times. Maximal and minimal individual titers are given, and the arithmetic mean is indicated in parentheses.

The results presented here indicate that muramyl peptides may respond satisfactorily to certain requirements for future vaccines and that there exist ways of overcoming certain problems raised by the utilization of carriers.

REFERENCES

Audibert, F., M. Jolivet, L. Chedid, R. Arnon, and M. Sela. 1982. Successful immunization with a totally synthetic diphtheria vaccine. *Proc. Natl. Acad. Sci.* **79**: 5042.

Audibert, F., M. Jolivet, L. Chedid, J.E. Alouf, P. Boquet, P. Rivaille, and O. Siffert. 1981. Active antitoxic immunization by a diphtheria toxin synthetic oligopeptide. *Nature* **289**: 593.

Beachey, E.H., J.M. Seyer, J.B. Dale, W.A. Simpson, and A.M. Kang. 1981. Type-specific protective immunity evoked by synthetic peptide of *Streptococcus pyogenes* M. protein. *Nature* **292**: 457.

Carelli, C., F. Audibert, L. Chedid, and J. Gaillard. 1982. Immunological castration of male mice by a totally synthetic vaccine administered in saline. *Proc. Natl. Acad. Sci.* **79**: 5392.

Chedid, L.A., M.A. Parant, F.M. Audibert, G.J. Riveau, F.J. Parant, E. Lederer, J.P. Choay, and P.L. Lefrancier. 1982. Biological activity of a new synthetic muramyl peptide adjuvant devoid of pyrogenicity. *Infect. Immun.* **35**: 417.

Ellouz, F., A. Adam, R. Ciorbaru, and E. Lederer. 1974. Minimal structural requirements for adjuvant activity of bacterial peptidoglycan derivatives. *Biochem. Biophys. Res. Commun.* **59**: 1317.

Herzenberg, L.A. and T. Tokuhisa. 1982. Epitope-specific regulation. I. Carrier-specific induction of suppression for IgG anti-hapten antibody responses. *J. Exp. Med.* **155**: 1730.

Sutcliffe, J.G., T.M. Shinnick, N. Green, and R.A. Lerner. 1983. Antibodies that react with predetermined sites on proteins. *Science* **219**: 660.

Inhibition of NCMC by Influenza Hemagglutinin-specific Monoclonal Antibody

Rosemonde Mandeville, Dominic M. Justewicz,
and Jacqueline Lecomte
Centres de Recherche en Immunologie et en
Virologie, Institut Armand-Frappier
Université du Québec
Laval, Québec, Canada H7N 4Z3

The induction or enhancement of natural cell-mediated cytotoxicity (NCMC or NK activity) by viruses and/or interferon has recently received some attention (Casali et al. 1981; Alsheikhly et al. 1983). We have shown that exposure of peripheral blood lymphocytes (PBL) in vitro to small amounts of bacterial (*Bacillus-Calmette-Guerin, Corynebacterium parvum, Brucella abortus*) or viral (influenza and polio vaccines) adjuvants augments their cytotoxicity to noninfected target cells (Mandeville et al. 1982a). We have also demonstrated that, unlike normal activity, this stimulation requires the integrity of the cellular membrane and de novo RNA and protein synthesis (Mandeville et al. 1982a,b).

Two possible mechanisms by which viruses could enhance the cytotoxic activity of PBL have been suggested, i.e., interferon production and/or direct induction by viral glycoproteins. Until now, the role of interferon in virus-induced NK activity has been controversial (Djeu et al. 1982) and unless otherwise proven, either very small amounts of interferon may suffice to induce important boosting of NCMC or the mechanism of boosting is truly interferon-independent. Actually, viral glycoproteins of lymphocytic choriomeningitis and measles (Casali et al. 1981), mumps (Harfast et al. 1980), and Sendai (Alsheikhly et al. 1983) viruses are efficient inducers of cytotoxicity to various uninfected target cells. In these studies it was demonstrated that the cytotoxic activity of PBL was primarily dependent on one of the two viral peplomers (HN glycoprotein) and that the removal of this glycoprotein by treatment with Pronase abrogated their capacity to stimulate cell-mediated cytotoxicity. More recently, Bishop et al. (1983) showed that blockage of viral protein synthesis of herpes simplex virus type 1 (HSV-1) inhibited the development of NK activity.

401

Because of the availability of a range of monoclonal antibodies specific for hemagglutinin (HA), nucleoprotein (NP), and matrix protein (M), we are able to present a more rigorous analysis of the mechanism of virus-induction of NCMC.

Dose-response Relationship

To determine the amount of intact influenza virus required to enhance NK killing of target cells and the kinetics of lysis, different concentrations of purified virus preparations were added directly to the test system (also described in Mandeville et al. 1983). By establishing a dose-response curve, we noted a linear relationship between the amount of virus present and the percentage of specific lysis of K-562 using an overnight Cr-release assay. A significant increase in NK activity was achieved by the addition of 5×10^{-1} to 5×10^{-5} μg HA per milliliter of both purified A/Brazil/11/78 and B/Singapore/222/79 (Fig. 1A), whereas no significant increase of spontaneous isotope release from virus-treated target cells was noted.

In Vitro Induction of NCMC

We next compared the effectiveness of the various influenza virus preparations (live or inactivated) to interferon by exposing target cells together with PBL to each of these mediators separately (Fig. 1B). We could demonstrate the following: (1) When used at similar concentrations, both types of influenza viruses, type A (A/Bangkok/1/79 and A/Brazil) and type B (B/Singapore), could enhance NCMC to an equivalent degree. (2) A given virus preparation and its corresponding monovalent vaccine stimulated the NK response in a similar manner. (3) Monovalent vaccines of the three strains included in the trivalent preparation induced an enhancement identical to that of the trivalent vaccine. (4) Virus preparations induced an enhancement of NK activity in a manner comparable to that of interferon.

Specificity of the Influenza-induced NCMC

To elucidate the role of the three viral proteins, we next investigated whether it was possible to inhibit the virus-induced cytotoxicity with monoclonal antibodies specific for HA, NP, and M proteins, respectively. Using radioimmunoassay, we have previously shown (D.M. Justewicz et al., in prep.) that the HA-specific monoclonal antibody is cross-reactive with both type-A and type-B influenza viruses, whereas NP-specific and M-specific monoclonal antibodies are type-A-specific. Moreover, using immunoblotting, the HA-specific monoclonal antibody reacted with the HA_1 subunit of the HA molecule. By virtue of its cross-reactivity with both type-A and type-B viruses, the fine specificity of the HA monoclonal antibody has been defined to the carbohydrate moiety of the HA molecule. When virus preparations were incubated with the different monoclonal antibodies before addition of PBL (or at the same time) to K-562, only the HA-specific monoclonal antibody could inhibit virus-induced cytotoxicity at the 100% saturating concentration (5×10^{-2} μg HA/ml) for the two viruses used: A/Brazil and B/Singapore (Fig. 1C). At 50% saturating concentration, however, no significant inhibition of virus-induced cytotoxicity could be elicited (data not shown). In comparison, monoclonal antibodies specific for NP and M proteins had little or no effect on virus-induced NCMC. Experiments were also conducted to determine

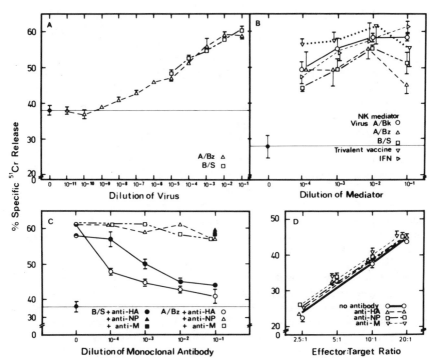

Figure 1
(A) Dose-response curve of virus-induced NCMC. PBLs from the same donor were exposed to purified A/Brazil/11/78 (H1N1) (A/Bz) and B/Singapore/222/79 (B/S). Dilutions of purified viruses were 10^{-1} to 10^{-11} μg HA/ml. The zero value indicates that no virus was used, representing normal NK activity at an effector:target (E:T) ratio of 10:1 (38% ± 1.3%). Vertical bars indicate standard deviation. (B) Induction of NCMC by various mediators. Aliquots of PBL from the same donor at an E:T ratio of 10:1 were exposed to purified virus preparations or a trivalent vaccine (formaldehyde A/BZ, B/S, and A/Bk [A/Bangkok/1/79 (H3N2)]) and interferon. (C) Specificity of the influenza-induced NCMC. Dilutions of each monoclonal antibody (0.015–15 μg IgG/ml) in a 10 μl volume were preincubated with virus preparations at 100% saturation of stimulation, for 1 hr at 37°C before adding to PBL and K-562 target cells at an E:T ratio of 10:1 in 18-hr assay. (D) Effect of monoclonal antibodies on spontaneous NK activity. Aliquots of PBL at four different E:T ratios were incubated with an undiluted sample of each of the three monoclonal antibodies.

whether any of these three monoclonal antibodies had any effect on normal NCMC. Figure 1D shows that none of these monoclonal antibodies had any direct modulating effect on the normal NCMC at any E:T ratio tested. These results were obtained repeatedly in all experiments performed.

DISCUSSION

Exposure of PBL to live influenza virus or its inactivated vaccine enhances their cytotoxic activity to uninfected target cells. This enhancement was, for a given individual, comparable to that obtained by interferon. Furthermore, only HA-specific monoclonal antibody could readily inhibit this virus-induced NCMC. The specific blocking suggests that an antigenic site present on HA_1, and not on HA_2, is responsible for NK stimulation. However, the HA_1-specific monoclonal antibody defines an antigenic site that has been previously identified as host carbohydrate, since it cross-reacts with type-A and type-B strains. It is suggested that NK effector cells detect a common antigenic determinant whose identity deserves more detailed analysis.

The present results therefore add to earlier reports showing that certain viral glycoproteins are efficient stimulators of NK activity (Casali et al. 1981; Ennis et al. 1982; Alsheikhly et al. 1983; Bishop et al. 1983). Furthermore, the cross-type reactive antigenic site(s) on viral HA recognized by NK effector cells provides an important avenue in the potentiation of the host immune response with vaccination. Current influenza vaccines are not fully efficacious (in terms of both humoral and cell-mediated immune responses), and annual revaccination is usually required to cope with either variation or waning immunity, or both. Thus, a better vaccine should stimulate all the components of the immune response and provide the same durable protection against minor antigenic drift as natural infection. The potentiation of the immune response to cross-reactive antigenic sites, in order to induce and activate cross-reactive humoral and local neutralizing antibodies, T lymphocytes, and NK effector cells, could be increased by favoring the expression of these sites on the HA molecule. This would no longer necessitate the requirement for strict anti-HA specificity to match the current strain(s) in the human population. A possible alternative would be to select an effective vaccine adjuvant to accentuate the expression of cross-reactive epitope(s).

ACKNOWLEDGMENTS

The authors express their gratitude to Mr. Marc Henrichon for his excellent technical assistance. This work was supported by a grant from the Institut Armand-Frappier.

REFERENCES

Alsheikhly, A., C. Orvell, B. Harfast, T. Andersson, P. Perlmann, and E. Norrby. 1983. Sendai-virus-induced cell-mediated cytotoxicity in vitro. The role of viral glycoproteins in cell-mediated cytotoxicity. *Scand. J. Immunol.* **17:** 129.

Bishop, G.A., J.C. Glorioso, and S.A. Schwartz. 1983. Relationship between expression of herpes simplex virus glycoproteins and susceptibility of target cells to human natural killer activity. *J. Exp. Med.* **157:** 1544.

Casali, P., J.G. Simons, M.J. Buchmeier, and M.B.A. Oldstone. 1981. In vitro generation of human cytotoxic lymphocytes by virus. Viral glycoproteins induce non-specific cell-mediated cytotoxicity without release of interferon. *J. Exp. Med.* **154:** 840.

Djeu, J.Y., N. Stocks, K. Zoon, G.J. Stanton, T. Timonen, and R.B. Herberman. 1982. Positive self regulation of cytotoxicity in human natural killer cells by production of interferon upon exposure to influenza and herpes viruses. *J. Exp. Med.* **156:** 1222.

Ennis, F.A., Q. Yi-Hua, and G.C. Schild. 1982. Antibody and cytotoxic T lymphocyte responses of humans to live and inactivated influenza vaccines. *J. Gen. Virol.* **58:** 273.

Harfast, B., C. Orvell, A. Alsheikhly, T. Anderson, P. Perlmann, and E. Norrby. 1980. The role of viral glycoproteins in mumps virus dependent lymphocyte mediated cytotoxicity in vitro. *Scand. J. Immunol.* **11:** 391.

Mandeville, R., N. Rocheleau, and J.-M. Dupuy. 1982a. In vitro modulation of NK activity by adjuvants: Role of interferon. In *NK cells and other natural effector cells* (ed. R.B. Herberman), p. 395. Academic Press, New York.

Mandeville, R., F.M. Sombo, and N. Rocheleau. 1983. Natural cell mediated cytotoxicity in normal human peripheral blood lymphocytes and its *in vitro* boosting with BCG. *Cancer Immunol. Immunother.* **15:** 17.

Mandeville, R., F.M. Sombo, N. Rocheleau, and D. Oth. 1982b. Effect of nitrobenzyne derivatives on natural and boosted human NK activity. *IRCS Med. Sci.* **10:** 927.

Inhibition of Transformation in a Cell Line Infected with a *ts* Mutant of Mo-MSV by Cytoplasmic Microinjection of Purified IgG from an Antiserum Generated against a Synthetic *v-mos* Peptide

Gary E. Gallick, David B. Brown,*
Edwin C. Murphy, Jr., and Ralph B. Arlinghaus†
Department of Tumor Biology
The University of Texas System Cancer Center
M.D. Anderson Hospital and Tumor Institute
Houston, Texas 77030

The preparation of successful vaccines using synthetic peptides as antigens requires not only that an immune response be elicited by the peptide antigen, but also that the antibodies to the peptide(s) be able to block specifically the biological function of the native protein. The transforming gene products of retroviruses offer an excellent model system for examining the capacity of antisera raised against synthetic peptides to neutralize specific functions of proteins. The pleiotrophic activities of these proteins result in tumor formation in animals, as well as in the dramatic changes that occur in transformation of cells in tissue culture. The latter changes are often easily detected by inspection of cell morphology under the light microscope. Thus, the ability to inhibit or reverse transformation will be reflected in the failure of cells to assume a "rounded" phenotype or by transition from a rounded to a morphologically normal ("flat") phenotype.

The purpose of this study was to assess the ability of an antiserum generated against a synthetic peptide representing part of the sequence of the transforming gene product P37*mos* of Moloney murine sarcoma virus (Mo-MSV) to inhibit the function of the complete transforming protein. The cells chosen for study are an established normal rat kidney cell line infected with a temperature-sensitive Mo-MSV mutant, designated Mo-MSV*ts110*, in which morphologic changes could be followed by altering the temperature. This infected cell line is termed 6m2 (Horn et al. 1981). Activity against the *mos*-gene product was measured by scoring for

Present addresses: *Yale University, Department of Biology, Kline Biology Tower, P.O. Box 6666, New Haven, Connecticut 06511; †Scripps Clinic and Research Foundation, Department of Molecular Biology, 10666 N. Torrey Pines Road, La Jolla, California 92037.

morphologic changes following cytoplasmic microinjection of purified IgG into cells infected with Mo-MSV*ts110*.

Preparation of Anti-*mos* Antiserum

Anti-*mos* antiserum was made by using a peptide comprising amino acids 37–55 of the predicted *v-mos* sequence (Van Beveren et al. 1981). The peptide was cyclized at the cysteine residues, conjugated to keyhole limpet hemocyanin, and injected into rabbits at 2-week intervals. After 2 months, antiserum was obtained that could specifically immunoprecipitate *mos*-related proteins. IgG from the antiserum was purified by column chromatography on a Bio-Rad DEAE Affi-Gel blue column.

The *ts110*-gene Product Is a Soluble Cytoplasmic Protein

Past studies from this laboratory have indicated that Mo-MSV*ts110* produces an 85-kD *gag-mos* fusion protein; i.e., sequences from the gene encoding core proteins are fused to sequences encoding the transforming protein (Junghans et al. 1982). The temperature-sensitive expression of the *gag-mos*-gene product results in infected cells assuming a transformed phenotype at 33°C, the permissive temperature, and a normal morphology at 39°C, the nonpermissive temperature (Blair et al. 1979; Horn et al. 1981). The changes in morphology following temperature shift allowed rapid determination of the effects of anti-*mos* antiserum. To determine the optimal cellular location in which the antiserum might exert the greatest potential effect on the Mo-MSV*ts110* gene product, localization studies were performed. Photomicrographs of *ts110*-infected cells, exposed to anti-*mos* IgG and then counterstained with fluorescein-conjugated goat anti-rabbit IgG, are shown in Figure 1. At 33°C, a diffuse cytoplasmic staining was observed throughout the cells (Fig. 1A). After a 24-hour shift to 39°C, most of the cytoplasmic staining disappears (data not shown). Distinct staining of a perinuclear ring, seen in 6m2 cells grown at both temperatures, as well as in other types of cells (Fig. 1B), is the result of reactivity of the anti-*mos* antiserum with a normal cellular protein (G.E. Gallick et al., in prep.). Thus, the indication that the *mos*-gene product produced by Mo-MSV*ts110* was primarily a soluble cytoplasmic protein suggested that it would be protected from antisera added directly to the culture media.

Microinjection of IgG

To overcome the problem of presenting the antiserum to the *gag-mos* antigen, purified anti-*mos* IgG was injected directly into the cytoplasm of Mo-MSV*ts110*-infected cells by glass-needle-mediated microinjection (Stacey 1981). Briefly, approximately 10 femtoliters of purified IgG in 1% KCl at a concentration of 43 mg/ml was injected into cells circumscribed by a small circle etched onto a coverslip. The cells were immediately returned to fresh growth media at the incubation temperature. Cultures to be shifted from 39°C to 33°C were allowed a half-hour recovery prior to shift. Approximately 80–90% of the cells survived injection. After incubation for various periods of time at the desired temperature, cells were

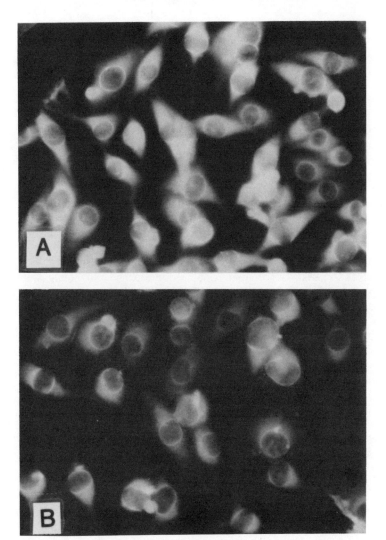

Figure 1
Localization of P85$^{gag\text{-}mos}$ in 6m2 cells by indirect immunofluorescence. Cells were grown on coverslips at 33°C (the permissive temperature for P85$^{gag\text{-}mos}$ expression) or at 39°C (the nonpermissive temperature), fixed in methanol, flooded with purified IgG from anti-*mos* 37-55 cyclic serum, and then reacted with fluorescein-conjugated goat anti-rabbit IgG. Cells were counterstained with Evan's blue stain and visualized under a fluorescent microscope. (A) 6m2 cells, 33°C; (B) NIH-3T3 cells, 33°C.

fixed with methanol, flooded with fluorescein-conjugated goat anti-rabbit IgG, and then counterstained with Evan's blue stain. Morphology was scored microscopically using a phase-contrast lens. Under these conditions, microinjected cells could not be distinguished from uninjected cells. Criteria for scoring cells were as follows: Cells determined to be morphologically "normal" had an appearance similar to that of cells observed in cultures maintained at 39°C, cells scored as morphologically "transformed" had the appearance of the majority of cells maintained at 33°C, and "semitransformed" cells were defined as those having more cytoplasm and extended pseudopodia than observed in most cells maintained at 33°C, although their morphology was not completely normal.

After scoring under phase contrast, the same field was viewed by fluorescence microscopy to determine which cells had been microinjected. As a result of the staining procedure, microinjected cells stained bright green, whereas uninjected cells stained red. Examples of the staining observed in infected cultures grown and microinjected at 39°C and then shifted for 4 hours to 33°C are shown in Figure 2. The microinjected (yellow-green) cells contained much more cytoplasm and appeared to be morphologically normal, whereas the noninjected (red) cells were rounded and assumed a transformed phenotype. The results of the microinjection studies are presented in Table 1. Two regimens of injection were studied: Cells were injected at 33°C, incubated at 33°C for 4 hours, and then fixed (see Fig. 2A) or, alternatively, cells were injected at 39°C and fixed 4 hours after a shift to 33°C (see Fig. 2B). To determine whether the process of microinjection might damage the cell or whether a nonspecific effect occurred due to the presence of rabbit IgG in the rat cell cytoplasm, purified rabbit anti-chicken ovalbumin IgG was injected as a control. The results shown in Table 1 demonstrate that the microinjected nonspecific IgG alone had no effect on the transformation process in virus-infected cells, the percentage of cells in each category being equivalent in both injected and noninjected cells, regardless of the regimen employed. In contrast, injection of anti-*mos* IgG at the permissive temperature resulted in striking changes in a large percentage of the cells. Whereas 97% of the noninjected cells were fully or partially transformed according to the above criteria, this percentage was reduced to 79% in injected cells. Only 17% of the injected cells were completely round and showed no evidence of adherence to the glass. Thus, the large majority of cells injected at 33°C had converted toward a more normal phenotype. Larger numbers of cells were injected at 39°C and examined after a 4-hour shift to 33°C because the more abundant cytoplasm in these cells made them easier to inject. Even more striking results were obtained by this regimen. The transition to the transformed phenotype was completely inhibited in 40% of the cells and partially inhibited in 47% of the cells, and only 13% of the cells underwent complete transformation. In marked contrast, 61% of the uninjected cells underwent complete transformation upon a shift to 33°C, with only 8% of the cells remaining morphologically normal when subjected to this regimen. These results strongly suggest that cytoplasmic injection of anti-*mos* IgG can inhibit the function of the *mos* protein in Mo-MSV*ts110*-infected cells.

To determine more precisely the effect of microinjection of anti-*mos* IgG into

Figure 2

Microinjection of anti-*mos* IgG into *ts110*-infected 6m2 cells. Cells were either grown and injected at 33°C and fixed 4 hr after injection (*A*) or grown and injected at 39°C and fixed 4 hr after shift to 33°C (*B*). Fixed cells were stained with fluorescein-conjugated goat anti-rabbit IgG and counterstained with Evan's blue so that microinjected cells appear yellow and noninjected cells appear red.

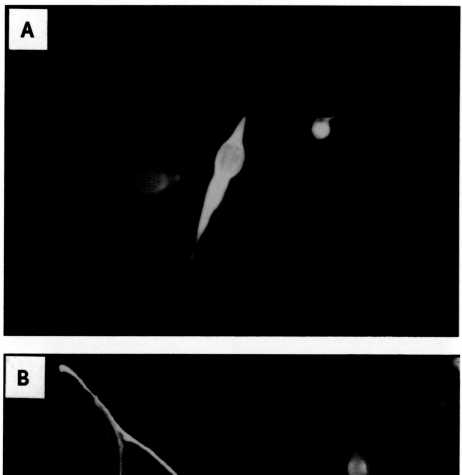

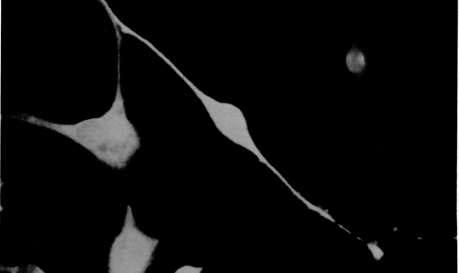

Figure 2 (*See facing page for legend.*)

Table 1
Microinjection of Purified IgG into 6m2 Cells

Antibody	Regimen	Injected			Noninjected		
		transformed[a]		normal	transformed		normal
		++	+		++	+	
Anti-ovalbumin	39°–33°C (4 hr)	77(58%)	50(37%)	7(5%)	98(52%)	69(37%)	21(11%)
Anti-37-55 cyclic	33°–33°C (4 hr)	5(17%)	18(62%)	6(21%)	48(53%)	41(44%)	2(3%)
Anti-37-55 cyclic	39°–33°C (4 hr)	10(13%)	36(47%)	30(40%)	67(61%)	33(31%)	9(8%)

[a](++) Cells completely round, no evidence of adherence; (+) cells contain pseudopodia or distended cytoplasm.

transformed cells, other parameters will be studied. For example, it would be interesting to determine whether or not microtubules and intermediate filaments, which are in disarray in transformed cells, can reorganize after microinjection with anti-*mos* IgG. Although these studies may have no direct bearing on the production of vaccines, the ability of the antiserum used in these studies to neutralize a biologically potent molecule bodes well for the efficacy of vaccines using synthetic peptides as antigens.

REFERENCES

Blair, D.G., M.A. Hull, and E.A. Finch. 1979. The isolation and preliminary characterization of temperature-sensitive transformation mutants of Moloney sarcoma virus. *Virology* **95**: 303.

Horn, J.P., T.G. Wood, E.C. Murphy, Jr., D.G. Blair, and R.B. Arlinghaus. 1981. A selective temperature-sensitive defect in viral RNA expression in cells infected with a *ts* transformation mutant of murine sarcoma virus. *Cell* **25**: 37.

Junghans, R., E.C. Murphy, Jr., and R.B. Arlinghaus. 1982. Electron microscopic analysis of ts110 Moloney mouse sarcoma virus: A variant of wild type virus with two RNAs containing large deletions. *J. Mol. Biol.* **161**: 229.

Stacey, D. 1981. Microinjection of mRNA and other macromolecules into living cells. *Methods Enzymol.* **79**: 76.

Van Beveren, C., J. Van Straaten, A. Galleshaw, and I. Verma. 1981. Nucleotide sequence of the genome of a murine sarcoma virus. *Cell* **27**: 97.

Immunodominant Region of EDP208 Pili: Antigen-Antibody Interaction

Robert S. Hodges,*† J.M. Robert Parker,*†
Ashok K. Taneja,*† Elizabeth A. Worobec,*
and William Paranchych*
*Department of Biochemistry, and the
†Medical Research Council Group in
Protein Structure and Function
University of Alberta, Edmonton, Canada T6G 2H7

The precise delineation of antigenic determinants serves as a powerful tool in the examination of structure-function relationships in biological macromolecules. This approach has also led to exciting developments in immunization strategies for diseases caused by a variety of infectious agents. Recent progress in immunological detection procedures, peptide synthesis methodology, and the elucidation of the primary structure of proteins from DNA and RNA sequence data has permitted the rapid characterization of antigenic sites in several microbial virulence factors. Indeed, many investigators are working toward the development of synthetic vaccines.

Studies in this laboratory have recently focused on the major antigenic determinant of an *Escherichia coli* pilus system encoded by the EDP208 conjugative plasmid (Armstrong et al. 1980). Bacterial pili are thin nonflagellar protein filaments found on the surfaces of many types of bacteria. These pili contain a single polypeptide subunit of 11,500 daltons with *N*-acetyl threonine (Ac-Thr) as the aminoterminal residue (Frost et al. 1983). The objective of these investigations is to identify specific functional groups within the antigenic region that promote antigen-antibody interaction.

The EDP208 pilus system is particularly suited for these studies, since bacteria carrying the EDP208 plasmid are highly piliated relative to other types of conjugative pili. Also, EDP208 pili are structurally similar to the well-studied F pilus system. The primary product released upon trypsin digestion of the EDP208 pilus monomer is the aminoterminal dodecapeptide. Although other tryptic cleavage sites exist in the protein, cleavage occurs only at Lys-12 to yield a fragment that is clearly the immunodominant domain (Worobec et al. 1983).

415

EXPERIMENTAL PROCEDURES

Peptide Synthesis and Purification

Peptides were synthesized on a Beckman synthesizer (model 990) using standard solid-phase methodology as reported for Ac-P(1-12) (Worobec et al. 1983), except that N^a-*t*-butyloxycarbonyl-β-O-benzyl-L-threonine (Boc-Thr) (Bzl) was coupled as the symmetrical anhydride. The solid support used was (copolystyrene 1% or 2% divinylbenzene) benzhydryl-amine-HCl resin. The programs used for the attachment of each amino acid were described previously (Hodges et al. 1981).

The peptides were purified on a reverse-phase high-performance liquid chromatography (HPLC) column (Beckman Ultrapore C3, 4.6 × 75 mm; solvent A = 0.1% trifluoroacetic acid (TFA)/H_2O, solvent B = 0.05% TFA/acetonitrile, gradient 1% B/min, flow rate 1 ml/min).

Preparation of Peptide Conjugates

The peptides were derivatized with the photoaffinity probe, *N*-hydroxy-succinimide ester of 4-azidobenzoic acid, as described previously (Watts et al. 1983; Worobec et al. 1983). These modified peptides were purified by reverse-phase HPLC as described above. A five- to tenfold molar excess of modified peptide to bovine serum albumin Fraction V (BSA) (1–2 mg of lyophilized probe peptide was dissolved in 75–150 μl of BSA stock solution prepared by dissolving 125 mg of BSA in 1 ml of 0.1 M KH_2PO_4 buffer, pH 6.8) was cross-linked to BSA by irradiating at 4°C, using a RPR 208 preparative reactor equipped with RPR 3500 Å lamps (Rayonet, The Southern New England Ultraviolet Co.). The peptide conjugates were purified by reverse-phase HPLC on a Synchropak RP-P column (250 × 10 mm; flow rate 4 ml/min, solvent A = 0.1% TFA/H_2O, solvent B = 0.05% TFA/acetonitrile, gradient 2% B/min).

RESULTS

To elucidate further specific residues responsible for antigenicity of the amino-terminal site, several synthetic analogs have been prepared by solid-phase peptide synthesis (Fig. 1). The relative avidity of these peptides was evaluated both as free peptides and peptide conjugates in ELISA and competitive ELISA procedures.

The peptide conjugates were prepared using the amino-directed photoaffinity probe, *N*-hydroxysuccinimide ester of 4-azidobenzoic acid, which in this case modifies the ε-amino groups of lysine. The reagent was synthesized as described by Chong and Hodges (1981). Based on hydrophilicity, one would predict that the carboxyterminal end of the dodecapeptide (residues 8–12) should contain the antibody-combining site. However, the coupling of the peptide to BSA through the ε-amino groups of Lys-8 and Lys-12 did not abolish the antigenic reactivity of the 12-residue peptide, suggesting that these residues were not involved in the antigen-antibody reaction. This was verified by the Ac-P(1-8) peptide conjugate that reacted strongly with anti-EDP208 pilus antisera, and the antisera to this conjugate reacted strongly with native pili. Comparison of the 8- and 12-residue

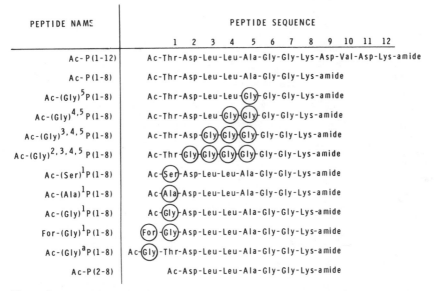

PEPTIDE NAME	PEPTIDE SEQUENCE
	1 2 3 4 5 6 7 8 9 10 11 12
Ac-P(1-12)	Ac-Thr-Asp-Leu-Leu-Ala-Gly-Gly-Lys-Asp-Val-Asp-Lys-amide
Ac-P(1-8)	Ac-Thr-Asp-Leu-Leu-Ala-Gly-Gly-Lys-amide
Ac-(Gly)^{5}P(1-8)	Ac-Thr-Asp-Leu-Leu-(Gly)-Gly-Gly-Lys-amide
Ac-(Gly)^{4,5}P(1-8)	Ac-Thr-Asp-Leu-(Gly)(Gly)-Gly-Gly-Lys-amide
Ac-(Gly)^{3,4,5}P(1-8)	Ac-Thr-Asp-(Gly)(Gly)(Gly)-Gly-Gly-Lys-amide
Ac-(Gly)^{2,3,4,5}P(1-8)	Ac-Thr-(Gly)(Gly)(Gly)(Gly)-Gly-Gly-Lys-amide
Ac-(Ser)^{1}P(1-8)	Ac-(Ser)-Asp-Leu-Leu-Ala-Gly-Gly-Lys-amide
Ac-(Ala)^{1}P(1-8)	Ac-(Ala)-Asp-Leu-Leu-Ala-Gly-Gly-Lys-amide
Ac-(Gly)^{1}P(1-8)	Ac-(Gly)-Asp-Leu-Leu-Ala-Gly-Gly-Lys-amide
For-(Gly)^{1}P(1-8)	(For)-(Gly)-Asp-Leu-Leu-Ala-Gly-Gly-Lys-amide
Ac-(Gly)^{a}P(1-8)	Ac-(Gly)-Thr-Asp-Leu-Leu-Ala-Gly-Gly-Lys-amide
Ac-P(2-8)	Ac-Asp-Leu-Leu-Ala-Gly-Gly-Lys-amide

Figure 1

Amino acid sequence of synthetic analogs of the immunodominant region of EDP208 pili. The circled residues represent changes from the native sequence.

free peptides in a competitive ELISA showed that both compete equally well with EDP208 pili (Fig. 2A). These peptides titrated more than 80% of the anti-pilus antibodies in the polyclonal anti-pilus antisera, confirming that this region is the major antigenic determinant. This result suggested that the aminoterminal amino acid residue Ac-Thr may play a significant role in the antigen-antibody interaction. Thus, a series of analogs were prepared by substituting the Ac-Thr with Ac-Ser, Ac-Ala, Ac-Gly, and formyl-Gly, as well as by removing the threonine residue to give Ac-P(2-8). The results of the competitive ELISA are shown in Figure 2A and are summarized in Figure 3.

The methyl group on the threonine side chain seems unimportant for antigenicity, with no decrease in binding affinity. However, the removal of the hydroxyl group results in a 220-fold decrease in I_{50} (Fig. 3). The effect of replacing Ac-Thr with formyl-Gly results in a 6670-fold decrease in I_{50}, suggesting the importance of the methyl group in the acetyl moiety. Removal of the threonine residue completely (Ac-P[2-8]) results in no inhibition, leading to the interpretation that the only residue responsible for antigenicity was the aminoterminal residue.

To verify this interpretation, a series of analogs were synthesized (Fig. 1), where the amino acid residues in the native sequence were progressively replaced by glycine residues from the carboxyl terminus. The results are summarized in Figures 2B and 3. The methyl group of Ala-5 contributes in a small way to the binding affinity of the peptide (fourfold decrease in I_{50}). However, the accumulative effect of removing the side chains of Leu-4 and Ala-5 (Ac-[Gly]^{3,4,5}P[1-8]) resulted in a 1380-fold decrease in I_{50}, suggesting the importance of the leucine side chain at position 4. The accumulative effect of removing the side chains of Leu-

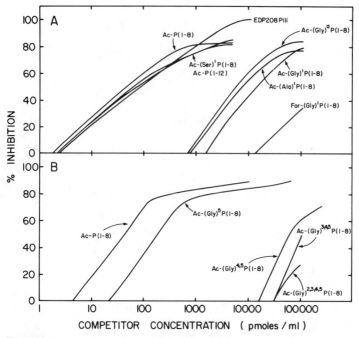

Figure 2
Competitive enzyme-linked immunosorbent assay (ELISA) of synthetic peptide analogs of the immunodominant region of EDP208 pili compared with native pili. Microtiter wells coated with EDP208 pili were incubated with appropriate dilutions of synthetic peptide-Fab fragment (Fab from IgG isolated from antisera to EDP208 pili). The Fab-pili complex was quantitated using goat anti-rabbit IgG conjugated to alkaline phosphatase. Substrate for alkaline phosphatase was *p*-nitrophenyl phosphate. Ac-P(2-8) showed no inhibition.

3, Leu-4, and Ala-5 (Ac-[Gly]^{3,4,5} P[1-8]) resulted in a 2220-fold decrease in I_{50}, suggesting that although the leucine side chain at position 3 contributes to the binding affinity, it does so very weakly compared with the leucine side chain at position 4. It looks as if two residues are contributing to the antigenicity in a major way, the most important residue being the aminoterminal Ac-Thr residue; without it the peptide will not bind to the antibody-recognition site. This can be explained by the loss of two potential hydrogen bonds to the acetyl amide bond (see 1b in Fig. 3) in addition to a hydrogen bond to the hydroxyl group and the hydrophobic interaction with the acetyl methyl. The second major contributor is the leucine side chain at position 4, which results in a hydrophobic interaction with antibody.

CONCLUSIONS

The EDP208 pilus system provides unique advantages for studying the details of antigen-antibody reactions. Use of synthetic peptides and a competitive ELISA procedure with a Fab antibody preparation has allowed us to identify several functional groups involved in the antigen-antibody interaction. These include ma-

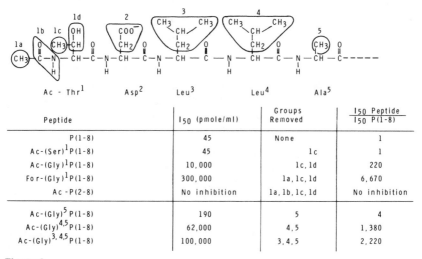

Figure 3
Relative contributions of amino acid side chains to the antigen-antibody interaction. I_{50} is the concentration of competitor required to give 50% inhibition in the competitive ELISA. I_{50} value for the peptide, Ac-(Gly)^{2,3,4,5} P(1-8), was not determined due to extremely weak binding (Fig. 2).

jor contributions from the acetyl methyl, acetyl amide bond, and hydroxyl moieties on the aminoterminal residue as well as the side chain of residue 4. Further studies are in progress to establish the minimum length of the antigenic region and the individual contributions of residues 2 through 5, although preliminary studies indicate that residues 1 through 5 constitute the entire antigenic determinant.

It is not known whether this aminoterminal region plays any structural or functional roles in the pilus protein. It is likely that at least ten additional gene products are involved in the synthesis, processing, and assembly of the EDP208 pilus. Is the aminoterminal domain required for any of these processes? Other functions of EDP208 conjugative pili include the mediation of phage infection by pilus-specific RNA- and DNA-containing bacteriophages and the bacterial conjugation process (Armstrong et al. 1980). Studies in progress are aimed at determining whether synthetic aminoterminal peptides can compete for any of these functions. Cloning and DNA sequencing studies on the EDP208 pilus gene are also in progress in this laboratory (Finlay et al. 1983). It is hoped that site-directed mutagenesis experiments will allow us to determine whether the aminoterminal domain is important for pilus synthesis and assembly and whether substitution of other antigenic determinants into this region could be tolerated by the assembly process.

REFERENCES

Armstrong, G.D., L.S. Frost, P.A. Sastry, and W. Paranchych. 1980. Comparative biochemical studies on F and EDP208 conjugative pili. *J. Bacteriol.* **141:** 333.

Chong, P.C.S. and R.S. Hodges. 1981. A new heterobifunctional crosslinking reagent for the study of biological interactions between proteins. I. Design, synthesis and characterization. *J. Biol. Chem.* **256:** 5064.

Finlay, B.B., W. Paranchych, and S. Falkow. 1983. Characterization of the conjugative plasmid EDP208. *J. Bacteriol.* **156:** 230.

Frost, L.S., G.D. Armstrong, B.B. Finlay, B.F.P. Edwards, and W. Paranchych. 1983. N-terminal amino acid sequencing of EDP208 conjugative pili. *J. Bacteriol.* **153:** 950.

Hodges, R.S., A.K. Saund, P.C. Chong, S.A. St-Pierre, and R.E. Reid. 1981. Synthetic model for two-stranded α-helical coiled-coils. Design, synthesis and characterization of an 86-residue analog tropomyosin. *J. Biol. Chem.* **256:** 1214.

Watts, T.H., P.A. Sastry, R.S. Hodges, and W. Paranchych. 1983. Mapping of the antigenic determinants of *Pseudomonas aeruginos* PAK polar pili. *Infect. Immun.* **42:** 113.

Worobec, E.A., A.K. Taneja, R.S. Hodges, and W. Paranchych. 1983. Localization of the major antigenic determinant of EDP208 pili at the N-terminus of the pilus protein. *J. Bacteriol.* **153:** 955.

High-performance Liquid Chromatography of Viral Proteins as a Tool in the Design of Synthetic Vaccines

Gjalt W. Welling, Gerda Groen,
Tineke Popken-Boer, Janine Nijmeijer,
Ruurd van der Zee, Jan B. Wilterdink,
and Sytske Welling-Wester
Laboratorium voor Medische Microbiologie
Rijksuniversiteit Groningen
9713 EZ Groningen, The Netherlands

Depending on the structural information available on the protein chosen for preparation of a synthetic peptide vaccine, three approaches can be used. First, if the tertiary and primary structures (i.e., the conformation and the amino acid sequence) are known, the accessibility of amino acid side chains—which would be a requisite for reaction with antibodies—can be determined and peptides can be selected for synthesis (Lerner 1983).

The second approach can be used when the tertiary structure of a protein is not available and specific parts of the amino acid sequence have to be selected in another way. Determination of the hydrophilicity profile of a protein reveals which parts of the amino acid sequence might be in contact with the outside environment and will be able to react with antibodies. The secondary structure (β-pleated sheet, a-helix, β-turn) can be predicted by a variety of methods, and together with the hydrophilicity profile, specific parts of the amino acid sequence can be selected for synthesis. Since many amino acid sequences have become available as a result of the progress in nucleotide sequencing, this approach is most commonly used.

The third approach can be used when no structural information on the protein is available. This approach uses the high resolution in separations that can be obtained by high-performance liquid chromatography (HPLC) of a mixture of proteins. HPLC of proteins has been possible during the past 4–5 years because of the availability of suitable column material (small particles with a large pore size of 30 nm) and appropriate bonded phases (Regnier 1983). This chromatographic method can be applied to the separation of membrane proteins when the strong tendency of such proteins to aggregate is taken into account. Solvents suitable

421

for separation of ordinary proteins often have to be redesigned for the separations of membrane proteins.

Briefly, the third approach consists of the purification of a membrane protein by an HPLC method (gel filtration, ion exchange, or reverse phase). The protein is then cleaved by cyanogen bromide or by proteolytic enzymes, and the resulting peptides are again purified by HPLC. At this stage or earlier, the aminoterminal amino acid sequences of the fragments and of the intact protein, respectively, can be determined by automated microsequencing (Hunkapillar and Hood 1983). However, it is also possible to investigate the immunological significance of a pure peptide in which the amino acid sequence is not yet known. When in vitro neutralization studies and protection studies have been carried out, the amino acid sequence of promising peptides can be determined. The last step will then be synthesis of these peptides.

Sendai Virus

Because Sendai virus, a paramyxovirus of mice, is readily available after growing in embryonated eggs, we have used it as a model. The virion has a diameter of about 100 nm, and two of its proteins, the fusion (F) protein and the hemagglutinin-neuraminidase (HN) protein, are partly embedded in the lipid bilayer and extend into the environment as spikes (Scheid and Choppin 1974). These two proteins are of interest for the preparation of a vaccine, since they play an important role in the infection process. The F protein consists of F_1 (m.w. 50,000) and F_2 (m.w. 13,000) that are connected by disulfide bridges. The HN protein has a molecular weight of 67,000.

Detergent Extraction and HPLC

HN and F proteins can be extracted from the lipid bilayer by mild nonionic detergents, e.g., Triton X-100, NP-40, and octylglucoside. We have used Triton X-100 (2% v/v, final concentration) for the extraction of 5–30-mg amounts of viral protein. After ultracentrifugation, the supernatant contains a mixture of HN and F proteins to which detergent molecules are attached. In addition, partly degraded HN molecules (HN$^-$) with a molecular weight of 55,000 are present. The detergent extract was subjected to three different modes of HPLC: gel filtration, ion-exchange, and reverse-phase HPLC.

Gel Filtration HPLC

The sample containing F, HN, and HN$^-$ in 4% SDS (w/v) was boiled for 2 minutes and applied to a TSK 4000 SW column. TSK 4000 was chosen instead of TSK 3000 since the molecular weight of the proteins increases by the attachment of SDS molecules. The solvent should contain 0.1% SDS. Since the sample was not reduced prior to chromatography, HN and HN$^-$ are present as dimers and tetramers, facilitating separation from the F protein which is present as a monomer (see Fig. 1). The separation was carried out with 100–200 µg of protein, and the yield was almost 100%.

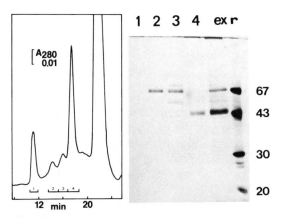

Figure 1

Gel filtration HPLC of detergent-extracted Sendai virions. The sample (ex) containing F, HN, and HN⁻ in 4% SDS (w/v) was heated at 100°C for 2 min, chromatographed on a TSK 4000 SW (600 × 7.5 mm) column (Toyo Soda Co.), and eluted with 50 mM sodium phosphate (pH 6.5) containing 0.1% SDS. The flow rate was 1 ml/min, and the absorbance was monitored at 280 nm. Peak fractions 1–9 were analyzed by SDS-polyacrylamide gel electrophoresis. The molecular weights of reference proteins (r) are indicated in kilodaltons.

Ion-exchange HPLC

We used an anion-exchange column (Mono Q) for the separation. Figure 2 shows that the proteins elute in the order HN⁻, HN, and F. HN and F can be separated, although multiple peaks containing either protein were observed. This is proba-

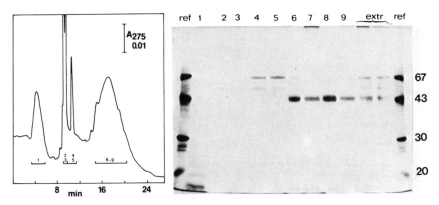

Figure 2

Anion-exchange HPLC of detergent-extracted Sendai virions. The protein mixture (extr) was fractionated on a Mono Q HR 5/5 (50 × 5 mm) column (Pharmacia), with a gradient from 20 mM Tris-HCl, (pH 7.8) to 0.5 M NaCl in 20 mM Tris-HCl (pH 7.8). Both buffers also contained 0.1% Triton X-100. The flow rate was 1 ml/min, and the absorbance was monitored at 275 nm. Fractions indicated by bars and numbers were analyzed by SDS-polyacrylamide gel electrophoresis. The molecular weights of reference proteins (ref) are indicated in kilodaltons.

bly due to the presence of charged carbohydrate attached to the proteins. To avoid aggregation during chromatography, 0.1% Triton X-100 was included in the solvent. Yields were 50% or higher.

Reverse-phase HPLC

In this case the detergent extract containing F, HN, and HN⁻ was reduced prior to chromatography, resulting in a mixture of HN, HN⁻, F_1, and F_2. In addition, a small amount of the matrix (M) protein (m.w. 38,000) was present. The proteins become attached to the hydrophobic column matrix and are eluted with a gradient of an increasing amount of organic solvent. We used a newly developed column material in which the bonded phase consists of a carbon atom attached to the column support, which has pores of 25 nm (TMS-250). Figure 3 shows that a considerable degree of purification can be obtained. Peak 1 contained the F_2 protein; peak 4 contained HN, HN⁻, and some unknown aggregate; peaks 5, 6, and 7 contained predominantly the F_1 protein; and M was present in peak 3. Yields using this mode of HPLC vary from 5% to 100%, depending on the protein (van der Zee et al. 1983).

DISCUSSION

The purification of viral membrane proteins is the first step toward the generation of viral peptide fragments, synthesis of viral peptides, and eventually a synthetic peptide vaccine. The first step alone, purification of viral proteins by HPLC, might be an alternative for the recombinant DNA approach for the preparation of sub-

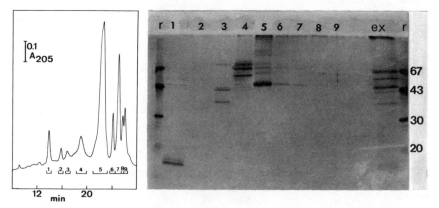

Figure 3
Reverse-phase HPLC of a detergent extract of purified Sendai virions reduced with dithiothreitol prior to chromatography on a TMS-250 (75 × 4.6 mm) column (Toyo Soda Co.). The detergent was removed by incubation with Amberlite XAD-2 (500 mg/ml) for 20 min at 37°C. The gradient used for elution consisted of 25% acetonitrile in water with 0.05% TFA to 75% acetonitrile in water with 0.05% TFA. The flow rate was 1 ml/min, and the absorbance was monitored at 205 nm. Peak fractions indicated by numbers were analyzed by SDS-polyacrylamide gel electrophoresis. The molecular weights of reference proteins are indicated in kilodaltons.

unit vaccines, provided sufficient quantities of viral protein can be isolated. Quantities (100–200 μg) of viral protein can be isolated relatively easily in one chromatographic step that takes less than 30 minutes, with yields varying from 5% to 100%, depending on the protein and the chromatographic system used. Repeated injections or changing from analytical columns (as used in our study) to preparative columns may provide larger quantities of purified viral proteins. However, when only small amounts of viral protein can be isolated, then the HPLC approach combined with automated microsequencing should be used. Amounts of viral protein as low as 20 ng have been detected by HPLC, and it has been shown by Hunkapillar and Hood (1983) that it is possible to sequence 13–68 amino acids from 5–850 pmoles of protein (50 ng of protein with a molecular weight of 50,000 = 1 pmole). This shows that such an approach might be feasible. Future progress in this type of approach will undoubtedly come from further improvement of HPLC column technology and refinement of microsequencing methods.

ACKNOWLEDGMENTS

This work was supported by grants GUKC 83-19 to S.W.-W. and IVh 81-8 to G.W.W. from the Netherlands Cancer Society (Koningin Wilhelmina Fonds). We thank Dr. J. Kato (Toyo Soda Company, Tonda, Japan) for providing the TMS-250 column. ·

REFERENCES

Hunkapillar, M.W. and L.E. Hood. 1983. Protein sequence analysis: Automated microsequencing. *Science* **219**: 650.

Lerner, R.A. 1983. Synthetic vaccines. *Sci. Am.* **248**: 48.

Regnier, F.E. 1983. High-performance liquid chromatography of proteins. *Methods Enzymol.* **91**: 137.

Scheid, A. and P.W. Choppin. 1974. Identification of the biological activities of paramyxovirus glycoproteins. Activation of cell fusion, hemolysis, and infectivity by proteolytic cleavage of an inactive precursor protein of Sendai virus. *Virology* **57**: 475.

van der Zee, R., S. Welling-Wester, and G.W. Welling. 1983. Purification of detergent-extracted Sendai virus proteins by reversed-phase high-performance liquid chromatography. *J. Chromat.* **266**: 577.

Enhancement of the Immune Response to a Cyclic Synthetic HBsAg Peptide by Prior Injection of Anti-idiotype Antibodies

Ronald C. Kennedy, James T. Sparrow, Yanuario Sanchez, Joseph L. Melnick, and Gordon R. Dreesman
Department of Virology and Epidemiology and Department of Medicine, Baylor College of Medicine, Houston, Texas 77030

Immunoglobulin idiotypes (Id) have been studied extensively since they were first characterized in 1963. Id, along with homologous anti-Id antibodies, are thought to be components of a network of complex reactions that regulates a given immune response. The idea that regulation can occur at the level of Id recognition via a series of Id-anti-Id reactions was first proposed by Jerne (1974). Id, located on or close to the antigen-binding site of both antibody molecules and lymphocyte antigen receptors, represent the components with which anti-Id react to control the immune response at both the afferent and efferent limbs. Numerous studies have implicated Id networks in regulating the immune response to a large variety of antigens. Manipulation of these networks by administration of anti-Id antibodies has been used to either enhance or suppress the normal response to antigen.

Antibody produced against hepatitis-B surface antigen (HBsAg), the lipoprotein envelope of hepatitis-B virus (HBV), provides protection against infection with HBV. Serologically, HBsAg has a cross-reactive group-specific *a* determinant and two sets of allelic subtype determinants referred to as *d* or *y* and *w* or *r*. Studies have indicated that the *a* determinant was responsible for the induction of protective antibody. Recently, we characterized a common Id shared by human antibodies to HBsAg (anti-HBs) (Kennedy et al. 1982; Kennedy and Dreesman 1983). The common Id was associated in part with the antibody-combining site because HBsAg and a nondenatured HBsAg-derived viral polypeptide isolated in a micelle form partially inhibited the common Id-anti-Id reaction. Further characterization revealed that the common Id was induced by a conformation-dependent group-specific *a* determinant because (1) three serotypes of HBsAg (*ayw,*

427

adw, and *adr)* inhibited the Id-anti-Id reaction equally well on a weight basis, (2) reduction of the disulfide bonds in HBsAg and alkylation of the free thiol groups abolished the ability to inhibit the Id-anti-Id reaction, and (3) denatured HBsAg viral polypeptides had a decreased inhibitor capacity when compared with native polypeptides. This common Id was also expressed on anti-HBs produced in BALB/c mice and six other species, indicating that an interspecies Id cross-reaction was detected (Kennedy et al. 1983a). In addition, the ability of anti-Id antibodies to enhance the anti-HBs response in vivo was demonstrated by the increase in the number of anti-HBs plaque-forming cells from spleens of BALB/c mice given anti-Id prior to HBsAg stimulation (Kennedy et al. 1983b).

DISCUSSION

Inhibition of the Id-anti-Id Reaction by a Cyclic Synthetic Peptide

A cyclic synthetic peptide containing amino acid sequences 122–137 of the major native HBsAg polypeptide was found to inhibit the Id-anti-Id reaction. On a molar basis, peptide 122–137 was 10^3 less efficient at inhibiting the reaction when compared with intact HBsAg particles. Reduction of the intrachain disulfide bond (Cys 124–137) and subsequent alkylation destroyed the ability of the peptide to inhibit the Id-anti-Id reaction. These data suggested that a conformation-dependent group-*a* epitope was associated with this cyclic peptide. Also, the inhibition of a common Id-anti-Id reaction by this peptide suggested that it was associated with antigenic determinants that induce protective anti-*a* antibodies in humans.

Induction of Anti-HBs by Injecting Anti-Id Antibodies

Previously, we demonstrated that BALB/c mice receiving anti-Id antibodies alone generated IgG anti-HBs plaque-forming cells (Kennedy et al. 1983b). These data indicated that anti-Id antibodies could induce an anti-HBs response without HBsAg stimulation. Injecting anti-Id alone in BALB/c mice produced a significant IgG anti-HBs response when compared with mice given similar injections of control antibodies (Table 1). The anti-Id anti-HBs was found to express the interspecies Id, since inhibition values of 38–54% were obtained with a group of four sera. Conversely, less than 10% inhibition of the Id-anti-Id reaction was obtained with the non-anti-HBs containing sera from the four mice injected with control antibodies and the preimmune sera from the anti-Id-induced anti-HBs. The antibody specificity of the anti-HBs produced by anti-Id injection was determined by a radioimmunoassay using microtiter plates coated with HBsAg subtypes *adw,* *adr,* and *ayw.* Each of the four mouse antisera bound the three different HBsAg subtypes equally well, indicating that the anti-Id anti-HBs was directed to the *a* determinant (Table 1). The fact that anti-HBs can be induced by injecting anti-Id alone suggests the potential use of anti-Id reagents as vaccines for HBV. In this regard, anti-Id-induced anti-HBs was directed against the *a* determinant of HBsAg and expressed an Id that was shared by anti-HBs produced in humans naturally infected with HBV.

Table 1
Induction of Anti-HBs by Injection of Anti-Id

First injection	Second injection	Anti-HBs titer[a]	% Inhibition of Id-anti-Id[b]	S/N[c]		
				adw	ayw	adr
Anti-Id	anti-Id	750	38	8.3	7.8	7.7
Anti-Id	anti-Id	1000	46	8.0	7.8	7.8
Anti-Id	anti-Id	1000	51	7.9	8.4	7.7
Anti-Id	anti-Id	1250	54	7.9	7.9	8.2
Pre-IgG[d]	pre-IgG	<5	0–9	<1.8	<1.6	<1.8

Each group of four mice received two injections of anti-Id or pre-IgG, 14 days apart. Mice were bled 12 days after the second injection.

[a]Reciprocal dilution of antisera that gave a positive (S) to negative (N) cpm ratio of 2.1 as determined by solid-phase radioimmunoassay.

[b]All sera were tested for the ability to inhibit the Id-anti-Id reaction at a 1:10 dilution.

[c]Positive (S) to negative (N) cpm ratio obtained with the three subtypes testing anti-Id-treated sera at 1:100 dilution and pre-IgG sera at 1:10 dilution.

[d]All four mouse antisera were negative at the dilution tested.

Priming the Anti-HBs Response by Anti-Id

In vivo injections of anti-Id antibodies were used to prime the immune system of mice to HBsAg (Table 2). Anti-Id reagents in conjugation with cyclic peptide 122–137 induced anti-HBs titers comparable to that obtained with a single injection of intact HBsAg particles. In addition, high anti-HBs titers were produced in mice injected with HBsAg following anti-Id immunization. These data indicate that anti-Id antibodies may be useful in priming the immune system of a host to HBV.

SUMMARY

Anti-Id antibodies were used to modulate the immune response to HBsAg in BALB/c mice. Injection of anti-Id antibodies alone induced anti-HBs that was directed against the *a* determinant and inhibited a common interspecies anti-HBs Id-anti-Id reaction. In addition, anti-Id treatment prior to HBsAg or synthetic pep-

Table 2
Priming the Anti-HBs Response by Prior Injection of Anti-Id Antibodies

First injection	Second injection	No. of mice	Anti-HBs response	
			range	mean
Pre-IgG	peptide 122–137	6	0–10	4.0
Anti-Id	peptide 122–137	7	10–50	38.6
Pre-IgG	HBsAg	5	10–50	34.0
Anti-Id	HBsAg	6	6,250–31,250	10,416

All mice received anti-Id or pre-IgG on day 0, followed by HBsAg or synthetic peptide on day 14, all by the intraperitoneal route. Serum was obtained on day 30, and the reciprocal of the endpoint dilution that gave a positive to negative cpm ratio of 2.1 was determined by radioimmunoassay.

tide stimulation enhanced the anti-HBs response. These data suggest that the immune response to HBV may be controlled via idiotype networks.

ACKNOWLEDGMENTS

This work was supported by National Research Service Award CA-09197 from the National Institutes of Health and by research contract DAMD 17-82C-2155 from the U.S. Army Medical Research and Development Command.

REFERENCES

Jerne, N.K. 1974. Towards a network theory of the immune system. *Ann. Immunol.* **125c:** 373.

Kennedy, R.C. and G.R. Dreesman. 1983. Common idiotypic determinant associated with human antibodies to hepatitis B surface antigen. *J. Immunol.* **130:** 385.

Kennedy, R.C., I. Ionescu-Matiu, Y. Sanchez, and G.R. Dreesman. 1983a. Detection of an interspecies idiotypic cross-reaction associated with antibodies to hepatitis B surface antigen. *Eur. J. Immunol.* **13:** 232.

Kennedy, R.C., Y. Sanchez, I. Ionescu-Matiu, J.L. Melnick, and G.R. Dreesman. 1982. A common human anti-hepatitis B surface antigen is associated with the group a conformation-dependent antigenic determinant. *Virology* **122:** 129.

Kennedy, R.C., K. Adler-Storthz, R.D. Henkel, Y. Sanchez, J.L. Melnick, and G.R. Dreesman. 1983b. Immune response to hepatitis B surface antigen: Enhancement by prior injection of anti-idiotype antibodies. *Science* **221:** 853.

Immunogenicity of Subunits from Influenza and Rubella Viruses

Michel Trudel, Pierre Payment,
Lise Thibodeau, and Armand Boudreault
Centre de recherche en virologie, Institut
Armand-Frappier, Université du Québec
Laval-des-Rapides, Québec, Canada, H7Y 1B7

Shirley Gillam
Department of Pharmacology
University of British Columbia 2176
Health Sciences Mall, Vancouver, Canada

One of the many approaches being pursued in the development of modern virus vaccines is the preparation of subunit vaccines that contain only the viral antigen(s) required to induce protection and are nucleic-acid-free. In the case of enveloped viruses, the surface glycoproteins are generally responsible for the induction of protection. One of the most effective methods to solubilize these membrane proteins relies on the use of the nondenaturing ionic detergent β-D-octylglucoside (Helenius et al. 1977). Use of this detergent permits a better control of the state of aggregation of the disrupted viral membrane proteins and also permits their reinsertion into the lipid bilayer of synthetic lipid vesicles by detergent dialysis. These viruslike structures have been termed virosomes or immunosomes by different authors. Evaluation of the immunogenicity of these structures has revealed marked differences in their efficiency, depending on the virus being studied. We present here the results obtained from the immunological evaluation of subunit preparations of two human enveloped viruses: influenza and rubella. These results underline some of the progress and also some of the problems encountered.

Influenza Subunits: Rosettes and Immunosomes

Influenza is a large enveloped virus of the Orthomyxoviridae family with subunits protruding from its surface (Fig. 1f). These subunits are composed of hemagglutinin (HA) and neuraminidase (NA). HA is thought to be responsible for induction of immunity. NA seems to play a lesser role in protection, although certain current studies are aimed at reevaluating its role. Two types of subunits, rosettes and immunosomes, were prepared and tested for their immunogenicity.

431

To prepare the rosette subunits, glycoproteins of purified influenza virus (A/Brazil/11/78 [H1N1]) were solubilized with 1% Triton N-101 and purified by rate-zonal ultracentrifugation on a 10–15% discontinuous and a 15–25% continuous sucrose gradient containing 30 mM β-D-octylglucoside (SW 40 rotor, 2 hr at 40,000 rpm). Fractions positive for hemagglutinating activity were pooled and used for reconstruction studies after dialysis. Electron microscopic observation of this material revealed mostly influenza HA and NA in rosette form (Thibodeau et al. 1981).

To prepare the immunosomes, liposomes were first prepared by slow injection, in phosphate-buffered saline, of a mixture of phosphatidylcholine, cholesterol, and lysolecithin solubilized in 50 mM β-D-octylglucoside in 16:2:1 molar ratios and dialyzed (Fig. 1a). The rosette subunits were adjusted to 7.5 mM octylglucoside, mixed with the liposomes, and dialyzed in a linear decreasing detergent gradient

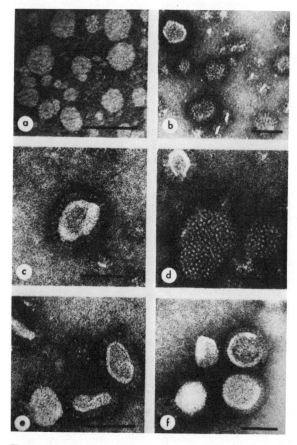

Figure 1
Electron micrographs of influenza immunosomes. (a) Liposomes; (b–e) immunosomes; (f) influenza virus, strain A/Brazil/11/78 H1N1. Bar, 100 nm.

for 48 hours. Electron micrographs of the virosomes (immunosomes) (Fig. 1b–e) show viruslike structures with the viral glycoproteins inserted into their surfaces. These virosomes are not as tightly packed as the virus (Fig. 1f); in some cases, we can observe virosomes showing "sea-urchin" morphology (Fig. 1d).

The humoral immunological efficiency of these structures, compared with that of the formol-inactivated virus, has been tested in mice by a single intraperitoneal injection of 6.0 μg of HA without adjuvant. Antibody titers were assayed by hemagglutination inhibition (HI). The results in Figure 2 show that subunits coupled to liposomes were nearly as efficient as the inactivated whole virus, whereas subunits in rosette form were less efficient. No adjuvant effect due to the presence of liposomes could be observed.

Rubella Subunits: Rosettes and Virosomes

Rubella is a small, spherical, enveloped virus 55–70 nm in diameter, and the immunogenic glycoprotein on the surface of the virus, which shows hemagglutinating activity, is 5–7 nm in diameter (Fig. 3A). Rubella is the only member of the genus *Rubivirus* of the Togaviridae family.

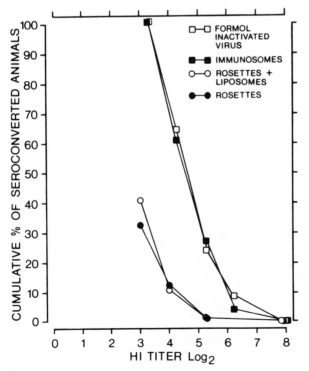

Figure 2
Cumulative percentage of seroconverted mice (HI titer) after intraperitoneal inoculation of 6 μg HA of influenza virus strain A/Brazil/11/78 H1N1 in different physical forms.

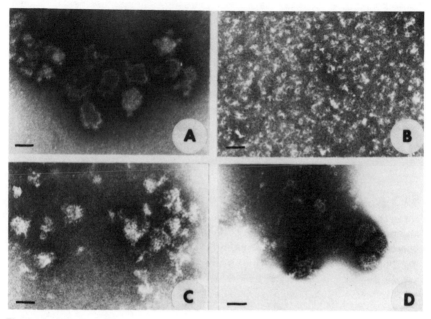

Figure 3
Electron micrograph of rubella virosomes. (*A*) Rubella virus, strain M-333; (*B*) rosettes;
(*C,D*) virosomes. Bar, 100 nm.

Using a procedure similar to that described for influenza, we have isolated HA
in rosette form and have characterized it as a 26S complex composed of eight
subunits of the E1, E2 glycoproteins (Fig. 3B).

The method developed for the influenza virosome preparation could not be
applied to rubella virus because the hemagglutinating activity was lost during the
48-hour dialysis and no subunits could adsorb on the liposomes. We adapted the
method of Helenius et al. (1977) and found that rubella rosettes could, at high
concentration in reduced volume, adsorb spontaneously into preformed homogeneous liposomes, prepared by sonication of phosphatidylcholine and dicetyl
phosphate (3.5:1) dried films resuspended in phosphate-buffered saline (Trudel
and Nadon 1981). After rate-zonal centrifugation on a 10–40% sucrose gradient
containing 0.5 M NaCl, we isolated a fast HA migrating fraction that showed reconstructed rubella virosomes (Fig. 3C,D). Electrophoresis patterns of these virosomes showed that they were composed of the two membrane glycoproteins
E1 and E2 (60K and 47K).

The immunogenicity of these rubella virosomes, compared with the immunogenicity of the rosettes and whole virus (live and β-propriolactone-inactivated),
was evaluated in a rabbit model. Only whole-virus particles, live or inactivated,
could induce HI (Fig. 4) or neutralizing antibodies at a dose of 0.16 μg HA, in a
single injection without adjuvant (Trudel et al. 1982). Virosomes were inefficient
at stimulating HI or neutralizing antibodies, even at the 100-μg HA level. These
results suggest that the antigenic sites responsible for the induction of HI anti-

bodies require a structural integrity that is found only on intact virions (live or inactivated) and that we have been unable to reconstruct by detergent dialysis. Unlike influenza, where even rosettes show some degree of efficiency, the important site for the induction of protective antibodies to rubella virus appears to be dependent on the quaternary structure of the subunits on the viral surface.

Spontaneous versus Detergent-mediated Adsorption

While studying the preparation of influenza and rubella virosomes, we spent some time looking into the question of spontaneous adsorption of viral glycoproteins on liposomes versus detergent-mediated adsorption during dialysis. In the absence of detergent, the influenza HA does not adsorb spontaneously, whereas the rubella HA can adsorb on liposomes in the presence or absence of detergent. We propose that this phenomenon is caused by the fact that the HA molecule of influenza is a transmembrane protein with a small hydrophilic segment capping the hydrophobic segment that is embedded in the viral membrane. The presence of detergent could mask this hydrophilic segment and could permit penetration into the lipid bilayer. Without detergent, the influenza HA is restricted from penetrating the liposome hydrophobic phase. Rubella HA is not a transmembrane

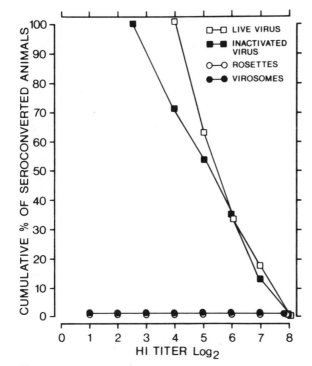

Figure 4
Cumulative percentage of seroconverted rabbits (HI titer) after intraperitoneal inoculation of 0.16 μg HA of rubella virus strain M-33 in different physical forms.

protein and has only a hydrophobic end that anchors readily on the lipid bilayer of the liposome.

Further Surface Analysis of Rubella Virus with Monoclonal Antibodies

Preliminary analysis of antigenic sites on the surface of rubella virus by a limited set of four monoclonal antibodies showing inhibition of biological activity (hemagglutination and/or neutralization) revealed at least three different sites on the molecule (Table 1). S1 can only neutralize the virus, S2 and S3 can both neutralize the virus and inhibit hemagglutination, and S4 shows only HI activity. The four monoclonal antibodies are capable of immunoprecipitating the virus and have been shown by electron microscopy to aggregate the surface proteins. Electrophoresis, blotting, and subsequent immunodetection reveal that these sites are lost when the proteins are solubilized, except for one reactive site located on the E1 (60K) glycoprotein reacting weakly with monoclonal antibody S1, which shows only neutralizing activity. This suggests that most of the important sites for HI or neutralization are related to the tertiary or quaternary structure of the rubella HA.

DISCUSSION

Our data on the immunogenicity of whole rubella virus (live or inactivated) and the subsequent loss of efficiency of the subunits in inducing HI or neutralization antibodies agree with our mapping studies with the monoclonal antibodies which show that these sites are related to the intact surface (see Table 1, Immunoprecipitation). Only S1 was capable of weakly reacting with dissociated E1, indicating that this protein in its native state is implicated in neutralization of the virus. Blotting studies with unreduced proteins are under way, as well as studies involving isolation and characterization of other monoclonal antibodies.

Our results also indicate that epitopes responsible for HI and neutralization are present on different sites on the virus surface. This phenomenon has recently been reported for other viruses, e.g., Japanese encephalitis, tick-borne encephalitis, and influenza virus (Kida et al. 1982; Kimura-Kuroda and Yasui 1983).

Table 1
Characterization of Monoclonal Antibodies Specific for Rubella Surface Proteins

Monoclonal antibody designation	Ig class	Biological activity[a]	Immunoprecipitation[b]	Protein blotting
S1	IgG2a	N	E1, E2, NP	E1
S2	IgG3	N, HI	E1, E2, NP	—
S3	IgG3	N, HI	E1, E2, NP	—
S4	IgG3	HI	E1, E2, NP	—

[a]N, neutralizing antibody; HI, hemagglutination-inhibiting antibody.
[b]E1, surface glycoprotein (60K); E2, surface glycoprotein (47K); NP, nucleoprotein (35K).

The influenza immunosome (virosome) preparations, on the other hand, are quite efficient. In clinical trials they should prove as good as formol-inactivated virus in inducing an immune response and should have fewer side effects.

ACKNOWLEDGMENT

We thank Francine Nadon and Sophie Gladu for their excellent technical assistance.

REFERENCES

Helenius, A., E. Fries, and J. Kartenbeck. 1977. Reconstitution of Semliki forest virus membrane. *J. Cell Biol.* **75:** 866.

Kida, H., L.E. Brown, and R.G. Webster. 1982. Biological activity of monoclonal antibodies to operationally defined antigenic regions on the hemagglutinin molecule of A/Seal/Massachussetts/1/80 (H7N7) influenza virus. *Virology* **122:** 38.

Kimura-Kuroda, J. and K. Yasui. 1983. Topographical analysis determinants on envelope glycoprotein Y3 (E) of Japanese encephalitis virus, using monoclonal antibodies. *J. Virol.* **45:** 124.

Thibodeau, L., P. Naud, and A. Boudreault. 1981. An influenza immunosome: Its structure and antigenic properties. A model for a new type of vaccine. *ICN-UCLA Symp. Mol. Cell. Biol.* p. 587.

Trudel, M. and F. Nadon.1981. Virosome preparation: Differences between influenza and rubella hemagglutinin adsorption. *Can. J. Microbiol.* **27(9):** 958.

Trudel, M., F. Nadon, R. Comtois, M. Ravaoarinoro, and P. Payment. 1982. Antibody response to rubella virus proteins in different physical forms. *Antiviral Res.* **2:** 347.

Summary

Robert M. Chanock
*Laboratory of Infectious Diseases, National
Institute of Allergy and Infectious Diseases
National Institutes of Health
Bethesda, Maryland 20205*

During the 4 days of this meeting, we learned of recent advances in understanding the genome of various viruses as well as the structure and function of viral protective antigens. This information, together with parallel advances in understanding immune mechanisms involved in resistance to virus diseases, provides us with eight new strategies for immunoprophylaxis, some of which will undoubtedly supplement or replace conventional methods previously used in developing vaccines that have been partially or completely effective in preventing disease caused by smallpox virus, rabies virus, yellow fever virus, poliovirus, influenza virus, measles virus, rubella virus, mumps virus, certain of the adenoviruses, and hepatitis-B virus.

Before evaluating these new strategies for immunoprophylaxis, consideration must be given to the special needs that exist for different virus groups based on their pathogenesis of infection and the immune mechanisms most important in recovery from disease and resistance to subsequent infection. A strategy suitable for prevention or modification of a systemic virus infection that can be interrupted at different sites of the body may not be effective for a localized mucosal virus infection. In the former, systemic antibodies are often sufficient or there may be an additional need for systemic cell-mediated immunity. However, resistance to viruses that cause infection limited to mucosal surfaces often requires effective local IgA immunity as well.

During this meeting, we also learned that an unbalanced immune response to measles virus antigens in which immunity was induced to the measles virus surface hemagglutinin (HA), but not the measles virus surface fusion protein, led to potentiation rather than prevention of disease. This observation indicates that

439

one of the goals of viral immunoprophylaxis should be a balanced immune response directed against all protective antigenic sites of the virus, in other words, a response that simulates that which occurs during natural infection. It is also desirable to stimulate a balanced response with respect to immunoglobulin immunity and cell-mediated immunity. The latter is stimulated most effectively when viral surface antigens are presented for recognition to the immune system in the context of cell-surface histocompatibility antigens. This is particularly important for enveloped viruses. As mentioned earlier, a balanced response also induces local immunity if the virus in question produces an infection limited to a mucosal surface. These admonitions should be kept in mind as new strategies for constructing vaccines are formulated and evaluated.

Eight new strategies for constructing virus vaccines were presented during this meeting. Four of these strategies are discussed immediately below under Nonreplicating Antigens, and the remaining four are discussed later under Attenuated Mutants for Use in Live Vaccines.

NONREPLICATING ANTIGENS

Expression of Protective Antigens in a Prokaryotic Host

The first strategy is one that shows the least promise at this time. It involves expression of viral protective antigens in a prokaryotic host, *Escherichia coli.* Poliovirus VP1, a capsid protein, has been produced as a fusion protein in *E. coli,* but this viral protein is processed rapidly and degraded to smaller peptides. The VP1 product has a half-life of less than 5 minutes and appears to be extremely toxic for *E. coli.* Influenza-A virus HA has also been expressed as a fusion protein that represents about 10% of the proteins produced by *E. coli;* however, this influenza protein does not stimulate appreciable amounts of neutralizing antibodies. Surface glycoproteins of TGE, a coronavirus pathogen of pigs, and herpes simplex virus type 1 (HSV-1) have also been expressed as fusion proteins in *E. coli,* but their protective efficacy has not been evaluated.

Expression of Protective Antigens in a Eukaryotic Host

A more impressive success in expressing immunogenic viral proteins in vitro has been made using a eukaryotic host such as yeast or a continuous line of mammalian cells. The impetus for these efforts has come mainly from the need to develop a less expensive vaccine for the prevention of infection with hepatitis-B virus (HBV). Although the currently licensed HBV vaccine, which contains purified 22-nm hepatitis-B surface antigen (HBsAg) derived from the plasma of chronically infected carriers, is protective, its high cost precludes its use in Third World countries where the need for effective immunoprophylaxis is greatest. This situation may soon be rectified because HBsAg has now been expressed in yeast in amounts apparently adequate for commercial production. Expression was achieved by transfection of yeast with a recombinant yeast expression vector containing the HBsAg gene inserted downstream from an inducible yeast promoter. Yeast-produced HBsAg is apparently not glycosylated, but it is immunogenic in chimpanzees. Yeast must be disrupted to release the antigen, but purification can be achieved by isopycnic and rate-zonal centrifugation. One procedure now being used for purification also includes immunoaffinity column chromatography.

Appreciable quantities of HBsAg can also be produced (1) in COS cells (a monkey cell line stably transformed by integrated SV40 that has a defective origin of replication) infected with an SV40-HBsAg recombinant and (2) in a line of continuous mouse cells transformed by a bovine papilloma virus–HBsAg (BPV-HBsAg) recombinant. Clinical evaluation of antigens generated in this manner is contingent upon approval by regulatory authorities for the use of continuous cell lines infected with recombinants bearing fragments of a transforming virus. At this moment, licensing of a yeast-produced HBsAg vaccine is probably more imminent.

Other immunogenic viral protective antigens have also been expressed in mammalian cells. For example, an HSV-1 surface glycoprotein, gD, has been successfully expressed in a continuous line of Chinese hamster ovary (CHO) dihydrofolate reductase (DHFR)-negative cells using a shuttle vector containing plasmid sequences, SV40 origin of replication, and a DHFR gene that facilitates selection of transformants. When the carboxyterminal region of the gD gene was deleted, the expressed glycoprotein was secreted into the culture medium. This product stimulated neutralizing antibodies and protected mice against a lethal challenge with HSV-1. Ultimately, it may be possible to use continuous cell lines, such as CHO or COS cells, and recombinants bearing fragments of transforming viruses for vaccine production because extremely sensitive methods are now available to verify the absence of cellular and viral DNAs from the final purified antigen.

Viral antigens produced in eukaryotic cells by recombinant DNA techniques will probably find their greatest usefulness in the control of systemic virus infections that are sensitive to the effects of neutralizing antibodies and that are not dependent on mucosal IgA antibody or cytotoxic T cells for their prevention or resolution. It is unikely that these antigens will prove to be more effective than inactivated whole virus or purified virus subunits against such infections, but recombinant-DNA-produced antigens should be easier to produce, less expensive, and inherently safer.

Synthetic Peptides as Immunogens

Within the past few years, major antigenic sites on protective proteins of a number of important viral pathogens have been identified. This has been achieved by a combination of methods that include (1) determination of the three-dimensional structure of the antigen (influenza-A-virus HA and neuraminidase [NA]), (2) comparison of amino acid sequences of viral antigens that had undergone antigenic change in nature (influenza-A-virus HA and NA and foot-and-mouth disease virus [FMDV] VP1), (3) sequence analysis of viral mutants selected to resist neutralization by monoclonal antibodies that neutralize virus infectivity (influenza-A-virus HA and NA, and poliovirus type-1 and type-3 VP1), and (4) identification of highly hydrophilic regions that should occupy an external and accessible location on the viral protein. The rapid development of information from these sources has stimulated considerable interest in producing synthetic peptides that represent the major antigenic sites of several important viral pathogens and in evaluating these peptides as immunogens.

Following the initial success in preparing immunogenic peptides of FMDV, it was thought that progress with peptides of other viruses would be equally swift. This has not proved to be the case, and the experience has been mixed. There have been some successes and some failures. For example, peptides representing many regions of the influenza HA, including the major antigenic sites, stimulated antibodies that bind to the HA, but these antibodies did not neutralize virus infectivity nor did they confer significant protection on hamsters. Other studies in mice revealed only partial protection. Failure of linear peptides to induce resistance may be due in part to the conformational nature of two of the major antigenic sites on the HA. These sites contain amino acids from distant regions of the linear polypeptide that are brought together during folding of the HA molecule.

A linear HBsAg peptide (amino acids 110–137) containing group-*a* and subtype-*d/y* determinants induced a low level of subtype antibody in chimpanzees, but it completely protected one of three animals from challenge with HBV and conferred partial resistance on another. The importance of conformation was demonstrated for a portion of this region of HBsAg (amino acids 122–137). A linear peptide containing amino acids 122–137 reacted only with monoclonal antibodies specific for subtype-*d/y* determinants, whereas a cyclic form of the peptide reacted with group-*a*-specific monoclonal antibodies as well as subtype-*d/y*-specific monoclonal antibodies. In other words, the group-*a* determinant present in this region was highly conformation-dependent.

In view of the success observed with FMDV and poliovirus type 3, it was surprising that peptides representing the major antigenic sites of poliovirus type 1 stimulated little if any neutralizing antibody. However, rabbits inoculated with these peptides were primed so that they responded to subsequent inoculation of subimmunizing amounts of whole virus by developing a high level of neutralizing antibodies. This priming effect may ultimately prove to be one of the most important new developments in immunoprophylaxis. For example, peptide priming may convert the moderate immune response that is usually observed following infection with an attenuated virus vaccine to a higher-level response resembling that induced by virulent virus. Similarly, the immune response to particulate antigens, such as HBsAg, may be potentiated by peptide priming.

Although the synthetic peptide approach has considerable potential, a number of real or theoretical obstacles remain to be resolved. In experimental studies in animals, the poor antigenicity of most synthetic peptides has necessitated the use of Freund's adjuvant to potentiate the immune response to these materials. Because Freund's adjuvant cannot be used in humans, clinical evaluation of synthetic viral peptides awaits the identification or development of an effective adjuvant that is acceptable for use in humans. Also, polymorphism of class II histocompatibility antigens that control immune response to individual synthetic peptide antigens may preclude the desired antibody response in a significant proportion of individuals in the general population.

Antigenic Mimicry with Anti-idiotype Antibodies

The idiotype of an antibody molecule is located on or close to its antigen-binding site. Antibodies directed against this site are designated anti-idiotype antibodies (anti-id). In some instances, anti-id is thought to mimic the conformation of the antigenic site of the antigen that induced the original antibody response. Anti-id directed against HBsAg antibodies or reovirus S1 capsid protein antibodies induce an immune response to these viral antigens. Anti-id can also prime an antibody response to HBsAg. These exciting observations suggest that it may be possible to immunize against virus diseases using defined anti-id, a product that is free of infectivity, viral proteins, and viral nucleic acid. However, before the practicality and effectiveness of this approach can be evaluated in humans, it will be necessary to produce anti-id in the form of human immunoglobulin so as to minimize an immune response to determinants other than anti-id. Most likely, human anti-id will be prepared in the form of monoclonal antibody. This raises a problem of safety because the production of human monoclonal antibodies involves fusion of human lymphocytes with human or animal myeloma cells. Perhaps this problem can be solved by removal of all DNA from the final anti-id preparation.

ATTENUATED MUTANTS FOR USE IN LIVE VACCINES

Advances in virus genetics and molecular biology provide a basis for construction of more stable attenuated mutants for use in immunoprophylaxis. Attenuation can be achieved by any mutation or sequence divergence that diminishes the capacity of virus to replicate in humans. Essentially, any gene of a small- or medium-size virus can serve as a target for attenuation because available information indicates that every gene product must function efficiently for these viruses to be virulent. The situation is probably similar for viruses with a large genome, such as herpesviruses and poxviruses. Although these viruses possess a few genes whose functions are not essential to replication, it is likely that most genes must operate efficiently for virus to grow well.

An essential property of any attenuated live-virus vaccine is stability of the attenuation phenotype. In many instances, this has been more difficult to achieve than satisfactory attenuation and immunogenicity. During the meeting, we learned of the genetic lability of poliovirus vaccine strains and the molecular basis for phenotypic "reversion" of the type-3 poliovirus vaccine strain. The type-3 strain sustained fewer mutations during its attenuation than did the type-1 poliovirus vaccine strain, and this may explain the greater genetic lability of the former virus. Comparison of sequences of the vaccine strain and a neurovirulent "revertant" suggested that phenotypic reversion occurred primarily by suppression, i.e., the development of second-site mutations that corrected the defects caused by the original mutations.

Our goal, except in the case of deletion mutants, should be to stabilize the attenuation phenotype by constructing vaccine strains that contain as many independent genetic determinants of attenuation as is consistent with viability and satisfactory immunogenicity. The more independent mutations or sequence divergences in a vaccine virus, the more new mutations required for restoration of virulence. In any case, it is likely that live-virus vaccine strains of the future will bear genes of defined nucleotide sequence that specify a satisfactory level of attenuation and immunogenicity. Once the nucleotide sequences responsible for attenuation have been identified, it will be possible to monitor attenuation in the laboratory during all phases of vaccine development, manufacture, and utilization in humans.

Attenuation by Gene Reassortment

Two approaches to attenuation that have yielded apparently stable mutants were described. The first approach applies only to viruses possessing a segmented genome, because this approach relies on gene reassortment to achieve attenuation. Initially, a virus that does not grow well in humans or lower primates is identified or produced in the laboratory. Subsequently, all of its genes except those coding for major protective antigens are transferred into a reassortant virus by gene reassortment during coinfection with a virulent human virus. Genes coding for the major protective antigens are derived from the virulent human parental virus.

Two influenza-A viruses that are restricted in humans show promise as donors of nonsurface protein genes that can be used to attenuate pandemic or epidemic viruses as they emerge. In one instance, an avian influenza-A virus that was restricted in primates was identified. Restriction probably resulted from evolutionary (and sequence) divergence of its genes from the corresponding genes of human influenza-A viruses. This divergence occurred as a consequence of long residence of avian influenza-A genes in viruses selected for their capacity to replicate efficiently in birds. The genes of the other donor virus, a human influenza-A isolate, sustained many mutations as a consequence of serial passage at suboptimal temperature in avian cells in culture. Influenza-A virus reassortants produced with either of the donors are satisfactorily attenuated and immunogenic in susceptible individuals and appear to retain the attenuation phenotype during replication in vivo. A similar approach is currently being pursued for attenuation of the human rotaviruses, major etiologic agents of diarrheal disease in humans and many animal species.

Attenuation by Deletion Mutation

Deletion mutation offers an attractive alternative to other approaches currently being investigated for stabilization of attenuation of live-virus vaccine strains. Such mutations should be stable because they are not subject to reversion, and it is unlikely that they would be easily suppressed by a new mutation at another site of the viral genome. A deletion mutant of HSV-1 lacking an early (a) gene was constructed and shown to be attenuated in experimental animals. Significantly, this mutant exhibited a reduced ability to be reactivated from ganglion cells. This is a property highly desirable for mutants of HSV because this virus frequently causes disease following reactivation from its site of latent infection in ganglia.

Construction of stable deletion mutants of negative-strand RNA viruses presents a more formidable challenge because of the need to transfer the information encoded in cloned DNA into negative-strand viral RNA and back into infectious virus. The most progress has been made with influenza-A virus, which has a segmented genome consisting of eight separate single-stranded RNA genes of negative polarity. Cloned DNA containing the complete sequence of individual influenza virus genes has been constructed by recombinant DNA techniques. When inserted into an appropriate viral vector, such as SV40, the cloned DNA is expressed in eukaryotic cells as functional influenza virus protein. Furthermore, deletion of certain strategic regions of cloned DNA can perturb function of the protein coded by the affected gene. Thus, the scene is set to produce deletion mutants of influenza-A virus and other negative-strand RNA viruses as well. What remains is the difficult task of developing a method for transferring the genetic information in cloned DNA back into an infectious virus.

Attenuated Vaccine Virus as a Vector for Heterologous Viral Protective Antigen

With recombinant DNA techniques, it is possible to insert genes for protective viral antigens into a heterologous virus that is attenuated for humans. This approach to immunoprophylaxis is currently being evaluated using vaccinia virus as the attenuated vector. Vaccinia virus has a long history of safe use in humans and the contraindications to its use are well known—infants with generalized skin conditions such as eczema and infants with profound T-cell defects. At least 22 kb of exogenous DNA can be inserted into vaccinia virus without diminishing its infectivity for cell culture. When genes for exogenous viral surface proteins are inserted into vaccinia downstream from a strong vaccinia promoter, the encoded viral surface antigens are expressed efficiently during infection in vitro or in vivo. This method for producing protective viral antigens in eukaryotic cells with a recombinant vaccinia vector offers considerable promise because glycoprotein antigens are expressed at the cell surface in the context of host histocompatibility antigens, thereby assuring an effective cellular as well as humoral immune response. Vaccinia recombinants have induced significant resistance to HBV and influenza-A virus in experimental animals. A vaccinia-HBsAg recombinant protected chimpanzees against challenge with HBV, whereas a vaccinia–influenza-A HA recombinant protected hamsters against an intranasal challenge of influenza-A virus. These observations should encourage further evaluation of this approach to immunoprophylaxis. Although currently there is considerable resistance to the use of vaccinia because of rare complications associated with this virus, the extremely favorable benefit-risk ratio of vaccinia recombinants able to protect against viruses with a high incidence of chronic morbidity as well as mortality may carry the day. This is particularly true for the prevention of neonatal and childhood infection with HBV in Third World countries because infection acquired early in life commonly becomes persistent and often leads to chronic liver disease and hepatic cell carcinoma.

Selection of Epitope Mutants Using Neutralizing Monoclonal Antibodies

Attenuation can also be achieved by selecting spontaneous mutants of rabies virus or reovirus that resist neutralization by neutralizing monoclonal antibodies directed against the viral surface protein involved in adsorption to host-cell receptors. Only a small proportion of neutralization-resistant rabies virus mutants exhibit attenuation in adult mice. These attenuated mutants are selected by monoclonal antibody that is directed against an epitope whose conformation is critical to virulence. The basis for attenuation of rabies mutants appears to be an amino acid substitution at a specific site within this epitope. Unfortunately, the attenuation phenotype is not stable because replication of these mutants in a permissive host, the suckling mouse, results in emergence of wild-type, virulent rabies virus. Also, attenuation of reovirus neurovirulence can be achieved by monoclonal antibody selection of viruses with a mutation affecting the adsorption function of the S1 capsid protein, but in this instance attenuation appears to be stable. Serial passage of attenuated reovirus mutants in vivo does not lead to the emergence of wild-type virus.

CONVENTIONAL APPROACHES TO ATTENUATION

Finally, it should be noted that conventional approaches to attenuation, such as serial passage in an unnatural host, are still useful for development of live-virus vaccine strains. Serial passage of a human virus in tissue culture derived from an unnatural host selects for multiple mutations, some of which restrict virus replication in human cells. Although this confounds attempts at understanding the genetic basis of attenuation, the final product is often satisfactory for use in immunoprophylaxis. Recent experience with hepatitis-A virus (HAV) can be cited as an example of this conventional approach yielding a promising vaccine candidate. Serial passage of HAV in African green monkey kidney cell cultures led to attenuation of this virus for chimpanzees, the experimental animal that most closely resembles humans in its response to HAV.

Posters

D.J.S. Arora, D.M. Justewicz, and R. Mandeville, Institut Armand-Frappier. Université du Québec, Canada: In vitro stimulation of NK cell activity with purified influenza virus surface antigens.

J. Bittle,[1] P. Worrell,[1] R. Houghten,[1] F. Brown,[2] and R. Lerner,[1] [1]Dept. of Molecular Biology, Scripps Clinic and Research Foundation, La Jolla, California; [2]Animal Virus Research Institute, Pirbright, England: Immunization with a chemically synthesized peptide derived from FMDV polypeptide VP1.

P. Casali, P.A. Rice, and M.B.A. Oldstone, Scripps Clinic and Research Foundation, La Jolla, California: Viruses perturb functions of human lymphocytes—Effects of measles virus and influenza virus on lymphocyte mediated killing and antibody production.

G.M. Fox, D. Langley, and S. Hu, Amgen, Inc., Thousand Oaks, California: Development of PPV subunit vaccine by recombinant DNA methods.

G.E. Gallick, D.B. Brown, E.C. Murphy, and R.B. Arlinghaus, University of Texas Science Center, M.D. Anderson Hospital, Houston: Inhibition of transformation in a cell line infected with a temperature-sensitive mutant of MSV by cytoplasmic microinjection of purified IgG from an antisera generated against a synthetic v-mos peptide.

P. Klemm, W. Gaastra, J. Josephsen, and J.K. Petersen, Dept. of Microbiology, Technical University of Denmark, Lyngby: E. coli fimbriae as basis for vaccines.

D. McCahon, A.M.Q. King, W.R. Slade, K. Saunders, and J.W.L. Newman, Animal Virus Research Institute, Pirbright, England: Study of the nature and extent of RNA recombination in a picornavirus (FMDV).

A.J. Morgan, A.R. Smith, R.N. Barker, and M.A. Epstein, Dept. of Pathology, University of Bristol Medical School, England: Progress in the development of an EBV subunit vaccine.

D. Moore,[1] D. Morgan,[1] B. Robertson,[1] P. McKercher,[1] E. Patzer,[2] S. Shire,[2] and D. Kleid,[2] [1]Plum Island Animal Disease Center, Greenport, New York; [2]Genentech, Inc., South San Francisco, California: A highly antigenic portion of FMDV O_1 VP_1 elicits bovine antibodies that protect mice but not cattle from FMDV infection.

B. Murphy,[1] N. Green,[2] S. Alexander,[2] R. Lerner,[2] and R. Chanock,[1] [1]NIAID, National Institutes of Health, Bethesda, Maryland; [2]Research Institute of Scripps Clinic, La Jolla, California: Evaluation in hamsters of synthetic peptides representing different antigenic sites of the influenza A virus hemagglutinin.

S.R. Petteway, J. Ray, L.A. Ivanoff, and B.D. Korant, E.I. Du Pont de Nemours and Co., Wilmington, Delaware: Expression of viral antigens in *E. coli*.

D.J. Rowlands,[1] B.E. Clarke,[1] A.R. Carroll,[1] F. Brown,[1] B.H. Nicholson,[2] J.L. Bittle,[3] R.A. Houghten,[3] and R.A. Lerner,[3] [1]Animal Virus Research Institute, Pirbright; [2]Biochemistry Dept., The University, Whiteknights Park, England; [3]Research Institute of Scripps Clinic, La Jolla, California: Comparative structural studies of the antigenic sites of FMDV.

M. Sela, C.O. Jacob, and R. Arnon, Dept. of Chemical Immunology, Weizmann Institute of Science, Rehovot, Israel: Synthetic approaches to vaccination against bacterial toxins.

P. van der Marel,[1] A.D.M.E. Osterhaus,[1] G. van Steenis,[1] A.L. van Wezel,[1] B. Sundquist,[2] and B. Morein,[2] [1]Rijksinstituut voor de Volksgezondheid, Bilthoven, The Netherlands; [2]Dept. of Virology, National Veterinary Institute, Uppsala, Sweden: Toward a measles virus subunit vaccine.

Author Index

Subject Index

*Refer to figure legend.